Occupational Health Psychology

Irvin Sam Schonfeld, PhD, MPH, is a professor of psychology at the City College of the City University of New York (CUNY), and is a professor of educational psychology *and* psychology at the Graduate Center of CUNY. He earned a BS at Brooklyn College, an MA at the New School for Social Research, a PhD at the CUNY Graduate Center, and a postdoctoral degree at Columbia University. He is on the editorial board of, and is a reviewer for, a number of journals. He has published in *Journal of Occupational Health Psychology, Journal of Clinical Psychology, Archives of General Psychiatry, Developmental Psychology, British Journal of Developmental Psychology, Journal of Abnormal Child Psychology, Clinical Psychology Review, Psychological Medicine, International Journal of Stress Management, Organizational Research Methods, Scandinavian Journal of Work, Environment & Health, Social Psychiatry and Psychiatric Epidemiology, Personality and Individual Differences, Pediatrics, Journal of Research in Science Teaching*, and elsewhere. He is also the founding editor of the *Newsletter of the Society for Occupational Health Psychology*. Among other subjects, Professor Schonfeld teaches courses on occupational health psychology, experimental psychology, and the epidemiology of mental disorders. When he is not working, he enjoys hiking and backpacking, and won an award from the Appalachian Mountain Club (AMC) for ascending the 48 highest peaks in New Hampshire. As an amateur photographer, he has had two of his photographs selected by the AMC for awards.

Chu-Hsiang (Daisy) Chang, PhD, is an associate professor at the Department of Psychology of Michigan State University. She received her PhD in industrial and organizational psychology from the University of Akron. Her research interests focus on occupational health and safety, leadership, and motivation. Specifically, she studies issues related to occupational stress, workplace violence, and the intersection of employee motivation and organizational leadership particularly with reference to employee health and well-being. Her work has been published in *Academy of Management Review, Academy of Management Journal, Journal of Applied Psychology, Journal of Organizational Behavior, Organizational Behavior and Human Decision Processes, Psychological Bulletin*, and *Work & Stress*. She has served as an associate editor at *Applied Psychology: An International Review* and *Journal of Organizational Behavior*, and is currently serving as an associate editor at *Journal of Applied Psychology*.

Occupational Health Psychology

Irvin Sam Schonfeld, PhD, MPH

Chu-Hsiang Chang, PhD

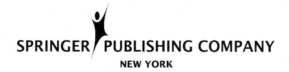

SPRINGER PUBLISHING COMPANY

NEW YORK

Springer Publishing Company, LLC
11 West 42nd Street
New York, NY 10036
www.springerpub.com

Acquisitions Editor: Nancy S. Hale
Compositor: S4Carlisle Publishing Services

ISBN: 978-0-8261-9967-6
e-book ISBN: 978-0-8261-9968-3
Instructor's Manual ISBN: 978-0-8261-9626-8

Instructors' Materials: Qualified instructors may request supplements by e-mailing textbook@springerpub.com

16 17 18 19 20 /5 4 3 2 1

The author and the publisher of this Work have made every effort to use sources believed to be reliable to provide information that is accurate and compatible with the standards generally accepted at the time of publication. The author and publisher shall not be liable for any special, consequential, or exemplary damages resulting, in whole or in part, from the readers' use of, or reliance on, the information contained in this book. The publisher has no responsibility for the persistence or accuracy of URLs for external or third-party Internet websites referred to in this publication, and does not guarantee that any content on such websites is, or will remain, accurate or appropriate.

Library of Congress Cataloging-in-Publication Data

Names: Schonfeld, Irvin Sam, author.
Title: Occupational health psychology / Irvin Sam
   Schonfeld, PhD, MPH, Chu-Hsiang Chang, PhD.
Description: New York : Springer Publishing Company, 2016. | Includes
   bibliographical references and index.
Identifiers: LCCN 2016041732 | ISBN 9780826199676
Subjects: LCSH: Psychology, Industrial. | Job stress. | Industrial safety. |
   Industrial hygiene.
Classification: LCC HF5548.8 .S3526 2016 | DDC 158.7—dc23
LC record available at https://lccn.loc.gov/2016041732

Special discounts on bulk quantities of our books are available to corporations, professional associations, pharmaceutical companies, health care organizations, and other qualifying groups. If you are interested in a custom book, including chapters from more than one of our titles, we can provide that service as well.

For details, please contact:
Special Sales Department, Springer Publishing Company, LLC
11 West 42nd Street, 15th Floor, New York, NY 10036-8002
Phone: 877-687-7476 or 212-431-4370; Fax: 212-941-7842
E-mail: sales@springerpub.com

Printed in the United States of America by Gasch Printing.

In memory of my parents, Ruth and George Schonfeld.
—Irvin Sam Schonfeld

Contents

Acknowledgments From Irvin Sam Schonfeld

The decision to write a book about occupational health psychology has a history, and that history illuminates why the book was written. The story of the book begins several years ago when Nancy S. Hale, who became my editor at Springer, made a surprise visit to my office at City College. She asked me to write a book about occupational health psychology.

I agreed to write the book because I have been conducting research in "occupational health psychology" (OHP) since before I knew the existence of such a term. I came to the subject matter of what would become OHP as a result of the convergence of a number of influences. One influence, naturally enough, was my own work experience. My first job was that of a math teacher in a dangerous urban public school. In that job, I had informally observed the corrosive effects of job stress, although at the time I had not imagined that one day I would be conducting research on job stress. The job stressors I observed were in the form of disrespectful behavior among students toward teachers, student-on-student violence, and student-on-teacher violence.

I left teaching to pursue a doctorate in developmental psychology. I was particularly interested in cognitive development, and conducted research on the foundations of children's cognitions about quantity. After earning a PhD, I failed to obtain the academic position I wanted, and took a job as the director of evaluation in the Office of Special Programs in a school district.[1] My job required me to evaluate grant-supported educational programs and, more importantly, to write grant applications to help support new district initiatives. The head of the office, the individual to whom I reported, was a man who was a very effective grant-writer—which meant that the superintendent would never fire him. He, unfortunately, was a screamer. With a ferocity I hadn't seen outside of a schoolyard, he once berated a secretary; as a result, she broke down in tears in the middle of the office. I observed another woman, the school district's administrator for math programs, someone whom I had personally tried to protect, begin to shake and stammer, and then break into tears *in anticipation* of a tongue-lashing from the office head. The head of the office had contempt for me because there I was, a new PhD, who had not one-tenth the grant-writing skills the office head had. In fact, I was more than a little confused about how to acquire those skills. Of course, screaming at people did not enhance skill acquisition. At the time, I shared with friends a comparison I made between my new job at the school

---

[1] I prefer not to disclose the name of the district and the names of the individuals involved.

district and a job that I had when I was in college. In college, I had a summer job in a South Brooklyn factory that manufactured ladies' slippers. I was a tool and die operator. Although the factory floor was hot, dirty, and dangerous, I joked with my friends who knew how much I disliked my job at the school district that the factory job was better than what I had in the Office of Special Programs. Between my job as a math teacher and my job at the school district, I got to know job stress very well.

In the middle of the school year, I expressed to the head of the office my dissatisfaction regarding how he treated the people who worked for him. My protest was useless. As the school year was ending, I was going to be released from my position. The district superintendent, who was perhaps feeling guilty about the awfulness of the Office of Special Programs, gave me an opportunity to teach math in his district. I rejected it and looked for another position.

The second influence was another work experience. This experience told me that a person can love his or her job. I had applied for a position in the Division of Child and Adolescent Psychiatry at New York State Psychiatric Institute, which has long been the Department of Psychiatry for Columbia University. I was, however, on a New York State line—the importance of this fact will become evident a little later. I started as a data analyst who soon enough got an opportunity to coauthor papers. In my new job, I made a discovery that rivaled that of Molière's Monsieur Jourdain. Monsieur Jourdain was shocked to learn that he was speaking in prose. I was almost equally surprised to learn that I was involved in research on the epidemiology of mental disorder. I loved the job. My colleagues and, especially, the head of the division, David Shaffer, were wonderful to work with.

The third influence was an embittering experience. This influence motivated me to write a section of Chapter 3 devoted to the impact of unemployment. After a year and a half on the job, the budgetary landscape became clouded. In 1983, Mario Cuomo had been elected governor of New York. He sharply cut the state's budget. Many state employees lost their jobs. Everybody on my budget line, the research associate line, was laid off. This event was doubly troubling to my wife and me because my wife was 4 months pregnant with our first child. There was also a special irony to this event. My wife, who worked for a labor union, worked together with her union colleagues to help Cuomo win the Democratic primary and the general election.

Although the layoff hurt very much, David Shaffer supported me for a couple of months with grant money and pushed me to apply for a postdoc in epidemiology at Columbia's School of Public Health (now known as Columbia's Joseph L. Mailman School of Public Health). With David's recommendation, I won a postdoctoral fellowship that enabled me to continue to support my family. The experience in the Psychiatric Epidemiology Training Program, my fourth influence, helped change the direction of my research interests away from children's cognition and away from child and adolescent psychiatry, although I continued, out of personal loyalty, to help David whenever I could. The epidemiology program mentors, Bruce Dohrenwend and Bruce Link, were leaders in research on life stress. The graduate courses in epidemiology and biostatistics and the program's highly stimulating weekly meetings immersed me in new content knowledge and new research strategies. The 2 years I spent in the Psychiatric Epidemiology Training Program formed a kind of chemical bond with my work history, triggering in me a realization that I want to say something important about work, stress, and health. When I got a job at City College, I immediately started to study job stress in teachers.

When Nancy Hale arrived in my office at City College, I was ready to write this book. But I wasn't ready to write the *whole* book. We agreed that I could select a coauthor to make the challenge of covering the field of OHP more manageable. My original coauthor dropped out of the project midstream. With the help of my colleague Paul Spector of the University of South Florida, I was fortunate to recruit Chu-Hsiang Chang, who is also known as Daisy, to join me in the writing. I thank Daisy for her work on Chapters 6, 8, 9, 10, and the sections of Chapter 7 devoted to agricultural and construction workers. Because I edited those chapters, if there are any errors to be found there—indeed, if there are any errors anywhere in the book—they are mine.

Along with the educated public, some of the book's readers will be undergraduates, graduate students, and faculty. To help those in the academy who will use the book in their courses, I wrote a short Instructor's Manual to provide sample essay questions that can be used in courses devoted to OHP. **Qualified instructors may request the Instructor's Manual by e-mail: textbook@springerpub.com**

As much as I love the field of occupational health psychology, I could not, even after managing to persuade Daisy to join this endeavor, ensure that the book covers every bit of the terrain that is OHP. I apologize to the readers that, for practical reasons, the book could not cover more territory. However, I hope that the book interests the reader in OHP, and stimulates the reader to pick up the *Journal of Occupational Health Psychology, Work & Stress*, and *Occupational Health Science*. Perhaps a reader would consider pursuing a career in OHP.

There are many people I thank for their help with the writing of the book. Without the capable staff of Springer Publishing Company, production of this book would not have been possible. My coauthor Daisy Chang brought her considerable expertise as a job stress researcher to the writing of the book. Several student volunteers provided me with thoughtful comments about various chapters. The students include Peter Luehring-Jones, Melanie Kleiner, Zuhair Reza, Elizabeth Spitz, Gail Swingler, Mia DiIanni, and Tanya Sidawi-Ostojic. Violeta Contreras read every chapter and gave me valuable feedback.

Richard Weiner and Milton Spett, two longtime friends, have been sounding boards for me. My CUNY colleague Mark Tausig discussed content-related matters with me. My friend Betty Groner gave me invaluable publishing advice.

A number of colleagues have enriched my academic life. These colleagues include Robert Melara, Brett Silverstein, Jon Horvitz, Glen Milstein, Tim Ellmore, Vivien Tartter, Naomi Nemtzow, and Ratna Sircar of the City College Psychology Department; Edwin Farrell, Hope Hartman, Andrew Ratner, and Sigmund Tobias of the City College School of Education; Ross Nehm of the Department of Ecology and Evolution at Stony Brook University; David Rindskopf, Jay Verkuilen, and Howard Everson of the Quantitative Methods program in the Department of Educational Psychology at the CUNY Graduate Center; and Eric Laurent of the Psychology Department of the University of Franche-Comté.

My friend and colleague Renzo Bianchi of the University of Neuchâtel helped me during the writing of the book. We collaborated on a series of research projects while I was working on the book. We continue to work together, often with Eric Laurent. Our combined efforts on those research projects, and our teamwork in writing the resulting papers, have constituted a kind of working respite for me from the labor—library research, writing, editing, fact checking—that this book required.

Another friend and colleague, Joseph Mazzola of Roosevelt University, and I have had a productive relationship working together on qualitative studies and a thought piece on qualitative research. My research collaboration with Joe has provided another kind of working respite from the labor required in producing this book.

My family has always been supportive of me. I include my sister Royce Schonfeld Katsir and her husband Zvi Katsir, my sister-in-law Marion Worenklein Cronen and her husband Arthur Cronen, my son Daniel Schonfeld and his wife Stacey Schumeister Schonfeld, and my daughter Emily Schonfeld and her husband Eric Greenbaum. In particular, Emily discussed scientific content with me and Daniel did computer troubleshooting for me. My wife, Pearl Knopf Schonfeld, encouraged my work on the book, and tolerated the mountains of paper copies of PDFs and assorted volumes resting on the dining room table. There were many times when we could have gone to a movie or a restaurant, but I sat pecking away at my computer on a Saturday night. On the rare occasion when I needed to sound off in response to a frustration about the book's progress, she was there to listen and be supportive. Let it be known that I appreciate and love my family much more than I can voice on this page.

Irvin Sam Schonfeld
Brooklyn, New York

Acknowledgments From Chu-Hsiang Chang

It's been a long and winding road for the publication of this book. I would first like to thank Irvin for inviting me to be part of this project. This invitation came to me right before I embarked on a challenging journey for work–life balance, which unfortunately did not work out as well as I had hoped. As a result, I was more difficult to work with than usual—not that this is a high bar to reach. This book reflects an accomplishment in the work domain that I will forever cherish. More importantly, it speaks to Irvin's infinite patience with and support for me during the writing period of the chapters.

I wish to acknowledge Aiya Jweihan and Mike Morrison for conducting the literature search and collecting the primary articles. Your efforts greatly reduced my workload, and I truly appreciated your assistance with the project.

I would like to thank my mentors, who guided me onto the path of occupational health psychology. Although this really started with me following a guy across the country, Paul Spector and Tom Bernard have both been instrumental in turning me into an OHP researcher. Both inspired me with their work ethic and their generosity with their time to mentor me. I appreciate their advice and value their feedback tremendously.

I also thank my family. My dear mother, Sabrina, who has shown me resilience and strength during the past 5 years, is a role model for me in every way. My late father, Wen, who always urged me to be an independent thinker, will always be in my mind as I conquer my fear. I'm thankful for the unconditional support and levelheadedness from my younger sister, Maggie. I'm nourished by your love and encouragement every step of the way.

Last but not least, I want to thank my husband, Russ Johnson, for standing by my side throughout this journey. Incidentally, he is the guy whom I followed across the country—so I must have done something right! I'm very fortunate to have someone who is a true partner in so many domains of my life. Professionally, Russ is a great sounding board for me to bounce ideas with. Personally, we share our love for music, food, and cats. Speaking of which, this is the first time (and probably the only time) that I can acknowledge our cats without having to use their initials. Oscar, Shatner, Espresso, Frappuccino, and Kitten: Thank you for the fun and joy you bring to our household, along with the lizards, snakes, and other critters that you generously share with us. I want to close this acknowledgment by thanking Russ for encouraging me to be who I want to be, for supporting my decisions even though he may not agree with them, for the comic relief he provides during the most difficult times, and for always being there for me.

Chu-Hsiang Chang

ONE

A Brief History of Occupational Health Psychology

KEY CONCEPTS AND FINDINGS COVERED IN CHAPTER 1

University of Nottingham
Journal of Occupational Health Psychology
ICOH-WOPS
European Academy of Occupational Health Psychology
Society for Occupational Health Psychology
Summary

"To love and to work" was Sigmund Freud's curt response when asked what a "normal person should be able to do well" (Erikson, 1963, pp. 264–265). This book is not about erotic love, the love to which Freud referred. Rather, the book is about the psychosocial aspects of work and how they bear on mental and physical health. Extensive research supports the view that the impact of working in a psychologically unrewarding job extends beyond work hours, and affects the individual's life situation and health (Gardell, 1976).

According to the Centers for Disease Control and Prevention (CDC, n.d.), occupational health psychology (OHP) involves "the application of psychology to improving the quality of work life, and to protecting and promoting the safety, health and well-being of workers." OHP is an interdisciplinary subfield of psychology that aims to improve our understanding of the impact of psychosocial working conditions on the health and well-being of people who work. This understanding can help us design interventions that make working conditions more healthful *and* economically productive (LaMontagne, Keegel, Louie, Ostry, & Landsbergis, 2007). An example of a psychosocial workplace characteristic that OHP researchers have investigated is the extent to which an organization affords workers autonomy in the performance of their jobs. OHP is interdisciplinary in that it borrows strength from such fields as industrial/organizational psychology, health psychology, occupational medicine, and epidemiology.

OHP is devoted to understanding the relation of work characteristics to *both* the psychological and the physical well-being of people who work. With regard to psychological effects, OHP research is concerned with the extent to which workplace characteristics affect depression, burnout, suicide, and psychological distress. Researchers also examine the impact of work characteristics on blood pressure, heart disease, musculoskeletal disorders, and accidents and injury. The OHP research umbrella extends even further, and includes the effects of job conditions on home life.

OHP research is concerned with what workers bring to their jobs. Investigators try to identify workers' coping responses that either fully or partly prevent job stressors from occurring or that mitigate the impact of stressors. Some coping responses are behavioral (e.g., a teacher taking direct action by initiating contact with the parent of a disrespectful student) and others, cognitive (e.g., mentally comparing oneself with a colleague who "has it worse than me"). In addition, OHP is concerned with how the psychological characteristics of a worker (e.g., preexisting psychological distress) pave the way for job stressors to occur.

The next section of this chapter examines the historical antecedents of OHP as well as its institutional history. The origins of such OHP-related themes that are developed later in the book, themes such as worker autonomy and support, and even the impact of combat on soldiers—people who work for the military—date well before OHP emerged as a recognizable subfield of psychology. This historical survey begins in the 19th century. The chapter works its way through the 20th century and into the 21st. In addition, it examines a few landmark studies as well as the development of important organizations that support OHP.

EARLY FORERUNNERS

Some of the readers of this book may remember the 1981 film *Chariots of Fire*. The film concerned the intense preparations of two British sprinters, Harold Abrahams and Eric Liddell, for the 1924 Olympic Games. The title of the film came from a poem written by the great English poet and visual artist William Blake (1808/1966), and was taken from the following stanza:

> Bring me my Bow of burning gold;
> Bring me my Arrows of desire:
> Bring me my Spear: O clouds unfold!
> Bring me my Chariot of fire!

It is a short poem known by its first line, "And did those feet in ancient time." The poem contemplated Jesus coming to England to create a heaven in that "green and pleasant land." Jesus, however, encounters the physical and spiritual destructiveness of the burgeoning Industrial Revolution. An earlier stanza reads:

> And did the Countenance Divine,
> Shine forth upon our clouded hills?
> And was Jerusalem builded here,
> Among these dark Satanic Mills?

Blake's poem reflected on the damage the Industrial Revolution caused not only to the physical landscape but also to the spiritual lives of its inhabitants. The poem reminds us of the harm rapid industrialization can do to human beings, their interpersonal relationships, and their relationship with their work. Karl Polanyi (2001/1944) noted that "writers of all views and parties, conservatives and liberals, capitalists and socialists, invariably referred to social conditions under the Industrial Revolution as a veritable abyss of human degradation" (p. 41).

Engels and Marx

In 1845, Friedrich Engels published *The Condition of the Working Class in England*. It is of note that this man who was so sympathetic to the working class was the son of a Prussian textile manufacturer. In 1842, his parents sent him to Manchester to work at one of his father's mills in the hope of spurring the young man to relinquish the pro–working-class sentiments he had already developed. His sojourn to England, however, further fueled his interest in the working class, and led to the research he conducted for the book on the English working class.

Engels wrote about how large and centralizing manufacturing was driving small traders and craftsmen out of business and creating a large industrial proletariat. He underlined the high rates of death from disease in industrial centers. He wrote:

> That a class which lives under the conditions already sketched and is so ill-provided with the most necessary means of subsistence, cannot be healthy

and can reach no advanced age, is self-evident. Let us review the circumstances once more with especial reference to the health of the workers. The centralisation of population in great cities exercises of itself an unfavourable influence; the atmosphere of London can never be so pure, so rich in oxygen, as the air of the country; two and a half million pairs of lungs, two hundred and fifty thousand fires, crowded upon an area three to four miles square, consume an enormous amount of oxygen, which is replaced with difficulty, because the method of building cities in itself impedes ventilation.

The 19th century saw the beginning of a growing concern for the impact of industrialization on the physical well-being of workers. The century also marked a growing concern for the link between industrial capitalism and workers' psychological well-being. In response to the Industrial Revolution, Karl Marx (1967/1844) developed the multilayered concept of alienation, a concept that had significant psychological meaning. In one sense, alienation refers to workers losing, with the rise of industrial capitalism, the ability to direct their own lives. Alienation reflects the individual's loss of conscious control over his or her creative labor. In another sense, alienation refers to the worker's estrangement from other workers as a result of the commodification of work. Workers become mere interchangeable, salable parts in a giant industrial flywheel. In another sense, alienation refers to industrial workers, in return for a wage, becoming distanced from what they create. During the Industrial Revolution, production lines reduced work to highly repetitive, monotonous tasks that offered little intrinsic satisfaction and almost no connection to the ultimate product the manufacturer produced. Marx wrote that, with the ever greater exertion demanded by the workplace, the more powerful the alien world around the industrial worker grows, "the poorer he and his inner world become."

Émile Durkheim

Émile Durkheim, the French thinker and sociologist, examined the business cycle in a new way, one that bore uniquely on psychological well-being. In his book *The Division of Labor in Society* (1984/1893), Durkheim advanced the idea that with industrialization, markets expand beyond local areas and become national (or international) in scope. With consumers so dispersed, the producer "can no longer figure out to himself [the market's] limits" with production lacking "any check or regulation," thus leading to miscalculations—upward or downward—of the size of demand (p. 305). The result is "crises that periodically disturb economic functions" (p. 305). This lack of regulation in the economy is an example of what Durkheim called "anomie."

In a later book, Durkheim (1951/1912) linked anomie to the risk of suicide. Using data from official records from a number of European countries, he found that increases in the number of suicides occurred during both the upward and downward phases of the business cycle. During the downward turn, the suicide rate increased. The suicide rate also increased during an uptick. He argued:

If therefore industrial or financial crises increase suicides, this is not because they cause poverty, since crises of prosperity have the same result; it is because they are crises, that is, disturbances of the collective order. Every disturbance of equilibrium, even though it achieves greater comfort and a heightening of general vitality, is an impulse to voluntary death. (p. 246)

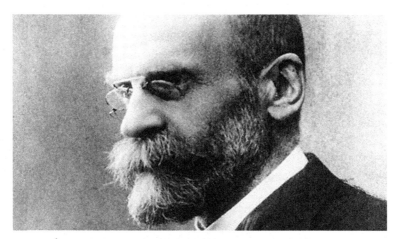

Émile Durkheim. (Photographer unknown. Copyright expired.)

He observed that poverty by itself is not related to increased risk of suicide. Rather, it is the cycling up and the cycling down that is associated with increased risk. Although not without methodological flaws, Durkheim's work on the business cycle is particularly important for OHP because his work closely links macroeconomic factors to intimate psychological outcomes.

Max Weber and the Iron Cage

The German sociologist Max Weber (1904–1905/1992) advanced a theory of the development of modern capitalism in the West. He viewed the growth of capitalism as an efflorescence of the Protestant faiths—particularly the Calvinist religions—that emerged in Europe with the Reformation.[1] In line with Calvinist religions such as Puritanism, work is seen as an ascetic "calling" that had religious significance. As this ascetic ethic of work became increasingly successful, it would largely strip itself of its religious significance. Weber wrote that this ethic

> began to dominate worldly morality, and did its part in building the tremendous cosmos of the modern economic order. This order is now bound to the technical and economic conditions of machine production which to-day determine the lives of all the individuals who are born into this mechanism. . . . Perhaps it will so determine [those lives] until the last ton of fossilized coal is burnt. (Weber, 1904–1905/1992, p. 181)

In Weber's view, what has become a highly rationalized, worldly morality dominates everyday life, and encloses the individual in "an iron cage."

Weber, in a book (1921/1947) published posthumously, described a theory of social and economic organization. He developed an idea for the advancement of

---

[1] The theory in some respects is wrong. For example, Belgium, a largely Catholic country, was faster to industrialize than Scotland, a largely Calvinist country. The rightness or wrongness of the theory is not the issue here. The issue is that Weber's ideas fueled thinking about the impact of work and the economy on people's lives.

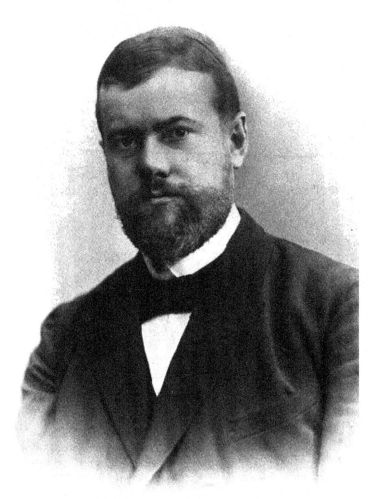

Photograph of Max Weber, circa 1894. (Photographer unknown. From the public domain, Wikipedia Commons.)

sociological theory that would resonate with theoretical developments in psychology. Weber's idea was that of the "pure type" or "ideal type." The ideal type is an abstraction that only imperfectly corresponds to any number of observable social phenomena. An example of an ideal type could be a perfectly rational course of action (in, say, a political campaign). A social theory encompasses a network of interconnections among ideal types. Because scientific theories concern the general rather than the particular, the ideal type serves as a device within the framework of a social theory that helps the theorist develop generalizations about social and economic life. Weber's ideal type can be thought to roughly correspond, in a general way, to the psychologist's idea of a construct, which is covered in Chapter 2.

Weber died in 1920 at a relatively young age, a victim of the Spanish flu pandemic, which swept a world exhausted by the Great War. His wife published a collection of his essays in 1922, one of which was devoted to a detailed analysis of the phenomenon of bureaucracy, a major feature of modern economic life. Weber (1922/1958) noted the division of labor, hierarchical arrangements, and rule-boundedness of bureaucracies. He further observed that a bureaucracy functions without sentiment.

> Its specific nature, which is welcomed by capitalism, develops the more perfectly the more the bureaucracy is 'dehumanized,' the more completely it succeeds in eliminating from official business love, hatred, and all purely personal, irrational, and emotional elements. . . . (p. 216)

Weber's thinking about economic life—its formalization, bureaucratization, and routinization—had a profound influence on later research on the impact of work on the workers themselves (Tausig & Fenwick, 2011).

Taylor and Ford

Although Durkheim (1951/1912) recognized the underside of the division of labor (e.g., isolation, inequality), he argued that the division of labor also provides value for society (e.g., congruence between the individual's abilities and his role, greater interdependence among citizens). Frederick Winslow Taylor and Henry Ford played important roles in the application of the division of labor to the factory system.

Frederick Winslow Taylor

Frederick Winslow Taylor (1911), in writing about *scientific management*, redirected the idea of the division of labor. Taylor compared an American worker playing baseball and an English worker on the cricket pitch to the same worker returning to his (Taylor was largely discussing men) job the next day. Taylor noted that on the playing field, the worker "strains every nerve to secure victory for his side." But on the job, "this man deliberately plans to do as little as he safely can." He labeled this lack of engagement at work "soldiering." Taylor advanced the idea that a worker "soldiers" because the worker believes that increasing his output will result in men being thrown out of work. Taylor also complained that workers overly rely upon "inefficient rule-of-thumb methods" that impede optimal production. By rule-of-thumb methods Taylor referred to inexact traditional knowledge with which the worker grew up (e.g., a worker using his thumb to estimate an inch instead of employing a ruler). Taylor's aim was to improve production efficiency by developing techniques to rid factories of soldiering and rule-of-thumb methods by installing scientific management.

According to Taylor:

> Under scientific management the "initiative" of the workmen (that is their hard work, their good-will, and their ingenuity) is obtained with absolute uniformity and to a greater extent than is possible under the old system; and in addition to this improvement on the part of the men, the managers assume new burdens, new duties, and responsibilities never dreamed of in the past. The managers assume, for instance, the burden of gathering together all the traditional knowledge which in the past has been possessed by the workmen and then of classifying, tabulating, and reducing this knowledge to rules, laws, and formulae which are immensely helpful to the workmen in doing their daily work. (p. 27)

Hughes (1989) observed that although there were examples of Taylor's methods leading to increased production, "there is also abundant evidence of failures" (p. 195). The application of scientific management at Bethlehem Steel, for example, led to intense worker opposition. According to Hughes, many workers, especially those in the skilled trades, found the Taylorist trade-off involving loss of autonomy for higher wages a bad deal. The work of Henry Ford and his associates can be seen as the continuation of Taylorism.

Henry Ford

Around the time Taylor published his work, American manufacturing firms were becoming more and more mechanized. Consistent with Taylorist principles, individual workers in those firms were increasingly slotted into doing highly discrete tasks that they would repeat many times during the work day. Henry Ford and his engineers were creative innovators in the area of industrial production (Hughes, 1989). They also developed their ideas of industrial management independently of Taylor (Sorensen, 1956). Nonetheless, the assembly lines at the Ford Motor Company were the apotheosis of scientific management. Charles E. Sorensen, who played multiple roles (engineer, executive) at the Ford Motor Company, wrote, "It was then that the idea occurred to me that assembly would be easier, simpler, and faster if we moved the chassis along, beginning at one end of the plant with a frame and adding the axles and the wheels . . ." (p. 115).

Ford's advocacy of a division of labor into discrete repetitive tasks is reminiscent of an idea associated with Adam Smith (1976/1776). Smith described a "small manufactory" in which 10 workers produced pins. The workers were very productive because, instead of each worker producing whole pins, each worker was assigned a discrete, but highly repetitive, task. The tasks formed a coordinated ensemble.[2] What Smith described, however, was preindustrial and limited to economies that were small in scale (Heilbroner, 1986). Ford and Taylor, and Marx for that matter, were concerned with large-scale industrial economies.

Ford's assembly line revolutionized production. He offered higher wages and an 8-hour day. Fordism, however, was not without an underside. Fordist (and by implication Taylorist) principles led to the "increasing dehumanization of workers" (Wallace, 2003). Ford's River Rouge plant was run like a "totalitarian state in miniature" (Wallace, 2003). Harry Bennett, one of Ford's lieutenants, directed Ford's Service Department, popularly known as "Ford's Gestapo." Bennett employed a small army of ex-convicts, former prize fighters, and ordinary informants who spied on workers. Workers who aroused suspicions at the Ford plant were beaten. Service Unit members attacked union organizers. Walter Reuther, the head of the United Auto Workers union, was one of those assaulted and severely injured (Nolan, 1997; Wallace, 2003). The fast pace of assembly line work with little time for rest or going

---

[2] Smith also foresaw that engaging in simple repetitive tasks hour after hour, day after day would have a deleterious effect on the mental functioning of the members of the vast laboring classes ("[the laborer] . . . generally becomes as stupid and ignorant as it is possible for a human creature. The torpor of his mind renders him, not only incapable of relishing or bearing a part in any rational conversation, but of conceiving any generous, noble, or tender sentiment" [p. 303, Vol. 2]). Smith went on to assert that in every civilized society, the state of mental torpor befalls "the laboring poor, that is, the great body of the people . . . unless government takes some pains to prevent it" (p. 303, Vol. 2).

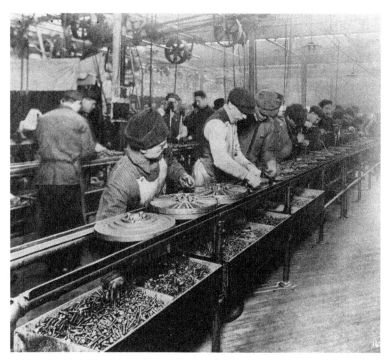

Ford assembly line, Highland Park, Michigan, 1913. (Photographer unknown, Copyright expired. Wikipedia Commons.)

to the toilet (Linder & Nygaard, 1998) had an adverse effect on workers. There were high rates of accidents at Ford's famous River Rouge plant, but Ford concealed the accident rate by creating a kind of conveyor system that dispatched accident victims to Ford's own hospital (Cruden, 1932). Cruden reported on the prevalent feelings of nervous tension among Ford's line workers.

It is not surprising that leaders of totalitarian regimes admired Ford and Taylor. Lenin, the exponent of scientific socialism, was smitten with scientific management (Hughes, 1989). Lenin, Trotsky, and Stalin expressed admiration for Ford's and Taylor's methods. In a 1924 address, Stalin (1940) expressed his high regard for Taylorist methods pioneered in the United States:

> American efficiency is that indomitable force which neither knows nor recognises obstacles; which with its business-like perseverance brushes aside all obstacles; which continues at a task once started until it is finished, even if it is a minor task; and without which serious constructive work is inconceivable. (p. 85)

Taylorist experts were brought from the United States to the nascent Soviet Union to help implement those methods in Russia (Hughes, 1989). The Ford Motor Company constructed a plant in Nizhny Novgorod. Ford, equally, had admirers in Nazi Germany (Wallace, 2003). In 1937, the Nazi government awarded Ford the Grand Cross of the German Eagle, the highest honor it could award a non-German, for his "humanitarian ideals" (Baldwin, 2001; Wallace, 2003).

Taylorism and Fordism became associated with dictatorial methods of improving workplace efficiency (Linder & Nygaard, 1998; Wallace, 2003). With this dictatorial focus on efficiency, the movements became associated with political dictatorships as well.

WORLD WAR I AND THE INTERWAR YEARS

It is expected that war would adversely affect the health in the civilian population, including that of workers. Using historical life insurance data, Winter (1977) found the opposite, at least for a country that was not invaded: "When the Prudential evidence of increased life expectation for civilian workers is also taken into account, it is clear that war conditions benefited in particular the non-combatant labouring population" (p. 502). After the outbreak of World War I, the British government was prompted to examine conditions of workers in munitions factories. The Health of Munition Workers Committee (1915) recommended that workers be given Sundays off. The Committee wrote,

> Continuous work is . . . a profound mistake, not only on social and religious grounds, but also economically, since it does not pay, the output not being increased. The output is not increased partly because men become bored and wearied with the monotony of the work. (p. 864)

In addition to rest periods, industrial canteens were established to ensure that munitions workers received nutritious meals (Health of Munition Workers Committee). By 1917, more than 700 of such canteens had been established (Winter, 1977).

Impact on Soldiers

War can have a terrible impact on the individuals in the military services. Siegfried Sassoon (1918), one of Britain's outstanding war poets, wrote:

> They leave their trenches, going over the top,
> While time ticks blank and busy on their wrists,
> And hope, with furtive eyes and grappling fists,
> Flounders in mud. O Jesu, make it stop!
> [Excerpted from the poem *Attack* by permission of the estate of Siegfried Sassoon]

Sassoon, who, while under fire, rescued a wounded soldier and later "single-handedly captur[ed] a German trench" on the Hindenberg Line, became an opponent of the War (Hochschild, 2011).

In the view of Freud (1956/1919), the emergence of so-called war neuroses involved an internal conflict, largely unconscious, between the conscript's "peaceful ego" and the former civilian's new, warlike one, superimposed on him by his military training and battlefield experience. The conscript's old peace ego "protects itself from a mortal danger by taking flight into a traumatic neurosis" (p. 209). Freud suggested (wrongly) that (a) war neuroses would be largely absent in a professional army and (b) those suffering from war neuroses would improve on the heels of the war's end. Freud opposed punishing soldiers suffering from war neuroses, declaring that the great majority of the casualties were not malingerers. He was particularly critical of German physicians "serving a purpose that was foreign to them," namely patching up psychologically wounded soldiers (often with electroconvulsive shock) and sending them back to the front. In Britain, Rivers (1918) advanced the view that the impact of the war on the mental health of soldiers can result from their repression of horrific war experiences. By repression, he did not necessarily mean the unconscious Freudian mechanism, although the influence of Freud on Rivers's thinking is clear. Rivers described a voluntary attempt "to banish from the mind the distressing memories of warfare or painful affective states which have come into being as the result of [soldiers'] war experience" (p. 173). The affective states to which he referred included feelings of shame that a soldier experiences when he thinks he may be deemed a coward by others.

Although he agreed with Rivers on the role of repression in war neuroses in soldiers, MacCurdy (1918) described a tension facing clinicians attempting to uncover the sources of mental health problems in soldiers engaged in trench warfare. On the one hand, MacCurdy believed that earlier "psychoneurotic tendencies" in individuals in civilian life are likely to predict later breakdown in warfare. On the other hand, he wrote that individuals with "a history of previous breakdowns or of having had tendencies toward psychoneurotic reactions in their past life [have] . . . nevertheless adapted themselves well to training and fought well" (p. 130). MacCurdy noted the great fatigue the experience of trench warfare often produced in soldiers. Fatigue was often a prelude to war neuroses. Although he did not mention brain injury, MacCurdy reported on the terrible role of the concussive impact of shells in precipitating anxiety reactions in soldiers in the trenches, who, if not killed were often buried under mounds of earth and had to be dug out by fellow soldiers.

These war neuroses should be viewed from within a larger context. Adam Hochschild (2011) documented the incredible stupidity and callousness with which the British high command threw men into the Battle of the Somme. On July 1, 1916, in the first hour of the attack, 19,000 British were dead. A total of 57,000 men were dead or wounded the first day. General Douglas Haig "doggedly, unyieldingly sent out order after order for more attacks on the Somme, and these would continue for an astonishing four and a half months" (p. 208). Operating under a "perverse logic," Haig associated German casualties with British losses, becoming angry when he considered British losses in an engagement to be too low. In the end, the British suffered 500,000 casualties and the French, 200,000. The command also failed to attain its territorial objectives.

The British author C. S. Lewis (1955), who served in France during the Great War, observed:

> But of the rest, the war—the frights, the cold, the smell of H.E.,[3] the horribly smashed men still moving like half-crushed beetles, the sitting or standing corpses, the landscape of sheer earth without a blade of grass, the boots worn day and night till they seemed to grow to your feet—all this shows rarely and faintly in memory. It is too cut off from the rest of my experience and often seems to have happened to someone else. (p. 185)

In his autobiography of his early life, from which the just-cited passage comes, Lewis wrote less about the appalling aspects of the war than about reading the essays of G. K. Chesterton while convalescing from an episode of trench fever; this passage, which is all that he wrote about combat, amounted to no more than an interjection. Perhaps given the physical and emotional pain he suffered, Lewis had largely fenced off his memories of combat. Lewis and two friends had been victims of friendly fire. In the Battle of Arras in 1918, a British shell aimed at the Germans landed on the three, killing the two friends, a highly competent sergeant whom Lewis venerated

---

[3] H.E. is an abbreviation for high explosives.

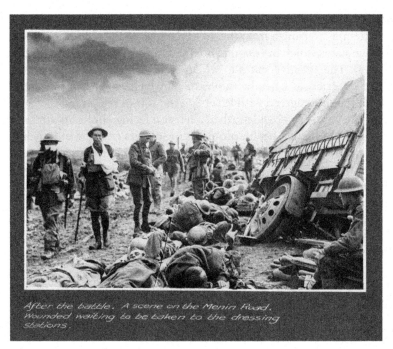

After the battle. A scene on the Menin Road. Wounded waiting to be taken to the dressing stations.

Wounded Australian soldiers, France, 1917. (Photographers James Francis [Frank] Hurley and George Hubert Wilkins. Official Australian War Photographs, produced by the Australian War Records Section, established by the British government in 1917. National Media Museum. Copyright expired. Creative Commons.)

and a fellow officer and intellect who Lewis believed would have become a lifelong friend; Lewis suffered multiple shrapnel wounds (Wilson, 1990). Lewis suffered another loss; his dear friend Paddy Moore went missing in action, and was presumed dead. In surviving the War, Lewis suffered headaches and nightmares (Jacobs, 2005).

Large numbers of surviving combatants became psychiatric casualties. "So many officers and men suffered shell shock, that, by the end of the war, the British had set up 19 military hospitals solely devoted to their treatment" (Hochschild, 2011, p. 242). In yet another example of supreme callousness, British military authorities sometimes accused shell-shocked soldiers of cowardice, and executed them (Hochschild). "Shell shock," a term that embraced a variety of conditions including the concussive effects of exposure to exploding ordnance and emotional disorders that develop in a variety of combat situations, was the term then commonly used (Great Britain. War Office, 2004/1922). In 1916, British physician Frederick W. Mott (1916a, 1916b) described an autopsy study he performed on two soldiers who died soon after having been exposed to explosive blasts. To take one of the two cases, Mott (1916b) observed that "there is no wound of any kind on his body or head, and no visceral lesion" (p. 442). He found hemorrhages in the brain's white matter and the basal ganglia. He surmised that the blast wave itself was the cause of the death.[4] The modern equivalents of shell shock include posttraumatic stress disorder and/or traumatic brain injury.

The early work on shell shock was important because there was now scientific discussion of psychological and neurological trauma resulting from exposure to war. This early work paved the way for later research during World War II. Eventually, OHP-related research, which embraces many occupations, would embrace research on exposure to war.

---

[4] See Chapter 11 for the most recent research on the impact of blast waves.

THE INTERWAR YEARS

Two important developments occurred during the interwar years that would influence the later emergence of OHP. The first was the appearance of efforts to understand the human relations side of organizations. Great Britain saw the institution of rest periods in munitions factories during World War I. The idea that rest periods would lead to improved productivity in U.S. workers, which was essentially a Taylorist notion, took root after the war. Ironically, this Taylorist idea precipitated a change in thinking that was more oriented to understanding the human side of organizational processes.

The second development was the Great Depression, which created mass unemployment. There was an impetus to conduct research designed to understand the psychological impact of unemployment.

Human Relations

Elton Mayo (1924), an Australian researcher working in the United States, closely studied a Philadelphia textile mill. The mill's spinning department had been suffering from a turnover rate of over 200% per year. Mayo observed that the repetitive nature of the work in the spinning department "make[s] for the development of pessimistic or other abnormal preoccupations" (p. 280). Mayo's solution was the implementation of a series of rest periods. Given Mayo's work in Philadelphia, it was natural for him to become involved in the Hawthorne studies.

Beginning in 1924, a number of studies were conducted at the Western Electric Company's Hawthorne plant in Cicero, Illinois, near Chicago. The Hawthorne studies had, at one time, so much prestige that one commentator (Hart, 1943) suggested that the research was the social science equivalent of the discoveries of Galileo and Mendel. From 1924 to 1927, the famous Hawthorne illumination studies took place at plant locations where workers (usually women) assembled relays. The studies are associated with the "Hawthorne effect," an effect that suggests that many different changes in working conditions or observer attention can lead to improvements in worker productivity. The effect turns out to be more myth than reality, given analyses of unearthed archived data (Levitt & List, 2011).

Another Hawthorne study began in 1927 and continued until 1932. It was on this study that Mayo (1933) focused much of his attention. The 1927 to 1932 study was better documented than the illumination studies. It involved five women who had been working in a large area with many other workers, assembling relays for the telephone company. The five were selected to work in a separate Relay Assembly Test Room (Mayo, 1933). During a sequence of 23 "experimental periods" (these periods did not really constitute an experiment with random allocation to treatment and control conditions), a series of changes was imposed on the five (two of the workers dropped out of the group, and were replaced midstream). The workers' output was measured during each period. The changes included the imposition of rest periods throughout the workday and alterations in their length and number. Another change that lasted through much of the study was that the workers' pay was tied to the output of the small group; formerly, their pay was tied to the output of the much larger group of workers from which the five were selected.

Mayo commented on the increases in the workers' output accompanying many (but not all) of the changes in the conditions in the Assembly Room:

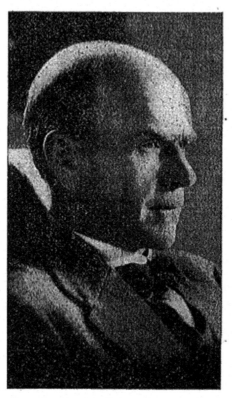

Elton Mayo (Photographer unknown. Undated photograph published in the University of Queensland Gazette, by permission of the Fryer Library, The University of Queensland Library.)

the individual workers and the group had to re-adapt themselves to a new industrial milieu, a milieu in which their own self-determination and their social well-being ranked first and the work was incidental. The experimental changes—rest-periods, food, and talk at appropriate intervals—perhaps operated at first mainly to convince them of the major change and to assist the re-adaptation. (p. 73)

Although this view is at most an exaggeration (Bell, 1947; Parsons, 1974), the idea advanced by Mayo is that improving working conditions, including psychosocial working conditions (e.g., "self-determination," opportunities to talk with fellow workers), has a beneficial impact on both worker well-being and productivity. Roethlisberger and Dickson (1939), other Hawthorne researchers, concluded that "the effects of the experimentally introduced changes in working conditions . . . proved to be carriers of social meaning rather than mere changes in physical circumstances" (p. 140).

The collective work of Mayo, Roethlisberger, and Dickson contributed to the development of the human relations movement in management. The movement recognized that "beneath the formalities of the organization chart was not chaos but a robust, informal organization, constituted by the activities, sentiments, interactions, norms, and personal and professional connections of individuals and groups that had developed over extended periods of time" (Anteby & Khurana, n.d.). At the Harvard Business School (HBS), where both Mayo and Roethlisberger were professors, the dominant Taylorist management principles that were once taught gave way to less mechanistic principles that stressed the fact that human relationships are an important part of the success of organizations. Bell (1947), expressing a dissenting view, advanced the idea that Hawthorne and studies like it reflected efforts at "greasing the skids" for factories and that command structures essentially continued to deny workers the kind of autonomy that humanizes workplaces.

Unemployment

Marie Jahoda was one of the first women to make a mark in the male-dominated social sciences. In 1933, Jahoda, Paul F. Lazarsfeld, and Hans Zeisel (1971/1933) published a groundbreaking book describing their research on residents of a small Austrian community. This community experienced very high levels of unemployment throughout the 1920s. The research team found that over time, unemployed community members became less engaged in everyday activities, becoming steadily more apathetic. Although Jahoda et al. collected a good deal of qualitative data, they also collected quantitative data that underlined the growing apathy. For example, from 1929 to 1931, the last year data were collected, the number of books the average resident borrowed from the library declined. Membership in the leading political party of that area also declined. Life history interviews with residents underlined the aimlessness of the residents' lives. Thus, Jahoda and her colleagues documented the psychological costs of unemployment and the Great Depression.

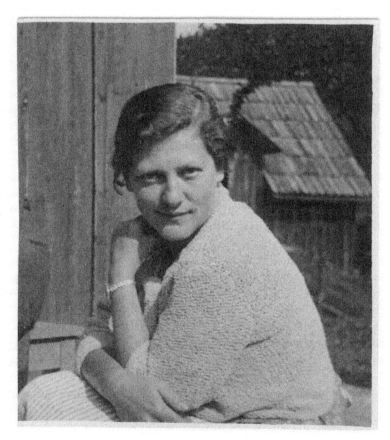

Marie Jahoda. (Photographer unknown. By permission of the Archiv für die Geschichte der Soziologie in Österreich, University of Graz.)

FROM THE WORLD WAR II ERA TO THE 1970S

The next section covers a period during which pioneering research and institution building took place. Some of the research took place during wartime, and concerned the impact of war on soldiers. After the war, investigators began to demonstrate that rigorous scientific methods could be applied to the study of the impact of psychosocial workplace factors on the health of workers in civilian jobs. The period was an era of institution building that has been relevant to OHP. It was also an era in which stress increasingly became the subject of articles and books.

World War II

During World War II, psychiatrists, psychologists, and sociologists took an interest in the so-called psychiatric casualties in the military. Samuel A. Stouffer and his colleagues (1949) published the watershed study of U.S. servicemen, *The American Soldier*, based on research conducted during the war, and involving large samples of Army personnel. Although anxiety problems and psychiatric casualties constituted just one part of their research, *The American Soldier* research was revolutionary in its application of social science methods to understanding the psychology of the soldier. Stouffer and his colleagues pioneered the development of instruments to ascertain the level of anxiety and psychosomatic symptoms experienced by the men. They anticipated the development of screening instruments that would be used in future research (Dohrenwend & Dohrenwend, 1982), particularly in research aimed at identifying probable psychiatric cases.

Stouffer et al. (1949) found that a higher proportion of breakdowns occurred in men during their first months in the service than during any other period of service. More importantly, they found that the intensity of exposure to combat was directly related to the men's risk of developing elevated levels of anxiety and psychosomatic symptoms. Even soldiers in the European Theater of Operations in April 1945, "when allied armies were advancing rapidly and the sense of imminent victory was in the air," experienced high levels of anxiety symptoms (p. 442). For example, 44% of the men aged 20 to 24 with some high school education experienced anxiety symptoms in the critical range. Stouffer et al. (1949) found extremely high rates of elevated levels of anxiety symptoms in veteran replacements who were about to return to combat in the central Pacific after a spell in the hospital (71% to 86%, depending upon age and educational level).

This is not to say that American servicemen experiencing high levels of combat stress were poor soldiers. They were not. Spiegel (1944), a psychiatrist who observed American troops in the Tunisian campaign, wrote that "not only was some of the gallant and heroic work done by men and officers in acute anxiety states, but a considerable amount of the ordinary combat accomplishment was performed by ordinary men experiencing rather severe anxiety" (p. 383). Good morale was related to the quality of company and platoon leadership. The capable leader

> saw to it that his men got the best possible food under the circumstances; sent blankets up to them at night if it were possible; made every effort to keep them well supplied with water and ammunition; saw to it that that promotions were fair; made certain that good work and gallantry were properly recognized; he got mail, news and information to them quickly. (Spiegel, 1944, p. 384)

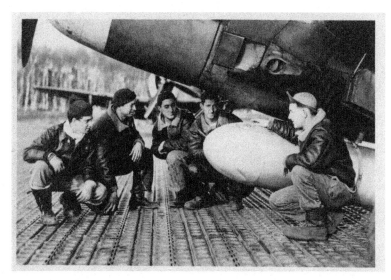

Members of the 356th Fighter Group, Eighth Air Force, U.S. Army Air Corps, Ipswich, England, 1943. The airman who is second from the left is George Schonfeld, the father of the first author. (Photographer unknown. Property of Irvin Sam Schonfeld.)

Roy Laver Swank (1949) was one of the first clinicians to examine the phenomenon then known as "combat exhaustion" using large samples of soldiers. He examined troops who served in the European Theater of Operations. In World War I, the term most commonly used was "shell shock." Swank observed among the casualties a great deal of fatigue. He also observed that the affected soldiers "lost their confidence, became irritable and agitated and appeared anxious. Later, other symptoms, namely, [psychomotor] retardation, preoccupation, mental defect and apathy," developed (p. 475). Swank found that combat exhaustion was severest and had earlier onsets in soldiers who served in units that suffered the highest casualty rates. Contrary to MacCurdy (1918), Swank also found that precombat stability was not related to combat exhaustion in men exposed to combat over long periods of time.

The research conducted by Stouffer and his associates (1949) and Swank (1949) on the impact of exposure to combat was superior to the research conducted during World War I. Research conducted during World War II did not blame the psychiatric causality. The hunt for causes identified the length and intensity of combat exposure and unit casualty rates. Research by Spiegel (1944) indicated that soldiers experiencing high levels of anxiety could acquit themselves well on the battlefield.

Institute for Social Research

OHP is quintessentially interdisciplinary. Interdisciplinary research requires robust institutional support. An example of the growth of institutional support comes from the history of the University of Michigan. In 1930, social scientists from eight different departments at Michigan organized the Social Science Research Council of Michigan (Frantilla, 1998; Institute for Social Research, n.d.). One of the aims of the Council was to advance cooperation across departmental lines.

Soon after the close of World War II, an institutional development affected the course of the social sciences. Rensis Likert, the creator of the famous Likert-type scale, founded the Institute for Social Research (ISR) at Michigan (Frantilla, 1998). Likert

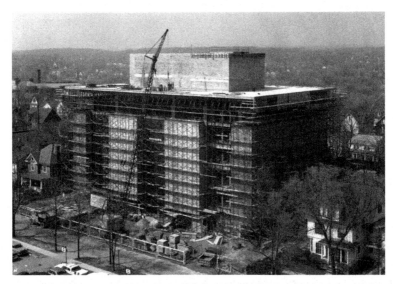

Undated photograph of the construction of a building to house the Institute for Social Research at the University of Michigan. (Photographer unknown. Photo courtesy of the University of Michigan, Institute for Social Research.)

initially founded the Survey Research Center in 1946. Then, in 1948, the Research Center for Group Dynamics moved from MIT to Michigan. In 1949, both Research Centers became divisions within the ISR umbrella organization (Cannell & Kahn, 1984). With time, other research centers were created, and came under the aegis of ISR. Research conducted by ISR staff has been supported by grants and contracts, and not out of the University's budget. ISR evolved into a kind of empyrean heaven for social science research. Although initially centered on social psychology, ISR research crossed disciplinary boundaries to include political science, sociology, and economics in addition to fields such as epidemiology, psychiatry, and statistics (Cannell & Kahn, 1984). ISR investigators have conducted research bearing on the interrelationships among work, well-being, and health (e.g., Caplan, Cobb, & French, 1975; House, 1980; Quinn & Staines, 1979).

Tavistock and Human Relations

The Tavistock Clinic, a psychoanalytically oriented psychiatric center, was established in London in 1920. During World War II, leaders of the clinic entered the Directorate of Army Psychiatry to use their skills to help troubled soldiers and to address problems related to morale in the British military. Trist and Murray (1990) underscored the emerging interdisciplinary character of the military-related efforts of the Tavistock Clinic group: "To meet these large-scale tasks the range of disciplines was extended from psychiatry and clinical psychology to social psychology, sociology and anthropology." In 1946, the leaders of the Tavistock Clinic organized the Tavistock Institute of Human Relations. Initially a division of the clinic, in 1947 the institute became independent. The institute promoted psychoanalytically oriented and social psychological research on human relations. In 1947, members of the institute and members of the Research Center for Group Dynamics established a new journal, aptly named *Human Relations*, for the purpose of furthering "the integration of psychology and the social sciences and relate theory to practice" (Trist & Murray, 1990; also see *Human Relations*, 2012).

Changes in the British Mining Industry

In 1951, Eric Trist and Kenneth Bamforth published in *Human Relations* an influential article on the effects of changes in the British coal mining industry on miners. Trist was one of the founding members of the Tavistock Institute, and Bamforth, a former coal miner, was a fellow there. Trist and Bamforth found that changes in the organization of work led to a reduction in the miners' autonomy:

> Superficially, borers, belt-builders, and belt-breakers look like pair structures that echo pre-mechanized days. But whereas the pairs of hand-got coal-getting had craft status and an artisan type of independence in working their own [coal] face, with the satisfaction of seeing through the whole coal-getting job, these longwall pairs are restricted to work tasks of singularly narrow component character. (p. 36)

Trist and Bamforth noted the "fractionated tasks" led to the miners losing a "sense of belonging" with the other members of their shift or production group. The research belied an early recognition of the importance of job-related autonomy for worker well-being.

Hans Selye

In 1956, endocrinologist Hans Selye published an influential book entitled *The Stress of Life*. Although not written with job stress in mind, his work influenced future research on general life stress as well as OHP research. His research since the 1930s was built on a foundation laid by scientists such as Walter B. Cannon. At this juncture, it is helpful to review some of what Cannon (1914) found before turning to Selye.

In a series of animal experiments, Cannon underlined the activation of the sympathetic adrenal-medullary (SAM) system in response to emotion-provoking challenges. Sensory impulses "aroused by the natural events in the course of an animal's life" (p. 357) are channeled to the adrenal glands, which rest atop the kidneys. The adrenal medulla, the central part of the adrenal glands (the adrenal cortex surrounds the adrenal medulla), in turn releases the hormone adrenaline (epinephrine) into the bloodstream. Adrenaline precipitates glycogenolysis, the conversion of glycogen stored in the liver and in muscle tissue into glucose, better preparing for the action of key muscles (e.g., the heart) that help the animal fight or flee a predator. Other muscles not important to fight or flight (e.g., muscles in the alimentary canal) experience a reduction in activity. Cannon (1929) later introduced the idea of homeostasis, which involves self-regulation and the maintenance of stable levels of temperature, protein, glucose, fat, oxygen, and so forth despite the presence of "continually disturbing conditions." Tendencies toward change are "automatically met."

Building on Cannon's research, Selye (1956), who also worked with animals, examined the response of the organism to foreign biological or chemical agents that potentially disturb homeostasis and to which the organism restoratively responds. Selye noted that the organism's responses are similar for many different disturbances. He also observed that people who were affected by a variety of diseases often shared many common symptoms. Selye used the term "stress" to describe a syndrome that includes "all the nonspecifically induced changes within a biologic system" in response to an aggressive outside agent, that is, the stressor (p. 54), and that some stress benefits the organism. He labeled the totality of the nonspecific response to a stressor the "general adaptation syndrome" (GAS). The syndrome comprises three stages: "(1) the alarm stage," "(2) the stage of resistance," and "(3) the stage of exhaustion." The GAS response involves the rapid mobilization and orchestration of the pituitary gland, the adrenal medulla and cortex, and the central and autonomic nervous systems.

Selye was concerned with the stress process as it unfolds in response to objective features of the environment: "physiological responses to environmental stimuli might occur without any subjective assessment of those stimuli" (Hurrell, Nelson, & Simmons, 1998, p. 369). Consistent with this view, Selye noted that "during World War II, veritable epidemics of 'air-raid ulcers' occurred in people living in some of the heavily blitzed cities in Great Britain" (p. 179).

Selye,[5] in the revised edition of his book (1976) and elsewhere (1985), amended the ideas about which he previously wrote. In his revised scheme, sensory input mediated by the cerebral cortex, the limbic system, and reticular formation reaches the hypothalamus. The hypothalamus, upon receiving the signals, produces corticotrophic hormone releasing factor (CRF). CRF, by way of the bloodstream, arrives at the pituitary gland, precipitating the pituitary's release of adrenocorticotrophic hormone (ACTH) into the circulatory system. In response to ACTH, the adrenal cortex releases glucocorticoids such as cortisol and corticosterone, which stimulate glycogenolysis, supplying energy for the muscles to respond to demands during an alarm state (glucocorticoids are not as important during the later resistance stage). ACTH also triggers the secretion of adrenaline and noradrenaline, that is, the catecholamines epinephrine and norepinephrine, in the adrenal medulla; nerve endings in the autonomic nervous system are also a site for catecholamine synthesis. Adrenaline triggers the formation of glucose from glycogen (as just mentioned) and from triglyceride stores; adrenaline also improves circulation to the muscles by increasing both pulse rate and blood pressure. What is outlined is the action of the hypothalamic–pituitary–adrenal (HPA) axis in the stress process.

Stressful Life Events

A line of research flowed out of Selye's work. His original 1956 book suggested that stressors can affect human health in nonspecific ways, and cause a variety of illnesses. In the 1960s, researchers began to examine the link between life events (LEs) and illness (Rahe, Meyer, Smith, Kjaer, & Holmes, 1964). LEs refer to events that cause different degrees of social readjustment (e.g., marriage, divorce, death of a loved one).

---

[5] There was also an underside of Selye's research. Selye received from the tobacco industry extensive support for his research on stress (Petticrew & Lee, 2011). Petticrew and Lee found that Selye advanced the ideas that (a) smoking can be beneficial as a stress-reducer and (b) antismoking campaigns can cause stress in members of the public. The authors observed that "Selye's expert evidence diluted existing evidence of the adverse effects of smoking and distracted attention from its harms. In failing to declare his receipt of tobacco funding when expressing his views against tobacco control, documents suggest he concealed a lack of scientific independence" (p. 414).

Some LEs are beneficial, others neither beneficial nor harmful to the individual, and still others are stressful. In the years after Holmes and Rahe's (1967) publication of their Social Readjustment Rating Scale (SRRS), research on the impact of stressful life events (SLEs) on health, particularly mental health, accelerated. Research on the health effects of SLEs largely concerned life in general, although a SLE such as getting fired would be included in LE inventories such as the SRRS. There was also a natural bridge from research interest in general life stress to research interest more specifically devoted to work-related stress (Karasek, 1979).

Stress Research in Sweden

Following Selye's research, investigators in Sweden studied the impact of work arrangements on SAM reactions. Sweden had become a center of stress research, with Lennart Levi founding the Stress Research Laboratory in 1959 and going on to establish the National Institute for Psychosocial Factors and Health in 1980 (Theorell, 1997). Levi (1972) found that a short-lived change from hourly wages to piece work was accompanied by increases in output as well as increases in adrenaline and noradrenaline. When returned to hourly wages, there were accompanying declines. Frankenhaeuser (1979; Frankenhaeuser & Gardell, 1976) found that compared with men in control jobs, men working at a sawmill in monotonous, machine-paced jobs showed high levels of adrenaline and noradrenaline excretion along with high levels of psychosomatic symptoms.

Developments in Sociology, Social Psychology, and Industrial Psychology

A number of social scientists including Ely Chinoy, a team made up mostly of ISR researchers, and Arthur Kornhauser, spurred interest in research on work, stress, and well-being. In 1955, sociologist Ely Chinoy published a book based on his research on blue collar workers. Having intensively interviewed 62 men who worked in a U.S. automobile manufacturing plant, he painted a picture of the monotony of the workers' blue collar jobs, and their search for satisfaction outside of work. Chinoy underlined two different ways in which the men experienced feelings of alienation. First, there is little opportunity for advancement. Second, the nature of the highly mechanized work required "the surrender of control over their own actions" (p. 85). The idea that control (or its absence) is an important feature of work reemerges with the research of Robert Karasek, which will be covered later in this chapter and in Chapters 3 and 4. Some of the men had pipe dreams such as fantasies of starting a farm. The dreams, however, were just that, dreams. The independence and autonomy that the dreams implied required more capital and training than the men, who were largely born into working class families, possessed. Chinoy anticipated the answer to a question later posed by Johannes Siegrist, whose work is discussed in Chapter 3, regarding why workers often remain in unrewarding jobs. Chinoy underlined the fact that costs of leaving and obtaining more satisfying jobs are major barriers.

In 1964, a team of social psychologists, three of whom were researchers at ISR, published a book describing innovative research on organizational stress. The book was published in an era when psychodynamic psychology was ascendant, and psychologists tended to locate the causes of psychopathology intrapsychically, and in the relationship of the individual with his or her parents. Kahn, Wolfe, Quinn, Snoek, and Rosenthal, however, were concerned with how organizational role relationships, combined with personality dimensions, affect job-related tension, job satisfaction, sense of futility at work, and so forth. They were also among the first researchers to study work-related coping. The team organized two studies, one of which was a survey of a nationally representative sample of U.S. workers, and the second an intensive investigation of 53 men in supervisory positions in "six industrial locations" in the United States. An innovation of the study was their interviewing the members of each focal person's "role set," that is, the collectivity of individuals in different roles, subordinates, supervisors, and individuals at the same level, whose own roles directly affected that of the focal person. The interviews assessed the pressures exerted on the focal person to change his performance; these pressures became the source for a measure of role conflict. Role ambiguity was assessed from data collected from the interview of the focal person. The authors found that conflict and ambiguity were linked to job-related tension. A methodological innovation of the study was that the investigators assessed role conflict and tension independently of each other; a methodological problem facing research on the psychological impact of working conditions has been how to assess the independent (e.g., psychosocial job stressors) and dependent variables (e.g., distress) without the assessment of one contaminating the assessment of the other. Although the study's results were far from eye-opening (e.g., role conflict and neurotic anxiety "combine additively" to affect tension), the research added momentum to psychology's efforts to evaluate the joint effects of job and person variables on health outcomes.

Arthur Kornhauser was a psychologist who became involved in industrial psychology. What distinguished him from his disciplinary colleagues who were "largely concerned with problems of increasing industrial efficiency" (Zickar, 2003, p. 366) was his interest in the plight of working people. In 1965, he published a book in which he described landmark research that combined qualitative and quantitative methods in a study of 407 male workers at 13 Detroit automobile manufacturing plants and a comparison sample comprising 248 men working outside of Detroit in manufacturing and nonmanufacturing jobs. Based on interview data, he found that the skill and responsibility required by a worker's job were inversely related to his mental health. In other words, workers with highly repetitive, semiskilled jobs were at risk for the worst mental health, and workers having jobs that required greater skill and responsibility tended to have better mental health. An innovation in his research included the development and validation of his measures of mental health. Another innovation was his concern for the possibility that the workers at risk for poor mental health had self-selected for the lowest-level jobs. Kornhauser adduced evidence to suggest that selection did not explain his findings. He also linked mental health to job satisfaction. In order to disentangle the effects of the worker's personality and the effects of the job, he advocated the use of longitudinal methods in future research on the mental health of workers. His study also pioneered efforts to examine "spillover" into life outside of work of negative feelings adverse work situations provoked.

The research by Kornhauser, Chinoy, and the team led by Kahn fueled interest in the impact of work on the health of workers. Contemporary research in OHP owes much to these investigators (Quick, 1999; Sauter & Hurrell, 1999). A number of themes emerged from their research, including concerns about worker autonomy, the impact of highly repetitive work, job-related conflict, the problem of selection, and the need for longitudinal studies.

Richard Lazarus

Although he has been a psychologist whose ideas apply to psychological stress in general, Richard Lazarus's 1966 book was influential in OHP circles. In Lazarus's model, an individual is informed by a number of antecedent characteristics, including motives, beliefs, and past learning. When confronted with a new "stimulus configuration," the individual appraises it for level of threat or anticipated harm; Lazarus called this initial evaluation "primary appraisal." Whether a circumstance is deemed a threat or not depends upon cognitions such as a person's judgment that the situation is likely to block the individual from attaining goals. The individual's personality and life history bear upon this appraisal. Threat appraisal comes between the stimulus configuration and the individual's reactions to it. Lazarus saw threat as being different from anxiety in that the latter is one of several potential affective consequences of a threat. OHP researchers with a Lazarus-type orientation have been concerned with the features of the work environment that are appraised as threatening.

In response to a threat, the individual often engages in coping behaviors. Coping refers to "strategies for dealing with threat" (Lazarus, 1966, p. 151). It includes action directly taken to change a threatening circumstance or the utilization of psychologically defensive maneuvers such as denying the threat or painting the threat picture in a rosier color. In addition to primary appraisal, Lazarus also developed the concept of secondary appraisal, which is another round of appraisal that refers to the individual's evaluation of the consequences of his or her coping actions. Along with Lazarus, Beehr and Newman (1978; Newman & Beehr, 1979) were particularly influential in encouraging research on work-related coping.

The appraisal idea has not been without its critics. Dohrenwend and Shrout (1985) found that a stressor measure developed by Lazarus and his colleagues (1985), one that relied on participant appraisal, was confounded with psychological symptoms. Dohrenwend and Shrout argued that measuring pure environmental events uncontaminated by appraisals and reactions is important to understanding the stress process. They suggested that researchers also assess an event's context, which includes vulnerability factors and resources, including the present social situation and personal dispositions that may modify the impact of the event on well-being.

Public health–oriented OHP researchers have been intent on characterizing objective features of the psychosocial work environment (Kasl, 1987) that affect the health of workers. Objective features of the environment are subject to change by way of interventions. Conversely, appraisals of events are personal, and put more of the burden of the environment's health effect on the worker.

Methodological Rigor in Research on Job Stress

Convincing evidence began to mount that researchers can employ rigorous methods to examine the link between work-related psychosocial conditions and physical health. Meyer Friedman, Ray Rosenman, and Vernice Carroll published perhaps the first such study in 1958. They examined fluctuations in serum cholesterol and blood clotting time as a function of stress in two groups of male accountants. One group, U.S. tax accountants, whose work chiefly involved completing tax returns, experienced severe job stress from April 1 to 15, the deadline for filing. The other group, specialized in corporate finance, experienced severe stress in the month of January (because of deadlines for corporate reporting) and from April 1 to 15. Friedman et al.

(1958) found that, independent of diet, weight, and exercise, periods of extreme occupational stress were related to faster blood clotting times and elevations in serum cholesterol, both risk factors for heart disease.

Some years later, two ISR researchers, Stanislav Kasl and Sydney Cobb (1970), published an influential paper concerning the impact of unemployment on blood pressure. Kasl and Cobb's study involved men experiencing plant closings and controls who were men continuously and comparably employed. The investigators were able to link job loss and unemployment to increases in blood pressure and reemployment to decreases.

In 1973, the ISR team of Sydney Cobb and Robert Rose published an article that linked job conditions to health outcomes in all-male samples. Cobb and Rose found that in comparisons with U.S. Air Force enlistees, air traffic controllers, an ostensibly high-stress job, showed higher rates of hypertension and peptic ulcer. Compared with men working in low-traffic towers, men working in high-traffic towers were at significantly higher risk for both hypertension and ulcer.

Thus, the studies conducted by Friedman et al. (1958), Kasl and Cobb (1970), and Cobb and Rose (1973) demonstrated to future investigators that rigorous research in which psychosocial workplace characteristics could be operationalized and linked to health outcomes could be conducted. Beehr and Newman (1978) observed that industrial and organizational (I–O) psychology had resisted research on work and health, and urged I–O and other psychologists to engage in rigorous research on work, stress, and health.

OSHA and NIOSH

A major legal milestone in the history leading up to the emergence of OHP came about when the United States Congress passed and President Nixon signed Public Law 91-596, the Occupational Safety and Health Act (Occupational Safety and Health Act of 1970). The purpose of the law has been to ensure safe and healthy working conditions for American workers. The Occupational Safety and Health Administration (OSHA), which the act created, and the Department of Labor (DOL) were assigned the responsibility of setting and enforcing health and safety standards at U.S. workplaces. OSHA became part of the Department of Health, Education, and Welfare, but is now part of the Department of Health and Human Services.

PL 91-596 also authorized the creation of the National Institute for Occupational Safety and Health (NIOSH), which eventually became a unit of the CDC. The law gave NIOSH a research mandate:

(1) to conduct such research and experimental programs as [the Director of NIOSH] determines are necessary for the development of criteria for new and improved occupational safety and health standards, and (2) after consideration of the results of such research and experimental programs make recommendations concerning new or improved occupational safety and health standards.

NIOSH does not write health and safety regulations. NIOSH's research findings inform the regulation process at OSHA and the DOL. NIOSH can also award grants to outside researchers such as professors at universities.

Another section of the law authorized NIOSH to conduct research pertinent to OHP. The law authorized research on job stress along with research on exposures

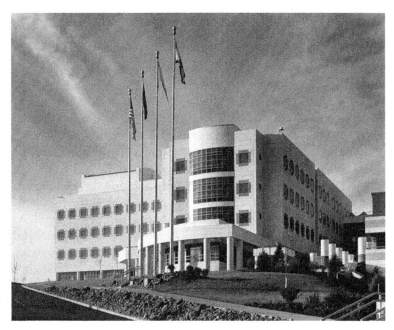

NIOSH facility in Morgantown, West Virginia. (Photographer unknown. Courtesy of NIOSH/CDC. Public Domain.)

to physical hazards: "the Secretary of Health and Human Services shall conduct and publish industry-wide studies of the effect of chronic or low-level exposure to industrial materials, processes, and stresses on the potential for illness, disease, or loss of functional capacity in aging adults." The law authorized NIOSH to support research on psychological factors that can be employed to improve worker safety and reduce accidents, including the modification of behavior and work habits (Cohen & Margolis, 1973).

J. Donald Millar, a physician who had become well known for his work for the CDC on the eradication of smallpox in Africa, became the director of NIOSH in 1981 (Fox, 2015). In the United States in the 1980s, the Social Security Administration saw the growth of disability claims for work-related psychological disorders (Sauter & Hurrell, 2016). While at the helm of NIOSH, the organization developed a list of the 10 leading work-related diseases and disabilities based on frequency, severity, and preventability; the list included psychological disorders (Millar, 1984). Millar took a leadership role in bringing to bear the weight of the organization in supporting research on work-related psychological disorders and developing a national prevention strategy (Sauter & Hurrell, 1999). NIOSH has gone on to award grants to OHP researchers. NIOSH's intramural research has also included an ambitious lineup of OHP-related studies (Caruso, 2009; Hitchcock, 2008; Murphy, 2002; Nigam, 2007; Streit, Nigam, & Sauter, 2011; Wallin, Considine, & Nigam, 2009).

P–E Fit

NIOSH's commitment to research on psychological factors was borne out in one of the first research endeavors the newly created agency supported, a study of the relation of psychosocial working conditions to physical and mental health (Caplan, Cobb, French, Harrison, & Pinneau, 1975; also see Caplan, 1987). This ISR study involved male workers in 23 U.S. occupational groups. An element of the study was loosely motivated by Darwinian theory, namely, the importance of the fit between the person and his or her environment. The authors advanced the view that "the goodness of fit" between the "characteristics of the worker" (e.g., needs and abilities) and the requirements of his or her work environment is likely to affect the individual's physical and mental health (p. 15).

Caplan, Cobb, French, Harrison, et al. (1975) were concerned with a methodological trap that would also be of concern to later OHP researchers, specifically, the potential problem that self-report stressor measures may be "contaminated" in that they tap more than one construct. For example, a self-report stressor scale is liable to assess stressors as well as personality dimensions and factors such as anxiety, depression, and job satisfaction, potentially inflating the correlation of the stressor scale with the other variables. Caplan et al. addressed the problem of contamination by employing measures that included bipolar vignettes of individuals in clearly described situations (e.g., "In Tom's job he works on many different tasks which are all in different stages of completion . . . Jim's job requires him to work on one job at a time. . . ." [p. 243]) and then have the worker indicate (a) where his current job fits on the continuum and (b) what kind of job he would like if he were looking for a new position. Although similar vignettes have not been widely used in OHP research, the seriousness of the ISR team's concern with the problem of confounding was a call for care in developing the methods required to study the impact of psychosocial work characteristics on strain, which is often operationalized by psychological symptoms.

An example of a person–environment (P–E) fit stressor is the discrepancy between the amount of complexity a job requires and the amount of complexity a worker prefers. The relation of P–E fit job complexity to depression was, as P–E theory suggested, curvilinear, with both too much and too little complexity related to elevated levels of depressive symptoms. For a period of time, P–E fit was a popular avenue of research, but since the late 1980s, interest in it has waned owing to difficulties specifying mathematical representations of P–E discrepancies and problematic statistical models of the relation of P–E discrepancies and strains (Ganster & Schaubroeck, 1991).

Burnout

Herbert Freudenberger (1974) was the individual who first identified the concept of burnout. Freudenberger admitted to having experienced burnout in the context of working in free clinics. He identified a number of physical signs of burnout that include feelings of exhaustion and fatigue, headaches, gastrointestinal problems, and sleeplessness. He also identified a number of behavioral signs. These signs included the reaction that the slightest pressure makes the individual feel overburdened; another is a suspicious attitude and the feeling that others—clients and colleagues—are out to take advantage of the individual. According to Freudenberger, the most dedicated and committed professionals working in free clinics, crisis intervention centers, and other arenas dedicated to helping people are at risk for burnout. The care the professional gives to a very needy clientele risks depleting the professional's reserves. Christina Maslach's (Maslach & Jackson, 1981; Maslach, Jackson, & Leiter, 1996) efforts to design an instrument to measure burnout helped to accelerate research on the subject. Over time, the concept of burnout has been extended beyond helping professionals to include almost all workers, and even to roles outside of work (Bianchi, Truchot, Laurent, Brisson, & Schonfeld, 2014).

Decision Latitude and Job Demands

Gardell (1971) examined mental health and alienation in a study of Swedish pulp and paper mill workers and engineers. He operationalized alienation in terms of the extent to which a worker "depreciates his work as a source of needs satisfaction" (p. 148). Gardell suggested that the problem of alienation at work was similar in both capitalist and socialist countries, with alienation emanating "from the industrial production system, and the causes should be chiefly sought in the authoritarian system of power and leadership" in the workplace (p. 148). Gardell found that the extent to which the workers exerted control and influence over their work was positively related to mental health and self-esteem, and negatively related to feelings of alienation.

In 1979, Robert Karasek published an article that became very influential in OHP circles. Using two large data sets, he showed the viability of a model in which the combination of low levels of decision latitude (i.e., control over job tasks conducted over the work day) and high levels of job demands adversely affects workers' mental health. The adverse mental health effects are often termed "psychological strains." The job demands component of the model largely comprised psychological workload, and not physical demands. The model was interactional, underlining that the combination of reduced latitude and high workload was particularly toxic for mental health.

Although prior research by Trist and Bamforth (1951) and Gardell (1971) underscored the impact of low levels of job-related autonomy on workplace morale and mental health, Karasek's model stimulated an outpouring of research, including research on both the independent and the interactive effects of decision latitude and workload on psychological symptoms and disorders. Karasek's model has been extended to examine the impact of the two factors on physical health (e.g., Karasek, Baker, Marxer, Ahlbom, & Theorell, 1981). The model was expanded to include another important variable, namely, coworker support (Johnson, Hall, & Theorell, 1989). The model has been a fountainhead of OHP research.

THE 1980S TO THE PRESENT

The rest of the chapter concentrates on institution building. Important organizations emerged during this period. These organizations became hubs for the coalescing of communities of OHP researchers and practitioners. The organizations have provided a network for the communication of OHP-related ideas. Many of the research developments that occurred in this period are covered in later chapters; however, two empirical studies are covered because of their groundbreaking nature. The chapter also examines the coining of the term "occupational health psychology." Having an effective term to subsume the work of researchers and practitioners in this field facilitates communication.

Two Groundbreaking Studies

The studies conducted by Friedman et al. (1958), Kasl and Cobb (1970), and Cobb and Rose (1973) demonstrated that the impact of psychosocial workplace characteristics on physical health could be rigorously studied. In a similar vein, two later studies demonstrated that the impact of psychosocial workplace characteristics on mental health could also be rigorously studied.

Katherine Parkes (1982) exploited a "naturally occurring work situation" involving female student nurses in the United Kingdom who were randomly assigned to different rotations (see the section on natural experiments in Chapter 2). One rotation group began in the surgical ward and ended in the medical ward; the other group rotated through the wards in the reverse order. Working in medical wards, with their "greater affective demands," was linked to markedly higher levels of depressive symptoms and lower levels of work satisfaction.

In the second study, Michael Frese (1985) followed male German industrial workers, using both subjective ratings of job stressors (e.g., ambiguities, conflict) and group-averages based on the ratings of three or more individuals doing the same job (but not necessarily working together). Controlling for psychosomatic symptoms (e.g., headaches, stomachaches) at baseline, baseline workplace stressors significantly predicted psychosomatic symptoms 16 months later. Reverse causality, a situation in which symptoms cause the hypothesized stressors, is difficult to rule out in cross-sectional studies, the most common type of study (see Chapter 2). In a test of a reverse causal hypothesis, symptoms at time 1, controlling for job stressors at time 1, failed to predict job stressors at time 2.[6]

Occupational Health Psychology

Although they did not use the term "occupational health psychology," Cooper and Marshall, in 1976, called for psychologists who conduct research on job stress to collaborate with other social scientists and medical professionals to advance what is essentially an interdisciplinary field. The term "occupational health psychology," first appeared in print in 1985 and 1986. In 1985, Robert Feldman, in a chapter in a book on workplace health promotion, a book that he and George Everly, Jr. edited, emphasized the need for interdisciplinary teamwork in health promotion: "Industrial hygienists, occupational physicians, occupational health psychologists, and occupational health educators all have a role to play to reduce and eliminate injuries and illnesses" (p. 286). Feldman also indicated that occupational health promotion and occupational health psychology share a role in improving workers' perceptions of risk and changing risky behavior in workers.

In 1986, George Everly, Jr., in an annual series on clinical practice, more fully acquainted readers with the term in an article entitled *An Introduction to Occupational Health Psychology*. Everly viewed OHP as a subspecialty of the older field of health psychology. For Everly, OHP involved the application of psychological theory and knowledge to prevent, diagnose, and treat "physical disease and dysfunction" that arise from workplace conditions. He was careful to note that workplace health promotion needs to be compatible with the organization's balance sheet, and went on to describe a systems approach to workplace health promotion that includes greater collaboration between an organization's health professionals and management. Everly

---

[6] One limitation of the study was that independent, expert-based objective ratings of stressors at time 1 failed to predict time 2 psychosomatic symptoms although such a finding does not impeach the main results because two different kinds of observers conducted the time 1 and time 2 objective ratings (engineers, psychology students). Because of imprecision in the objective measures of job stressors, correlations between objective measures and strain represent a kind of "lower bound of the true correlation" (p. 325). The imprecision reflects the fact that the raters, in the relatively short time (at most an hour and a half) they had to observe each of the various positions, imperfectly captured the job stressors an individual worker encountered in his lived workplace experience.

also suggested that for OH psychologists, training include counseling or clinical psychology, "industrial psychology," biomedical preparation, and public health.

The next time the term would appear in a publication was in 1990. Raymond, Wood, and Patrick published a paper in the *American Psychologist*, a journal received by every member of the American Psychological Association (APA). The authors enunciated the view that psychologists have an obligation to ensure healthy work environments. Raymond et al. (1990) called for doctoral-level training in OHP, training that would be strongly interdisciplinary. Unlike Feldman and Everly, Raymond et al. were concerned with training that would enable psychologists to deal with disorders arising from work-related stress.

Work & Stress

Journals are an important vehicle for communication in science. In 1987, Tom Cox and Phillip Dewe of the University of Nottingham founded the first journal devoted to OHP-related topics (Cox, 2011). At the time of its founding, the journal did not use the term "occupational health psychology," for the term had not yet had wide currency. Cox named the journal *Work & Stress*. The name of the journal is telling because "interest in work-related stress was accelerating and the contents of the first volumes reflect the fact that the main interest in those years was on that specific subject" (Cox, Taris, & Tisserand, 2009, p. 17). In the 1990s, as the field of OHP widened, the journal began to expand its focus beyond workplace stress (Cox et al., 2009), publishing papers on the relation of psychosocial working conditions to musculoskeletal symptoms, the relation of learning opportunities to decision-authority, organizational factors that affect accident risk, and so on.

APA–NIOSH Conference Series

With NIOSH supporting the addition of psychological disorders to its portfolio of work-related disorders, a number of scientists at NIOSH in the late 1980s made common cause with the APA. The prevention of work-related psychological disorders was on the agenda of a 1986 symposium sponsored by NIOSH (Quick, Murphy, & Hurrell, 1992). In 1989, individuals at NIOSH (Steven Sauter, Joseph J. Hurrell, Jr., and others) and APA (Gwendolyn Keita, Heather Roberts Fox, and others) began a collaboration that included planning for the APA/NIOSH Work and Well-Being Conference that would be held the next year in Washington, DC. J. Donald Millar, the then-director of NIOSH, approved funding to help underwrite the cost of the conference (Sauter & Hurrell, 2016). This international conference included panels of interdisciplinary experts on "stress and job design, the surveillance of occupational stress and psychological disorders, and enhancing occupational mental health" (Quick et al., 1992). Conferences were also attended by industrial/organizational, experimental, and developmental psychologists, physicians, nurses, social workers, human resources personnel, economists, and labor leaders. In the beginning, the conferences ran every 2 to 3 years, but by 2006, the conference series became biennial. The conferences provided a congenial setting for OHP professionals to get to know one another and to get to know each other's work.

Doctoral Programs in OHP

In order for OHP to sustain itself, a flow of new researchers and practitioners into the field was needed. APA and NIOSH collaborated in a new way; they began to provide seed money to help underwrite the creation of postdoctoral programs in OHP. Leaders in the two organizations, however, soon acknowledged that the best route to bringing more professionals into the field was to support doctoral training in OHP (Hammer & Schonfeld, 2007). At the time of the writing of this book, there are 11 OHP graduate programs in the United States.

University of Nottingham

In 1988, through a merger of two research groups, Tom Cox helped found the Centre for Organizational Health and Development (COHD) at the University of Nottingham (Leka, 2016 and personal communication, April 2016). Through a later merger and name change and a reemergence under its original name, the Centre has played an important role in research, practice, and policy bearing on the management of psychosocial risk in workplaces (Leka, 2016). In 1996, Cox developed a curriculum for an OHP master's program at the University of Nottingham. It was the first master's degree program of its kind. The founding of the program was consistent with the call by Raymond et al. (1990) for the training of psychologists in the science needed to ensure healthy work environments. Today the University of Nottingham offers a doctorate in Occupational Health—Psychology and Management.

Journal of Occupational Health Psychology

In the context of their organization's efforts to develop a strategy for prevention of work-related psychological disorders (NIOSH, 1988), two NIOSH researchers, Steven Sauter and Joseph J. Hurrell, Jr., together with NIOSH colleagues, conceived of a new kind of journal devoted to work, stress, and health. After several years of exploratory and developmental effort, Sauter and Hurrell invited James Campbell Quick of the University of Texas, Arlington, to serve as the first editor. The three worked collaboratively with Gary VandenBos of APA's Publications Office to establish the *Journal of Occupational Health Psychology* (*JOHP*) (Hurrell & Sauter, personal communication, May 2013, September 2016; Quick, 2010). NIOSH funding helped underwrite the journal's start-up costs. APA published the first volume in 1996. Like *Work & Stress*, *JOHP* has had an international presence, with contributors from many different countries.

ICOH–WOPS

A goal of the International Commission on Occupational Health (ICOH), an important international organization founded in 1906, has been to ensure progress toward safer and healthier workplaces. In 1993, the organization began to concern itself with OHP. ICOH formed a preliminary working committee devoted to understanding work organizations and psychosocial factors (S. Leka, personal communication, April 1, 2014). In 1996, the organization formally founded the 35th of its 35 scientific committees, the Scientific Committee on Work Organisation and Psychosocial Factors (WOPS). The goals of ICOH–WOPS include exchanging, accumulating, and disseminating "information relevant to psychosocial factors at work and health among workers, and also to facilitate research and practice in the field" (Kawakami, 2009, p. 9). Beginning with its inaugural conference in Copenhagen in 1998, ICOH–WOPS has organized a triennial conference series on psychosocial factors in the workplace.

European Academy of Occupational Health Psychology

In 1997, representatives of the University of Nottingham and representatives of two departments of occupational medicine in hospitals in Denmark, Skive Syghus and Herning Syghus, completed the preparatory work needed for the convening of a committee, the purpose of which was to lay the foundation for an international body devoted to research, practice, and teaching in OHP (European Academy of Occupational Health Psychology, 1999; Houdmont, 2009). That international body, the European Academy of Occupational Health Psychology, was formally founded in 1999. Within a year, the EA-OHP was headquartered at the Institute of Work, Health & Organisations at the University of Nottingham and led by Tom Cox.

The organization helped to advance research, teaching, and practice in OHP by creating working groups in each domain (Houdmont, 2009). In 2000, the Academy became the home of the journal *Work & Stress*. The EA-OHP organized a conference series that became biennial. In 2004, Paul Flaxman, Joanna Pryce, and Fehmidah Munir published the Academy's first newsletter, the purpose of which has been to report on research and practice and keep the readers up to date on organizational news. The organization also created an Internet listserv to help members get in touch with each other for the purpose of sharing information and providing research and practice advice. In 2009, the EA-OHP initiated a book series, *Contemporary Occupational Health Psychology: Global Perspective on Research and Practice*, devoted to reviews and empirical research.

Society for Occupational Health Psychology

As mentioned earlier, beginning in 1990, APA and NIOSH organized what turned into an international conference series devoted to work and well-being. A sentiment that emerged among individuals attending the APA/NIOSH conferences was that it was important to identify "ways of growing the field" (Hammer & Schonfeld, 2007). A series of meetings devoted to the subject were held between 2001 and 2004. Meeting participants discussed plans for creating an organization in the United States that would be devoted to advancing OHP. In 2004, at the APA's offices in Washington, DC, the Society for Occupational Health Psychology (SOHP) was founded and its first officers elected (Hammer & Schonfeld, 2007). Leslie Hammer of Portland State University was named the first president of SOHP.

SOHP provides members with resources pertaining to research, practice, and teaching. In 2006, the Society assumed a role together with APA and NIOSH in organizing the, by then, biennial conference series on work, stress, and health. In 2008, SOHP began to coordinate benefits with EA-OHP. The two organizations arranged the conference series to take place in alternate years. In 2006, although still published by APA, *JOHP* became associated with the Society. The Society, together with APA, developed a listserv to help members communicate with each other. In 2007, SOHP began a newsletter under the editorship of Irvin Schonfeld. The newsletter serves multiple purposes including communicating organization-related news to members, publishing OHP-relevant articles of general interest (e.g., innovative statistical applications, the impact of economic downturns), showcasing graduate programs in OHP, and publishing articles on the history of OHP. In 2017, SOHP will have taken an even bigger step, and, under the editorship of Robert Sinclair, begin to publish a new journal, *Occupational Health Science*.

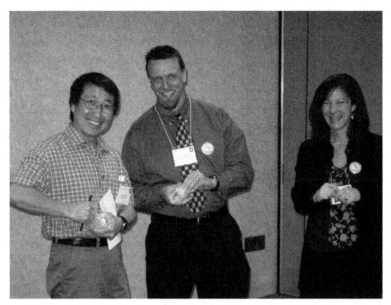

Contributors to the APA/NIOSH/SOHP Work, Stress, and Health Conference in 2006 in Miami. From left to right Peter Chen, Robert Sinclair, and Leslie Hammer. (Photographer, Irvin Sam Schonfeld.)

We make one additional observation that bears on both EA-OHP and SOHP is worth noting. This observation underlines something important about OHP, namely, the interdisciplinary character of OHP research. Although most of the organizations' members come from psychology, both organizations welcome members from disciplines outside of psychology because those members, like their psychologist brethren, contribute to OHP research. EA-OHP has had a president who is a physician.

SUMMARY

OHP is concerned with the relation of workplace psychosocial characteristics to the physical and psychological well-being of people who work. The reader of this chapter can follow the development of the OHP from its forerunners to the emergence of organizations that sustain the field. The chapter began with a celebrated poem that reflected on the physical and spiritual impact of the Industrial Revolution in England. Engels's (1969/1845) work on the physical effects of industrialization on workers was underlined. Marx (1967/1844) employed the multilayered concept of alienation to describe the psychological impact of industrial capitalism on workers. Durkheim (1951/1912) linked upward and downward changes in the business cycle to suicide risk. Weber (1993/1904–1905) observed how work, which was once thought of as a calling, turned on itself, and became what for many individuals is an "iron cage." The early 20th century saw the rise of Taylorism and Fordism with their focus on efficiency. Taylorism and Fordism became associated with dictatorial methods of improving workplace efficiency (Cruden, 1932; Hughes, 1989; Linder & Nygaard, 1998; Nolan, 1997; Wallace, 2003) although Taylorist research helped spur the use of rest periods as a means to improve productivity. In the context of the Hawthorne study, Taylorist research gave way to concerns about the impact on workers of psychosocial aspects of the workplace (Mayo, 1933; Roethlisberger & Dickson, 1939). An Austrian research team led by Marie Jahoda examined the psychological hardships of unemployment. The chapter also examined the psychological impact of combat on soldiers in two world wars (e.g., Stouffer et al., 1949; Swank, 1949).

After World War II, a number of developments emerged from both research and organizational standpoints that contributed to the development of OHP. Research conducted by Trist and Bamforth (1951), Chinoy (1955), Kahn et al. (1964), and Kornhauser (1965) added to research on work and psychological well-being. Selye (1956) provided an impetus for biological research on stress. His research implicated the hypothalamus, adrenal glands, and autonomic nervous system in responding to environmental stressors. Increased interest in worker autonomy and workload emerged (Karasek, 1979). Investigators demonstrated that rigorous methods could be used to study the impact of psychosocial workplace conditions on both physical (e.g., Cobb & Rose, 1973; Friedman et al., 1958; Kasl & Cobb, 1970) and psychological functioning (e.g., Frese, 1985; Parkes, 1982). Between 1985 and 1990, the term "occupational health psychology" began to appear in print (Everly, 1986; Feldman, 1985; Raymond et al., 1990).

After World War II, a number of organizational developments helped sustain research in OHP, including the ISR at the University of Michigan. The Tavistock Institute for Human Relations was founded in 1946. Tavistock researchers and colleagues at MIT launched the journal *Human Relations* in 1947.

In the United States, Public Law 91-596 was passed in 1970, authorizing the creation of OSHA and NIOSH. NIOSH would go on to support OHP-related research. APA and NIOSH organized a series of international conferences, beginning in 1990. The conference series was an important ingredient in getting OHP-oriented researchers and practitioners to know each other. APA and NIOSH began to provide seed money for doctoral programs in OHP. Beginning in 1996, the University of Nottingham pioneered graduate training in OHP in Europe. The journal *Work & Stress* was organized in 1987, and *JOHP* in 1996. ICOH-WOPS was founded in 1996, EA-OHP, in 1999, and SOHP, in 2004.

Like other branches of science, OHP was built on research efforts that antedate the founding of the discipline. The field has since become an established specialty within psychology, but with interdisciplinary currents. It is represented by dedicated journals and has organizational support.

REFERENCES

Anteby, M., & Khurana, R. (n.d.). *A new vision* (Historical collections). Boston, MA: Harvard Business School, Baker Library. Retrieved from www.library.hbs.edu/hc/hawthorne/anewvision.html#e

Baldwin, N. (2001). *Henry Ford and the Jews: The mass production of hate.* New York, NY: Public Affairs.

Beehr, T. A., & Newman, J. E. (1978). Job stress, employee health, and organizational effectiveness: A facet analysis, model, and literature review. *Personnel Psychology, 31,* 665–699. doi:10.1111/j.1744-6570.1978.tb02118.x

Bell, D. (1947, January). The study of man: Adjusting men to machines. *Commentary, 3,* 79–88.

Bianchi, R., Truchot, D., Laurent, E., Brisson, R., & Schonfeld, I. (2014). Is burnout solely job-related? A critical comment. *Scandinavian Journal of Psychology, 55,* 357–361. doi:10.1111/sjop.12119

Blake, W. (1966). And did these feet in ancient time. In J. Bronowski (Ed.), *William Blake: A selection of poems and letters.* Hammondsworth, England: Penguin. (Original work published 1808)

Cannell, C. F., & Kahn, R. L. (1984). Some factors in the origins and development of the Institute for Social Research, the University of Michigan. *American Psychologist, 39,* 1256–1266. doi:10.1037/0003-066X.39.11.1256

Cannon, W. B. (1914). The emergency function of the adrenal medulla in pain and the major emotions. *American Journal of Physiology, 33*, 356–372.

Cannon, W. B. (1929). Organization for physiological homeostasis. *Physiological Review, 9*, 399–431.

Caplan, R. D. (1987). Person-environment fit theory and organizations: Commensurate dimensions, time perspectives, and mechanisms. *Journal of Vocational Behavior, 31*, 248–267. doi:10.1016/0001-8791(87)90042-X

Caplan, R. D., Cobb, S., & French, J. R. P., Jr. (1975). Relationships of cessation of smoking with job stress, personality, and social support. *Journal of Applied Psychology, 60*, 211–219. doi:10.1037/h0076471

Caplan, R. D., Cobb, S., French, J. R. P., Jr., Harrison, R. V., & Pinneau, S. R., Jr. (1975). *Job demands and worker health: Main effects and occupational differences* (U.S. Department of Health, Education, and Welfare, Publication No. [NIOSH] 75-160). Washington, DC: U.S. Government Printing Office. [Also published by the Institute for Social Research, University of Michigan, Ann Arbor, 1980.]

Caruso, C. C. (2009). NIOSH OHP activities. *Newsletter of the Society for Occupational Health Psychology, 5*, 16–17.

Centers for Disease Control and Prevention. (n.d.). *Occupational health psychology (OHP)*. Retrieved from www.cdc.gov/niosh/topics/ohp

Chinoy, E. (1955). *Automobile workers and the American dream*. Boston, MA: Beacon.

Cobb, S., & Rose, R. M. (1973). Hypertension, peptic ulcer, and diabetes in air traffic controllers. *Journal of the American Medical Association, 224*, 489–492. doi:10.1001/jama.224.4.489

Cohen, A., & Margolis, B. (1973). Initial psychological research related to the Occupational Safety and Health Act of 1970. *American Psychologist, 28*, 600–606. doi:10.1037/h0034997

Cooper, C. L., & Marshall, J. (1976). Occupational sources of stress: A review of the literature relating to coronary heart disease and mental ill health. *Journal of Occupational Psychology, 49*, 11–28. doi:10.1111/j.2044-8325.1976.tb00325.x

Cox, T. (2011). *Professor Thomas Cox CBE*. Retrieved from https://proftcox.com/occupational-health-psychology

Cox, T., Taris, T., & Tisserand, M. (2009). Across the pond: The journal *Work and Stress*. *Newsletter of the Society for Occupational Health Psychology, 6*, 17–18.

Cruden, R. L. (1932, March 16). The great Ford myth. *The New Republic*, pp. 6–9.

Dohrenwend, B. P., & Dohrenwend, B. S. (1982). Perspectives on the past and future of psychiatric epidemiology. *American Journal of Public Health, 72*(11), 1273–1277.

Dohrenwend, B. P., & Shrout, P. E. (1985). 'Hassles' in the conceptualization and measurement of life stress variables. *American Psychologist, 40*, 780–785. doi:10.1037/0003-066X.40.7.780

Durkheim, É. (1951). *Suicide: A study in sociology* (J. A. Spaulding & G. Simpson, Trans.). Glencoe, IL: Free Press. (Original work published 1912)

Durkheim, É. (1984). *The division of labor in society* (W. D. Halls, Trans.). New York, NY: Free Press. (Original work published 1893)

Engels, F. (1969). *The condition of the working class in England*. Moscow, Russia: Panther Edition. Retrieved from www.marxists.org/archive/marx/works/1845/condition-working-class/index.htm (Original work published 1845)

Erikson, E. H. (1963). *Childhood and society*. New York, NY: W. W. Norton.

European Academy of Occupational Health Psychology. (1998). *Enabling document*. Retrieved from www.ea.ohp.org

Everly, G. S., Jr. (1986). An introduction to occupational health psychology. In P. A. Keller & L. G. Ritt (Eds.), *Innovations in clinical practice: A source book* (Vol. 5, pp. 331–338). Sarasota, FL: Professional Resource Exchange.

Feldman, R. H. L. (1985). Promoting occupational safety and health. In G. S. Everly, Jr. & R. H. L. Feldman (Eds.), *Occupational health promotion: Health behavior in the workplace* (pp. 188–207). New York, NY: Wiley.

Fox, M. (2015, September 3). Dr. J. Donald Millar, 81, dies; Led C.D.C. mission that helped eradicate smallpox. *The New York Times*, p. B14.

Frankenhaeuser, M. (1979). Psychoneuroendocrine approaches to the study of emotion as related to stress and coping. In H. E. House, Jr. (Ed.), *Nebraska Symposium on Motivation* (Vol. 26, pp. 123–161). Lincoln: University of Nebraska–Lincoln.

Frankenhaeuser, M., & Gardell, B. (1976). Underload and overload in working life: Outline of a multidisciplinary approach. *Journal of Human Stress, 2*, 35–46. doi:10.1080/0097840X.1976.9936068

Frantilla, A. (1998). *Social science in the public interest: The fiftieth year history of the Institute for Social Research*. Bentley Historical Library Bulletin, 45. Ann Arbor: University of Michigan.

Frese, M. (1985). Stress at work and psychosomatic complaints: A causal interpretation. *Journal of Applied Psychology, 70*, 314–328. doi:10.1037/0021-9010.70.2.314

Freud, S. (1956). Introduction to psycho-analysis and the war neuroses. In J. Strachey (Ed. & Trans.), *The standard edition of the complete psychological works of Sigmund Freud* (Vol. XVII, pp. 207–215). London, England: The Hogarth Press. (Original work published 1919)

Freudenberger, H. J. (1974). Staff burn-out. *Journal of Social Issues, 30,* 159–165. doi:10.1111/j.1540-4560.1974.tb00706.x

Friedman, M., Rosenman, R. H., & Carroll, V. (1958). Changes in the serum cholesterol and blood clotting time in men subjected to cyclic variation of occupational stress. *Circulation, 17,* 852–861. doi:10.1161/01.CIR.17.5.852

Ganster, D. C., & Schaubroeck, J. (1991). Work stress and employee health. *Journal of Management, 17,* 235–271. doi:10.1177/014920639101700202

Gardell, B. (1971). Alienation and mental health in the modern industrial environment. In L. Levi (Ed.), *Society, stress and disease* (Vol. 1, pp. 148–180). Oxford, England: Oxford University Press.

Gardell, B. (1976). Technology, alienation and mental health: Summary of a social psychological research programme on technology and the worker. *Acta Sociologica, 19*(1), 83–94.

Great Britain, War Office. (2004). *Report of the War Office Committee of Enquiry into "shell-shock."* London, England: Imperial War Museum. (Original work published 1922)

Hammer, L., & Schonfeld, I. S. (2007). Historical perspective: The historical development of the Society for Occupational Health Psychology. *Newsletter of the Society for Occupational Health Psychology, 1,* 2.

Hart, C. W. M. (1943). The Hawthorne experiments. *The Canadian Journal of Economics and Political Science, 9*(2), 150–163.

Health of Munition Workers Committee. (1915). *British Medical Journal, 2*(2867), 863–864.

Heilbroner, R. L. (1986). *The essential Adam Smith.* New York, NY: W. W. Norton.

Hitchcock, E. (2008). NIOSH OHP activities. *Newsletter of the Society for Occupational Health Psychology, 3,* 10.

Hochschild, A. (2011). *To end all wars: A story of loyalty and rebellion, 1914–1918.* Boston, MA: Houghton Mifflin Harcourt.

Holmes, T. H., & Rahe, R. H. (1967). The social readjustment rating scale. *Journal of Psychosomatic Research, 11,* 213–218. doi:10.1016/0022-3999(67)90010-4

Houdmont, J. (2009). Across the pond: A history of the European Academy of Occupational Health Psychology. *Newsletter of the Society for Occupational Health Psychology, 7,* 4–5.

House, J. S. (1980). *Occupational stress and the mental and physical health of factory workers.* Ann Arbor, MI: Survey Research Center, Institute for Social Research, University of Michigan.

Hughes, T. P. (1989). *American genesis: A century of invention and technological enthusiasm, 1870–1970.* New York, NY: Viking.

Human Relations. (2012). *About the journal.* Retrieved from www.tavinstitute.org/humanrelations/about_journal/aims.html

Hurrell, J. J., Jr., Nelson, D. L., & Simmons, B. L. (1998). Measuring job stressors and strains: Where we have been, where we are, and where we need to go. *Journal of Occupational Health Psychology, 3,* 368–389. doi:10.1037/1076-8998.3.4.368

Institute for Social Research. (n.d.). *Our history.* Retrieved from http://home.isr.umich.edu/about/history

Jacobs, A. (2005). *The Narnian: The life and imagination of C.S. Lewis.* San Francisco, CA: HarperCollins.

Jahoda, M., Lazarsfeld, P. F., & Zeisel, H. (1971). *Marienthal: The sociography of an unemployed community.* Chicago, IL: Aldine. (Original work published 1933)

Johnson, J. V., Hall, E. M., & Theorell, T. (1989). Combined effects of job strain and social isolation on cardiovascular disease morbidity and mortality in a random sample of the Swedish male working population. *Scandinavian Journal of Work, Environment & Health, 15,* 271–279. doi:10.5271/sjweh.1852

Kahn, R. L., Wolfe, D. M., Quinn, R. P., Snoek, J., & Rosenthal, R. A. (1964). *Organizational stress: Studies in role conflict and ambiguity.* Oxford, England: Wiley.

Karasek, R. A. (1979). Job demands, job decision latitude, and mental strain: Implications for job redesign. *Administrative Science Quarterly, 24*(2), 285–307.

Karasek, R. A., Baker, D., Marxer, F., Ahlbom, A., & Theorell, T. (1981). Job decision latitude, job demands, and cardiovascular disease: A prospective study of Swedish men. *American Journal of Public Health, 71*(7), 694–705.

Kasl, S. V. (1987). Methodologies in stress and health: Past difficulties, present dilemmas, future directions. In S. V. Kasl & C. L. Cooper (Eds.), *Stress and health: Issues in research methodology* (pp. 307–318). Chichester, England: Wiley.

Kasl, S. V., & Cobb, S. (1970). Blood pressure changes in men undergoing job loss: A preliminary report. *Psychosomatic Medicine, 32*(1), 19–38.

Kawakami, N. (2009). The ICOH Scientific Committee of Work Organization and Psychosocial Factors. *ICOH Newsletter, 7*(2), 9.

Kornhauser, A. (1965). *Mental health of the industrial worker: A Detroit study*. New York, NY: Wiley.

LaMontagne, A., Keegel, T., Louie, A., Ostry, A., & Landsbergis, P. (2007). A systematic review of the job-stress intervention evaluation literature, 1990–2005. *International Journal of Occupational and Environmental Health, 13*(3), 268–280.

Lazarus, R. S. (1966). *Psychological stress and the coping process*. New York, NY: McGraw-Hill.

Lazarus, R. S., DeLongis, A., Folkman, S., & Gruen, R. (1985). Stress and adaptational outcomes: The problem of confounded measures. *American Psychologist, 40,* 770–779. doi:10.1037/0003-066X.40.7.770

Leka, S. (2016). OHP at the Centre for Organizational Health & Development (COHD), University of Nottingham, U.K. *Newsletter of the Society for Occupational Health Psychology, 15,* 8.

Levi, L. (1972). Stress and distress in response to psychosocial stimuli: Laboratory and real life studies on sympathoadrenomedullary and related reactions. *Acta Medica Scandinavica, 528*(Suppl.), 1–166.

Levitt, S. D., & List, J. A. (2011). Was there really a Hawthorne effect at the Hawthorne plant? An analysis of the original illumination experiments. *American Economic Journal: Applied Economics, 3,* 224–238. doi:10.1257/app.3.1.224

Lewis, C. S. (1955). *Surprised by joy: The shape of my early life*. London, England: Geoffrey Bles.

Linder, M., & Nygaard, I. (1998). *Void where prohibited: Rest breaks and the right to urinate on company time*. Ithaca, NY: Cornell University Press.

MacCurdy, J. T. (1918). *War neuroses*. Cambridge, MA: Cambridge University Press.

Marx, K. (1967). Economic and philosophical manuscripts. In L. D. Easton & K. H. Guddat (Eds. & Trans.), *Writings of the young Marx on philosophy and society* (pp. 283–337). Garden City, NY: Anchor Books. (Original work published 1844)

Maslach, C., & Jackson, S.E. (1981). The measurement of experienced burnout. *Journal of Occupational Behavior, 2*(2), 99–113.

Maslach, C., Jackson, S. E., & Leiter, M. P. (1996). *Maslach Burnout Inventory manual* (3rd ed.). Palo Alto, CA: Consulting Psychologists Press.

Mayo, E. (1924). Recovery and industrial fatigue. *Journal of Personnel Research, 3,* 273–281.

Mayo, E. (1933). *The human problems of an industrial civilization*. Cambridge, MA: Harvard.

Millar, J. (1984). The NIOSH-suggested list of the ten leading work-related diseases and injuries. *Journal of Occupational Medicine, 26*(5), 340–341.

Mott, F. W. (1916a). The effects of high explosives upon the central nervous system. Lecture 1. *The Lancet, 4824,* 331–338.

Mott, F. W. (1916b). The effects of high explosives on the central nervous system. Lecture 2. *The Lancet, 4826,* 441–449.

Murphy, L. R. (2002). Job stress research at NIOSH: 1972–2002. In P. L. Perrewé & D. C. Ganster (Eds.), *Research in occupational stress and well-being, Vol. 2, Historical and current perspectives on stress and health* (pp. 1–55). Amsterdam, The Netherlands: Elsevier Science.

National Institute for Occupational Safety and Health. (1988). A proposed national strategy for prevention of psychological disorders. In *Proposed national strategies for the prevention of leading work-related diseases and injuries (Part 2)* (NTIS No. PB-89-130348). Cincinnati, OH: Author.

Newman, J. E., & Beehr, T. A. (1979). Personal and organizational strategies for handling job stress: A review of research and opinion. *Personnel Psychology, 32,* 1–43. doi:10.1111/j.1744-6570.1979.tb00467.x

Nigam, J. A. S. (2007). NIOSH OHP activities. *Newsletter of the Society for Occupational Health Psychology, 1,* 5–6.

Nolan, J. (1997, August 7). The battle of the overpass. *The Detroit News*. Retrieved from http://apps .detnews.com/apps/history/index.php?id=172

Occupational Safety and Health Act of 1970, as amended through January 1, 2004. Retrieved from www .osha.gov/pls/oshaweb/owasrch.search_form?p_doc_type=OSHACT&p_toc_level=0

Parkes, K. R. (1982). Occupational stress among student nurses: A natural experiment. *Journal of Applied Psychology, 67,* 784–796. doi:10.1037/0021-9010.67.6.784

Parsons, H. M. (1974). What happened at Hawthorne? *Science, 183*(4128), 922–932. doi:10.1126/science.183.4128.922

Petticrew, M. P., & Lee, K. (2011). The "Father of Stress" meets "Big Tobacco": Hans Selye and the tobacco industry. *American Journal of Public Health, 101,* 411–418. doi:10.2105/AJPH.2009.177634

Polanyi, K. (2001). *The great transformation. The political and economic origins of our time*. Boston, MA: Beacon. (Original work published 1944)

Quick, J. C. (1999). Occupational health psychology: Historical roots and future directions. *Health Psychology, 18*, 82–88. doi:10.1037/0278-6133.18.1.82

Quick, J. C. (2010). The founding of the *Journal of Occupational Health Psychology. Newsletter of the Society for Occupational Health Psychology, 9*(13), 15–16.

Quick, J. C., Murphy, L. R., & Hurrell, Jr., J. J. (1992). *Stress & well-being at work: Assessments and interventions for occupational mental health.* Washington, DC: American Psychological Association.

Quinn, R. P., & Staines, G. L. (1979). *The 1977 Quality of Employment Survey: Descriptive statistics with comparison data from the 1960–70 and the 1972–73 surveys.* Ann Arbor: Institute for Social Research, University of Michigan.

Rahe, R. H., Meyer, M., Smith, M., Kjaer, G., & Holmes, T. H. (1964). Social stress and illness onset. *Journal of Psychosomatic Research, 8*, 35–44. doi:10.1016/0022-3999(64)90020-0

Raymond, J. S., Wood, D. W., & Patrick, W. K. (1990). Psychology doctoral training in work and health. *American Psychologist, 45*, 1159–1161. doi:10.1037/0003-066X.45.10.1159

Rivers, W. H. R. (1918, February. 2). The repression of war experience. *The Lancet, 194*, 72–77.

Roethlisberger, F. J., & Dickson, W. J. (1939). *Management and the worker.* Cambridge, MA: Harvard.

Sassoon, S. (1918). *Attack.* Retrieved from www.bartleby.com/136/5.html

Sauter, S. L., & Hurrell, J. J., Jr. (1999). Occupational health psychology: Origins, context, and direction. *Professional Psychology: Research and Practice, 30*, 117–122. doi:10.1037/0735-7028.30.2.117

Sauter, S. L., & Hurrell, J. J., Jr. (2016). Tribute to J. Donald Millar: 1934-2015. *Newsletter of the Society for Occupational Health Psychology, 15*, 2.

Selye, H. (1956). *The stress of life.* New York, NY: McGraw-Hill.

Selye, H. (1976). *The stress of life* (Rev. ed.). New York, NY: McGraw-Hill.

Selye, H. (1985). The nature of stress. *Basal Facts, 7*(1), 3–11.

Smith, A. (1976). *An inquiry into the nature and causes of the wealth of nations.* Chicago, IL: University of Chicago Press. (Original work published 1776)

Sorensen, C. E. (1956). *My forty years with Ford.* New York, NY: Collier Books.

Spiegel, H. X. (1944). Psychiatric observations in the Tunisian campaign. *American Journal of Orthopsychiatry, 14*(3), 381–385. doi:10.1111/j.1939-0025.1944.tb04892.x

Stalin, J. (1940). Foundations of Leninism. *Leninism.* London, England: George Allen & Unwin. (Original work published 1924)

Stouffer, S. A., Lumsdaine, A. A., Lumsdaine, M. H., Williams, R. M., Jr., Smith, M. B., Janis, I. L., . . . Cottrell, L. S., Jr. (1949). *The American soldier: Combat and its aftermath* (Vol. 2). Princeton, NJ: Princeton University Press.

Streit, J. M. K., Nigam, J. A. S., & Sauter, S. L. (2011). The NIOSH Work Organization and Stress-Related Disorders (WSD) Program. *Newsletter of the Society for Occupational Health Psychology, 9*, 14–15.

Swank, R. L. (1949). Combat exhaustion: A descriptive and statistical analysis of causes, symptoms and signs. *Journal of Nervous and Mental Disease, 109*, 475–508. doi:10.1097/00005053-194910960-00001

Tausig, M., & Fenwick, R. (2011). *Work and mental health in social context.* New York, NY: Springer. doi:10.1007/978-1-4614-0625-9

Taylor, F. W. (1911). *Principles of scientific management.* New York, NY: Harper & Brothers.

Theorell, T. (1997). Future work life—special issue, in honor of Lennart Levi: Introduction. *Scandinavian Journal of Work, Environment & Health, 23*(Suppl. 4), 5–6.

Trist, E. L., & Bamforth, K. W. (1951). Some social and psychological consequences of the longwall method of coal getting. *Human Relations, 4*, 3–38. doi:10.1177/001872675100400101

Trist, E. L., & Murray, H. (1990). *The social engagement of social science: A Tavistock anthology.* Philadelphia: University of Pennsylvania Press. Retrieved from http://moderntimesworkplace.com/archives/archives.html

Wallace, M. (2003). *The American axis: Henry Ford, Charles Lindbergh, and the rise of the Third Reich.* New York, NY: St. Martin's Press.

Wallin, J., Considine, K., & Nigam, J. A. S. (2009). Solutions for engaging businesses and their employees in research studies. *Newsletter of the Society for Occupational Health Psychology, 7*, 16–17.

Weber, M. (1947). *The theory of social and economic organization* (A. M. Henderson & T. Parsons, Trans.). New York, NY: Free Press. (Original work published 1921)

Weber, M. (1958). *From Max Weber: Essays in sociology* (H. H. Gerth & C. W. Mills, Trans.). New York, NY: Oxford University Press. (Original work published 1922)

Weber, M. (1993). *The Protestant ethic and the spirit of capitalism* (T. Parsons, Trans.). London, England: Routledge. (Original work published 1904–1905)

Wilson, A. N. (1990). *C. S. Lewis: A biography*. New York, NY: Fawcett Columbine.

Winter, J. M. (1977). The impact of the First World War on civilian health in Britain. *Economic History Review, 30*, 487–503. doi:10.1111/j.1468-0289.1977.tb00278.x

Zickar, M. J. (2003). Remembering Arthur Kornhauser: Industrial psychology's advocate for worker well-being. *Journal of Applied Psychology, 88*, 363–369. doi:10.1037/0021-9010.88.2.363

TWO

Research Methods in Occupational Health Psychology

KEY CONCEPTS AND FINDINGS COVERED IN CHAPTER 2

A goal of occupational health psychology (OHP) researchers is to generate and organize knowledge bearing on the relationship between work-related psychosocial factors and the health of workers. Like researchers in other branches of psychology, OHP researchers elaborate theories, develop hypotheses, and devise ways to test those hypotheses. The testing of hypotheses can give rise to new knowledge. That knowledge can help in the development of interventions to improve occupational health.

One task of OHP researchers is to elaborate scientific theories. A scientific theory is a logically consistent model that describes and explains relationships among constructs. Constructs are higher-order abstractions, which are discussed more fully later in the chapter. An example of a construct from another branch of psychology is intelligence. Examples of prominent constructs in OHP include decision latitude and psychological distress. A scientific theory in OHP describes and explains relations among the constructs that are the foci of OHP. Theories in OHP explain relationships among constructs such as decision latitude at work, psychological job demands, psychological distress, and so forth. It is unlikely that a single theory can address all the relationships that are the subject of OHP research; a theory, however, should address the interrelationships among some of those constructs.

Karl Popper (1963) developed the idea that a scientific theory must be able to generate hypotheses. According to Popper, a hypothesis is a conjecture that is falsifiable. In other words, a hypothesis is a statement that, when gauged against observations a scientist assembles, can be shown to be false. Alternatively, a hypothesis can be shown to be consistent with the assembled observations. Popper, in fact, criticized psychoanalytic theory, asserting that it is not a *scientific* theory because it does not generate these falsifiable statements called hypotheses.[1] An example of a theory generating a statement that is falsifiable comes from Karasek (1979). His theory was built on the idea that the constructs decision latitude and psychological job demands, dimensions that characterize work roles, contribute to (another construct) distress in workers. Decision latitude refers to the amount of autonomy a worker has to decide on the means to achieve work-related demands. Psychological workload refers to aspects of a job such as the complexity of work-related tasks. A hypothesis that follows from Karasek's theory is that compared with other workers, workers having jobs that combine little latitude with heavy demands will experience higher levels of psychological distress. Research on decision latitude and psychological workload will be discussed at length in Chapters 3 and 4.

Science can depart from the Popperian view. Hypotheses can derive from accumulated observations, that is, induction, and not necessarily from a theory (Ng, 1991). In other words, induction can help build a foundation of observations that leads to hypothesis generation (and theory development). Durkheim's research on suicide was inductive. His research connecting suicide risk to the business cycle (see Chapter 1) was built on "social facts" or accumulated observations rather than hypotheses that derived

---

[1] Popper's critique of Freudian psychology is instructive. If a Freudian encounters a man attempting to hurt a child, the Freudian would explain that man's behavior in terms of repression stemming from some aspect of the Oedipal complex. A Freudian who learns of a man who sacrifices his life to save a child would explain the man's self-sacrifice in terms of sublimation. According to Popper, every configuration of human behavior is a verification of a preconceived set of ideas. No human behavior contradicts psychoanalytic ideas. What the Freudian fails to do is "go out on a limb" to use psychoanalytic ideas to predict behavioral differences among individuals that will occur in the future. In other words, what the Freudian fails to do is to come up with testable hypotheses.

from a theory. One can observe departures from the Popperian ideal in contemporary research. Spector and Zhou (2014) took an inductive approach to studying gender differences in counterproductive workplace behaviors (harms employees inflict on coworkers and workplaces). Occasionally, a researcher taking an inductive approach to a problem will employ a work-around when dealing with Popperian journal reviewers by "inventing a theory leading to hypotheses," as if the hypotheses were generated beforehand (P. Spector, personal communication, March 2014).

Susser (1979) wrote that "the most cogent test of a hypothesis . . . is to attempt disproof" (p. 54). Before attempting disproof through hypothesis testing, a distinction must be made between conceptual hypotheses and operational hypotheses (Kleinbaum, Kupper, & Morgenstern, 1982). A conceptual hypothesis reflects ideas, for example, that the abstractions (constructs) decision latitude and psychological job demands influence another construct, psychological distress. To conduct empirical research, one needs operational hypotheses. To create operational hypotheses that are the real-world analogues of conceptual hypotheses, constructs have to be operationalized, that is, reflected in real-world measures. Operationalizations are imperfect, but they can capture enough of what constructs represent to allow investigators to conduct research. Decision latitude may be represented by averaging a worker's responses to a small number of specially written, highly focused questionnaire items that ask workers to estimate how much freedom they have to make decisions about the tasks they ordinarily perform on the job. Or one may operationalize decision latitude by averaging independent experts' judgments regarding the amount of latitude workers with certain jobs are allowed. Only after a researcher decides how to operationalize the constructs targeted for research can a study be planned, data collected, and operational hypotheses tested.

A reader may react to the hypothesis just described by alternatively hypothesizing that job demands and latitude play no role in the development of psychological distress *even if* research reveals that workers in high-demands–low-latitude jobs experience high levels of distress. The Karasek hypothesis (the combination of high demands and low latitude leads to distress) may have a rival hypothesis that better explains the relationship between work and psychological distress.

Researchers observe that high-demand–low-latitude jobs tend to be low paying. Perhaps it isn't that high-demand–low-latitude jobs drive distress. Rather, it may be that the earnings attached to jobs play a decisive role in the development of distress. Compared with workers in higher latitude positions, workers with little latitude tend to be employed in lower paying jobs. Job-related economic and social disadvantages could be the drivers of psychological distress. OHP researchers concern themselves with rival hypotheses, and make it a practice to evaluate alternative hypotheses (Platt, 1964).

When a theory generates hypotheses researchers find to be consistent with observations, the theory gains prestige in the research community. Conversely, a theory that generates hypotheses found to be inconsistent with the relevant observations loses prestige. Theories themselves are neither proven nor disproven. They are insulated from direct testing or falsification. A hypothesis is the currency that is tested. As hypotheses go, the theories behind them gain or lose favor.

RESEARCH DESIGNS

There are a variety of research designs. Specific circumstances pertaining to each line of research narrow the choices for OHP investigators. These designs include the experiment, quasi-experiment, cross-sectional study, various longitudinal study designs, and so forth. In this section, a number of research designs used in OHP research are explored. The research designs are presented with a minimum of statistical exposition, although there will be some, recognizing that this section is devoted to research designs themselves and not to statistics. Apart from a description of each research design, there is an example of the design as it has been implemented in practice.

Experiment

As in the biomedical sciences, in the psychological sciences the experiment is a vehicle used in assessing cause–effect relations (in biomedical research, an experiment designed to test the efficacy of a treatment for a disease or disorder is called a "randomized controlled trial" or "clinical trial"). An experiment has at least two key features that should be underlined.[2] One feature is that the effects of two or more rival treatments or interventions are compared. Ordinarily, the experimental group comprises research participants (also known as "research subjects") who are assigned to a special treatment or a control condition. In OHP research, the special treatment can be a new, potentially health-improving way of managing one or more units within an organization. The treatment could be "special" because it is a new intervention or a modified version of an existing treatment. The control condition could be a condition in which participants are exposed to no treatment, a waiting list control condition, or an existing treatment. An OHP investigator can compare the efficacy of multiple rival treatment conditions that reflect different modifications of the standard way the targeted work organization operates and a treatment that is equivalent to the standard way the organization operates.

The second feature of an experiment involves allocating experimental units to the rival treatments. The term "experimental unit" often refers to research participants, but it can also refer to clusters of individuals such as work units. The experimental units must be randomly assigned to the rival treatments. Random assignment means that every participant in a participant pool (e.g., workers in an organization) has the same probability of being assigned to any of the rival treatments. The advantage of random assignment over other methods of assigning participants is that, on average, the participants in the rival treatment groups will be similar on most background characteristics. These background characteristics include factors that were measured at the outset of the experiment and factors that went unmeasured. There are many unmeasured background characteristics. Random assignment ensures that the groups will, on average, be similar on those background characteristics (measured and unmeasured). The groups will thus differ in one way—exposure to one of the two or more rival treatments. The groups will not differ on most other characteristics. Thus, the rival treatments are *not* likely to be *confounded* with other factors that could potentially explain the effect of the treatments on the participants.

Randomization works best when there are large numbers of participants to allocate to the rival treatment groups. For instance, it is more advantageous to allocate 200 participants per treatment group than 10 participants per group. Consider the statistic

---

[2] These features are not necessarily features of experiments in the physical sciences (e.g., chemistry or physics). The experiment as described here applies to biomedical and psychological research.

known as the "standard error of the mean." The standard error is the standard deviation of a sampling distribution. Without being overly technical, the standard error of the mean reflects how much treatment means would vary if the researcher would repeatedly draw same-size random samples from the population of interest (e.g., workers in the manufacturing sector), expose each of those samples to a particular treatment, and graph the means of all those samples. Compared with means drawn from large samples (where standard errors tend to be small), means obtained from small samples would vary to a much greater extent (the standard error would be large). Put another way, as sample size increases, the standard error of the mean decreases. The result is that means obtained from large samples would be more reliable—more stable—than means obtained from small samples. In general, it is a good practice to conduct experiments using large samples because the estimates of treatment effects are more stable.

Flaxman and Bond's (2010) research on stress management training is an example of an OHP-related experiment. They randomly assigned London government workers to two rival treatments, stress management training and a waiting list control group. A waiting list control group is usually scheduled to be exposed to the experimental treatment after the treatment has been completed in the first group, which was the case in this study. When the first group has completed the treatment but the members of the waiting list control group have not yet begun the treatment, the two groups are compared on the dependent variables. One dependent variable in Flaxman and Bond's study was psychological distress, which they operationalized by mean scores on a self-reported, psychological symptom scale. Flaxman and Bond found that at the end of the 6-month period the study was in the field, members of the experimental group experienced significantly less distress than members of the waiting list control group (who had not yet begun the promised treatment). Flaxman and Bond found that among the workers in either group who experienced the highest levels of psychological distress at the study's outset, those in the experimental group improved by a "clinically significant degree."

As mentioned earlier, the term "experimental units" applies not only to individuals; the term can also refer to clusters of individuals. In Flaxman and Bond's experiment, individual workers were the experimental units that were randomized into experimental and control groups. But sometimes it is not practical to randomize individual workers into rival treatments. Instead, OHP researchers randomize larger units. For example, organizational units can be randomly assigned to rival treatments. In a study that involved 16 Los Angeles schools, Siegel, Prelip, Erausquin, and Kim (2010) randomly assigned each school to an experimental intervention or a control condition. Employees at the eight experimental schools were provided a health-promotion intervention (e.g., to encourage healthy eating, walking). The eight control schools received a stipend but not the intervention. Compared with employees in the control schools, employees in the intervention schools showed statistically significant reductions in body mass 2 years after the experiment began.

Quasi-Experiment

The quasi-experiment is similar to an experiment; both are used to compare the effects of rival treatments on dependent variables. The quasi-experiment, however, differs from the experiment in an important way. In the experiment, research units are randomly allocated to rival treatment groups. By contrast, in the quasi-experiment, intact or preexisting groups are exposed to the rival treatments or a treatment and a no-treatment control condition (e.g., a stress-reduction intervention, such as a yoga class, is introduced in one administrative office but not in an administrative office elsewhere in the same city). There is no random assignment to the rival treatment groups in a quasi-experiment.

The absence of random assignment of participants to rival treatments places a limitation on quasi-experiments. In a quasi-experiment, a researcher cannot assume that the participants in the rival treatments are similar on most background characteristics. In response to this limitation, researchers who conduct quasi-experiments often assess the study participants on many background factors before the individuals are exposed to treatments. The researchers conduct statistical tests to ascertain whether the groups differ on any of the *measured* background factors. If a researcher finds that the treatment groups differ on a background factor that could potentially explain the hypothesized effects of the treatment, the researcher can implement statistical adjustments to equate the treatment groups. A fundamental problem with the quasi-experiment, however, is that one or more *unmeasured* background factors may explain potential differences in the outcome variables, differences that ostensibly appear to have emerged as a result of the impact of the treatment. The best way to control the impact of unmeasured background characteristics on treatment outcomes is to conduct an experiment with random assignment. However, sometimes there are obstacles to randomly assigning workers to different groups (e.g., manager resistance), making a quasi-experiment the most viable option for investigators.

An example of an OHP-related quasi-experiment is Bond and Bunce's (2001) study of the impact of work reorganization in a sample of British government employees. The intervention consisted of employee-driven action research, in which employees collaboratively researched work-related problems, and then developed and implemented research-informed organizational changes. The purpose of these changes was to increase employee control over work processes that would reduce stress-related problems. In order to reduce the chance of cross-unit contamination (i.e., members of the experimental group disclosing to control workers elements of the treatment, potentially precipitating change in the control group), Bond and Bunce employed a wait-list control group consisting of a work group located in a different building. The researchers took steps to select a control group comprising workers who were similar in age, gender, and education to the workers in the experimental group. Bunce and Bond found that the workers in the experimental group showed better mental health and lower absence rates than workers in the control group.

Internal Validity of Experiments and Quasi-Experiments

In discussing their study's limitations, Bond and Bunce (2001) wrote that "we have inevitably had to use a quasi-experimental design and are, therefore, left open to various threats to internal validity" (p. 300). Internal validity, which is distinct from scale validity (a topic discussed later), refers to the extent to which a study's design allows researchers to draw cause–effect conclusions. One prominent threat to a quasi-experiment's internal validity is that some unmeasured factor, and not the treatments, may have affected the dependent variables. The beauty of a true experiment is that random allocation of participants into rival treatment groups evens out potential background differences among the members of the rival groups. Ordinarily, the true experiment, in comparison with the quasi-experiment, has greater internal validity.

Cross-Sectional Study

The most commonly employed research design in OHP—and probably all of psychology—is the cross-sectional study. In a cross-sectional study, the researcher obtains measures on a sample at one point in time. The cross-sectional study is ill-equipped to answer questions about cause and effect. If cross-sectional research finds that two factors are related, that finding does not ensure that one factor caused the other. Because the two factors were assessed at the same point in time, and a cause must antedate the effect (temporal precedence of the cause), the cross-sectional study can rarely establish temporal precedence of one factor over the other.

Schonfeld (1990) conducted a cross-sectional study of coping in teachers. He found that two types of coping were related to lower levels of distress. One type of coping, positive comparisons, involves such psychological strategies as comparing oneself favorably to another teacher. Another type, direct action, involves such behavioral strategies as making pronounced efforts to turn a failing student around. Higher levels of each type of coping were related to lower levels of distress. Because coping and distress were measured at the same point in time, it is not clear which came first. It is possible that distress influenced coping patterns or that one or more unmeasured third factors gave rise to both psychological distress and the coping patterns. Thus, a cross-sectional relation between distress and coping is compatible with any of three conditions: (a) coping affects distress, (b) distress affects coping, and (c) third factors give rise to both distress and coping. Although cross-sectional research cannot ordinarily help us draw cause–effect conclusions, such research can be helpful because researchers can learn that certain factors are related. The pattern of correlations found in a cross-sectional study can offer clues investigators would like to follow up using other study designs.

Case-Control Study

A case-control study is often conducted for the purpose of identifying factors that are associated with a disorder. A case-control study involves at least two groups of individuals. The members of one group, or the cases, have a disorder to be studied. The members of the second group, or the controls, are free of the disorder. The study design, however, is more aptly termed a "case-comparison study" (MacMahon & Pugh, 1970). The term "control group" as it is used here is not an apt term because the group is not a control group in the way we understand the term as it applies to an *experiment*.

Information on the backgrounds and histories of the group members is ascertained through interviews, questionnaires, medical exams, and record checks to determine whether one or more factors are more common in the backgrounds of members of the cases or controls. If the researcher intends to identify factors that are *specific* to a particular disorder, he or she would include a third group that has a disorder other than the disorder that is the focal concern of the investigators. Some factors, such as low socioeconomic status, are related to a great many disorders. If a researcher plans to identify risk factors that are specific to a disorder such as schizophrenia, it would be helpful to include a second control group with a different mental disorder in addition to a disorder-free control group.

Link, Dohrenwend, and Skodol (1986) conducted a case-control study to identify risk factors specific to schizophrenia. The study comprised three groups: a case group consisting of schizophrenic patients; two control groups, one comprising individuals suffering from depression, and the other, community residents with no evidence of psychopathology. Link et al. found that compared with the depressed and healthy controls, the schizophrenic participants were significantly more likely to have had first-time jobs (which were likely to antedate their first schizophrenic episodes) that exposed the cases to noisome work characteristics. Noisome work characteristics not only refer to frequent exposure to loud noise, but also include adverse air quality, high levels of heat, cold, or humidity, or hazards. The schizophrenic and depressed participants did not differ in the average occupational prestige of their initial jobs or in their levels of education.

Because case-control research is retrospective, individuals suffering from a disorder may attempt to find the meaning of their current condition (Tennant, Bebbington, & Hurry, 1981). In this "effort after meaning," the cases may magnify some experiences, diminish others, and fail to recall yet others, misleading investigators trying to identify risk factors for the disorder being studied. Link et al. (1986) surmounted this difficulty. The researchers linked the participants' first full-time jobs to independent, objective data that characterized the working conditions associated with the jobs. Those objective data were derived from the Dictionary of Occupational Titles (DOT), a document that was periodically published by the U.S. Department of Labor (now replaced by an online database). To create the DOT, analysts evaluated a large number of characteristics of thousands of U.S. jobs. Link et al. (1986) used DOT evaluations, which, of course, were obtained independently of the participants in the case-control study, to characterize the participants' jobs. Thus, the noisome job characteristics were ascertained independently of the personalities of the study participants.

Longitudinal Study

The defining characteristic of a longitudinal study is that data are obtained from the same sample at two or more points in time (sometimes called a "panel study"). Because it is not ethical to conduct experiments in which investigators knowingly assign workers to better and worse job conditions, longitudinal studies, by assessing existing working conditions and worker health at different points in time, can be valuable in testing hypotheses that certain working conditions are related to future worker health. In conducting longitudinal research, it is often helpful to assess the health problem and the hypothesized risk factors for the problem at every data collection point. For example, if an OHP researcher is studying risk factors (e.g., heavy psychological workload) for depression, it is often helpful to assess the risk factors and depression at each wave of data collection.

Some longitudinal research does not follow this pattern. In a 1-year longitudinal study of Canadian teachers, Burke and Greenglass (1995) used multiple linear regression (MLR) to predict burnout (time 2) from work stressors assessed 1 year earlier (time 1). Although the authors found that time 1 workload predicted emotional exhaustion (a core component of burnout) at time 2, the analysis was problematic in a way that is instructive. The design of the study does *not* take into account the stability of exhaustion between times 1 and 2. By statistically adjusting for time 1 exhaustion, the investigator adjusts for the stability of exhaustion over time, and as a result, the regression of time 2 exhaustion on time 1 exhaustion and work stressors will help ascertain how much exhaustion increases or decreases from its baseline, if at all, as a function of work stressors (Kelloway & Francis, 2013). Because Burke and Greenglass did not statistically control for time 1 exhaustion, the study was problematic. The analysis resembles cross-sectional analyses in which it is not clear which factor developed first. Kasl (1983) called such a study a "phoney" longitudinal study.

A more effective regression analysis would examine the impact of time 1 workload on time 2 emotional exhaustion, while statistically controlling for time 1 exhaustion (among workers who remained in the same job for the length of the study). In this way, the OHP investigator could learn whether workload predicts future exhaustion adjusting for any confounding of workload and exhaustion at time 1 as well as the relation of time 1 exhaustion to exhaustion 1 year later. It would be equally important to conduct an analysis in which time 1 exhaustion predicts time 2 workload, while controlling for time 1 workload. Such an analysis evaluates the *reverse* causal hypothesis that emotional exhaustion contributes to higher workload (e.g., burned-out teachers getting into a rut in which they work with little respite).

Kivimäki, Elovainio, Vahtera, and Ferrie's (2003) 2-year longitudinal study of personnel working in 10 hospitals was methodologically sounder than the study conducted by Burke and Greenglass. Kivimäki et al. assessed the relation of time 1 organizational justice (e.g., fairness of workplace procedures) to time 2 health indicators (e.g., certified sickness absence), statistically controlling for the health indicators at time 1. Organizational justice still predicted health indicators at time 2. In other words, lower levels of justice were related to increased health problems, controlling for health problems at time 1. The researchers also found that health indicators at time 1 were *not* related to organizational justice at time 2, suggesting that the direction of the effect is from justice to health and not the reverse. Kivimäki et al. were able to establish the temporal precedence of a risk factor over health outcomes. Temporal precedence is an important piece of evidence, although not the only evidence needed, supporting the hypothesis that low levels of organizational justice contribute to ill health in workers.

In addition to controlling for the time 1 health outcomes in research on the impact of time 1 working conditions on time 2 health outcomes, other quality-control concerns bear on longitudinal studies. One concern is timing. How much time should elapse between time 1 and time 2? Should there be a 10-year lag between measurement periods? Probably not, because: (a) the nature of the job of an individual who remains in the same position can change over time; (b) people often change jobs given a sufficiently long follow-up period. What about a 6-month lag? It depends. The timing of data collection in a longitudinal study depends on the nature of the jobs being studied and the investigators' preliminary knowledge of the impact of risk factors on health outcomes (Kasl, 1983; Kelloway & Francis, 2013).

Cohort Studies

A particular type of longitudinal study has been employed in epidemiological research, namely, the "prospective cohort study," which is often more simply called a "prospective study." A cohort is an identifiable group of people. They may be people born at a certain time and in a certain place. They may be British civil servants aged 35 to 55 working in 20 departments in London in 1985, as in a study described by Kuper and Marmot (2003). In studies that follow a fixed cohort, which largely reflects the types of cohorts seen in OHP research, "no entries are permitted into the study after the onset of follow-up" (Kleinbaum et al., 1982, p. 56).

In a prospective cohort study, the research participants are initially assessed for the presence or absence of the risk factors or exposure variables. For example, Kuper and Marmot initially ascertained who in their sample was exposed to jobs with low decision latitude and high demands, a combination that has been hypothesized to be harmful to coronary health. A key feature of the prospective study is that participants who are found to have the target disorder during an initial screening are excluded from the longitudinal follow-up. The study strategy is designed to ensure that exposure to the risk factor occurs *before* the disorder develops in any of the participants (the temporal precedence of the cause). Researchers test hypotheses regarding whether newly incident cases of the target disorder that emerge over the course of the follow-up period are more likely to develop in initially healthy participants who were exposed to putative risk factors than in initially healthy participants who were not exposed. Kuper and Marmot found that over approximately 11 years, heart disease was more likely to develop in civil servants who were exposed to low-latitude–high-demands jobs than in civil servants who were not exposed. Kuper and Marmot also statistically adjusted for differences between the exposed and the nonexposed groups on confounding variables such as age, salary grade, and so forth.[3]

Meta-Analysis

The next two sections describe different approaches to meta-analyses, methods that have gained considerable attention in the research community. Meta-analyses are methods for obtaining results by combining numerous data sources. The two-stage meta-analysis is older than the one-stage meta-analysis. When reading older research reports, two-stage meta-analyses are often simply referred to as "meta-analyses."

Two-Stage Meta-Analysis

Because meta-analyses pull together diverse studies with their many different samples, they provide a foundation for making generalizations that is broader than the conclusions OHP researchers can draw from results involving a specific sample. Compared with the statistical power to detect effects in any single study, statistical power is greater in a meta-analysis. A meta-analysis works differently from the research designs the reader already encountered in the chapter. The "participants" in a two-stage meta-analytic study, that is, the traditional meta-analysis, are individual studies. Like most OHP studies, a meta-analysis begins with a hypothesis. Typically, the meta-analyst attempts to identify every study that sheds light on the hypothesis of interest (e.g., compared with control interventions or a waiting list control, a certain type of intervention leads to better worker health). To identify relevant studies in journal articles, book chapters, dissertations, and theses, the analyst searches databases such as PsycINFO and PubMed. The analyst also reviews the reference lists of reports already identified (Box 2.1).

---

[3] The "retrospective cohort study" is another type of cohort study, although rarer in the OHP literature. To conduct such a study, one needs to identify archival data that can be reassembled for the purpose of constructing a retrospective cohort. The structure of a retrospective cohort study is similar to that of the prospective cohort study except that in a retrospective study all the events have already taken place. Initially healthy workers are identified at a point in time. Some were exposed to a risk factor, and some were not. All the workers are followed over time using existing records to identify the occurrence of a target health event. In a classic retrospective cohort study (Case, Hosker, Mcdonald, & Pearson, 1954), workers in the chemical dye industry and control sectors were followed using documentary records. Dye workers were found to be at extremely high risk for bladder cancer.

BOX 2.1 Databases

OH psychologists use a number of databases when identifying studies for a meta-analysis as well as for locating previous research that is relevant to an intervention they are initiating or new research they are planning. One database is PsycINFO. PsycINFO, which is a resource provided by the American Psychological Association, covers the world literature in psychology as well as a large fraction of the literature in allied disciplines (e.g., psychiatry, education, sociology). Most university libraries and many public libraries provide access to PsycINFO.

The reader can learn more about PsycINFO at the following website: www.apa.org/pubs/databases/psycinfo/index.aspx

PubMed is another database OH psychologists consult for meta-analyses and other purposes. PubMed covers the world literature in the life sciences. PubMed is sustained by the United States National Library of Medicine of the National Institutes of Health, and can be directly accessed by anyone with a computer and the Internet.

The website is: www.ncbi.nlm.nih.gov/pubmed

A database that largely parallels PubMed is MEDLINE, which can be found online in university and public libraries.

EMBASE is a biomedical database that can supplement PubMed and MEDLINE. EMBASE covers the proceedings of many conferences.

It should also be noted that sometimes the same publication is indexed in two or more databases. For example, the *Scandinavian Journal of Work, Environment & Health* is indexed in PsycINFO, PubMed, MEDLINE, and EMBASE. However, when conducting an OHP-related literature search, it is often helpful to search multiple databases to get the best coverage. Even if a journal is covered in more than one database, there are omissions in one database that are covered in another. By searching multiple databases, the chance that a relevant paper will be missed is reduced.

The analyst broadcasts alerts on Internet-based "listservs" that ask listserv participants for relevant studies they conducted or know about, including unpublished studies on the topic of interest. Some studies do not get published because investigators with null results are discouraged from publishing. It is important to conduct a broad search for research reports, even those with null or unanticipated negative findings. Unanticipated findings can include results in which the health of the experimental group became worse than that of the control group; however, these studies should still be considered for use in the meta-analysis. Doctoral dissertations and master's theses are scoured because dissertation and thesis writers with negative findings have less incentive than writers with positive findings to publish results (Box 2.2).

BOX 2.2 Listservs

OH psychologists communicate with each other by in-person meetings, e-mail, and telephone. Another method of communication that has become popular in OHP is the listserv. The American Psychological Association (APA) hosts a listserv relevant to OHP, and the European Academy of Occupational Health Psychology (EA-OHP) hosts one.

(continued)

> **Box 2.2 Listservs (*continued*)**
>
> The listservs provide a forum for discussions, and members can use them to broadcast requests for information and receive replies. Conference announcements and requests for papers are also broadcast on the listservs. Anyone can join a listserv.
>
> To join the APA's OHP listserv, visit this website:
>
> http://lists.apa.org/cgi-bin/wa.exe?A0=OHPLIST
>
> To join the APA's other listservs, please write to the following e-mail address: listserv@lists.apa.org
>
> To join the EA-OHP listserv, go to www.jiscmail.ac.uk/cgi-bin/webadmin?A0=EA-OHP

The meta-analyst develops criteria to judge the quality of each of the identified studies. The analyst uses these criteria to decide what studies to include in the meta-analysis. The decision to include or exclude a study is based solely on the quality of the study, and not a study's results. For a meta-analysis to assess the efficacy of an intervention, the analyst may decide that he or she will include only randomized experiments, and exclude quasi-experiments and intervention studies that lack a control group. In a meta-analysis of the impact of a psychosocial job factor such as decision latitude on a later health outcome, the analyst may include only (a) longitudinal studies for which time 1 measures of the health outcome are controlled and (b) prospective cohort studies. The analyst often excludes cross-sectional studies or conducts a separate meta-analysis of the methodologically weaker studies.

From the results section of each study, the meta-analyst extracts important findings. One kind of finding is the number of standard deviations the mean of an experimental group is above or below the mean of a control group. The statistic is called "Cohen's *d*." It is a measure of effect size, that is, how much better (or worse) the experimental group is compared with the control group or how much worse a group of workers exposed to a risk factor is compared with a group not exposed. Cohen's *d* is used when the dependent variable is measured on a continuous scale. The Pearson correlation coefficient, *r*, between the predictor and the health outcome can also serve a meta-analysis. Other statistics that can be extracted for the purpose of a meta-analysis are the odds ratio (*OR*) and the adjusted *OR*. These latter statistics are used when a dependent variable is a disease endpoint, which is binary (a participant was either diagnosed with the target disorder or was not). The adjusted *OR* reflects the influence of the risk factor on the disease endpoint, statistically controlling for other factors.[4] By converting the result of every study to be included in a meta-analysis into Cohen's *d*s or *OR*s, the meta-analyst has taken studies that may have assessed risk factors and dependent variables with a variety of different measures, and made those measures comparable by creating a common metric (Cohen's *d* or an *OR*). Although effect sizes can be classified as large, medium, and small, it

---

[4] Without being overly technical, an *OR* of 1.50 means that the risk of a disorder is approximately 50% greater in individuals exposed to a factor than in nonexposed individuals; an *OR* of 2.00 means that the risk of a disorder is approximately twice (or 100% greater) in exposed individuals than in the nonexposed. An *OR* of 0.50 means that the risk of a disorder in those exposed to a factor is half of that in the nonexposed; instead of a risk factor, we have a protective factor. An adjusted *OR* of 1.50 means that the risk of a disorder in the exposed group is approximately 50% greater, statistically adjusting for the other predictive factors.

should be noted that small effect sizes do not necessarily reflect minor or unimportant effects (Rosnow & Rosenthal, 1989), particularly when the effects bear on health or mortality (see Chapter 4).

Once the meta-analyst has extracted the relevant statistics from the results sections of the highest quality research reports, the analyst averages the relevant effect sizes regardless of whether they were statistically significant or not. Lack of statistical significance reflects effect size within the constraints of sample size. It is important to average effect sizes over many high-quality studies. The analyst may average every Cohen's *d* bearing on a dependent variable such as psychological distress. For example, for every randomized experiment in which (a) an experimental intervention was pitted against a control condition and (b) a continuous measure of distress was the dependent variable, Cohen's *d* is extracted, and all the *d*s are averaged (Cohen, 1992). All other things being equal, the results of larger studies are more reliable than the results of smaller studies. Study findings based on larger samples are weighted more heavily than study findings based on smaller samples.[5] In a meta-analysis in which they converted the findings from each of 55 randomized treatment-control contrasts to Cohen's *d*s, Richardson and Rothstein (2008) found that job-related stress management programs had, in terms of mental health, an average effect size of a little more than half a standard deviation when compared with control conditions. Larger, more beneficial, effects were found for cognitive behavioral interventions in comparison with the effects of other interventions. In a meta-analysis that averaged adjusted *OR*s from five longitudinal studies, Stansfeld and Candy (2006) found that low workplace social support was related to a 30% higher risk of later depression or severe psychological distress.

One-Stage Meta-Analysis

The aforementioned approach to meta-analysis is a two-stage approach. In the first stage, individual data from any one study are analyzed at the level of the individual study, typically by the original study team. The study's results are found in the results sections of journal articles, dissertations, and so forth. The meta-analyst extracts the relevant findings from the results sections of the studies that meet preestablished quality criteria. Then the meta-analyst converts the relevant findings to *d*s or *OR*s, which, in turn, become the input into the second stage of the two-stage meta-analysis, the averaging of the results of the original research reports.

A different kind of meta-analysis, a one-stage approach, has begun to gain adherents. In the one-stage meta-analysis, researchers obtain the raw data from all contributing studies, and analyze the data at the level of each individual participant rather than at the study level (Stewart et al., 2012). One-stage studies require cooperation from the original study teams, whereas in two-stage studies, the data needed are often found in existing results sections and ordinarily don't require cooperation from the original investigators.

Studies that contribute to one-stage meta-analyses, like studies that contribute to two-stage meta-analyses, can use different measures of key variables. In two-stage meta-analyses, study results are converted into a common metric like Cohen's *d* or adjusted *OR*s. By contrast, in one-stage meta-analyses, a different kind

---

[5] The weighting scheme differs depending on whether the meta-analysis uses a fixed effects or random effects model (Borenstein, Hedges, & Rothstein, 2007).

of "harmonization" must take place because the data are merged at the level of the individual participants. If workplace autonomy, an important workplace psychosocial factor in OHP, is measured differently in the original studies to be used in a one-stage meta-analysis, researchers may decide to operationally define individuals in a semiconsistent manner from study to study. For example, the meta-analysts could operationally define individuals with scores above a study sample's mean on an autonomy scale score as high in autonomy, and individuals below that mean as low in autonomy, and then repeat the algorithm for each contributing study even if contributing studies use different scales composed in different languages. In a one-stage meta-analysis involving more than 56,000 individuals from six different longitudinal studies, Fransson et al. (2012) found that among physically active workers, those who held high-workload–low-latitude jobs, compared with other physically active workers exposed to more favorable job conditions, were about 20% more likely to become inactive 2 to 9 years later.

One- and two-stage meta-analyses tend to yield similar results. One-stage meta-analyses, however, provide more statistical power in the context of assessing interactions (Stewart et al., 2012).

Final Comment on Meta-Analyses

Meta-analyses are not without shortcomings. Research on the quality of two-stage meta-analyses of biomedical treatment studies suggests that results are not always in agreement with large ($n > 1,000$), well-controlled clinical trials that were run subsequent to the meta-analyses with similar foci (LeLorier, Grégoire, Benhaddad, Lapierre, & Derderian, 1997). Large, well-controlled clinical trials are the gold standard in biomedical research on clinical interventions. One-stage meta-analyses are subject to information loss owing to procrustean harmonization procedures that require the chopping of different scales at different midpoints, depending on the sample and the measures used.

Other Research Designs in OHP

The next sections examine other research designs that have earned considerable attention. These include the diary study, the natural experiment, and the interrupted time-series. Another category is a broad family of qualitative research methods.

Diary Studies

As the name suggests, diary studies often involve the collection of data on a sample of workers every day over a period of time, such as 1 or 2 weeks. Some diary studies (e.g., Marco, Neale, Schwartz, Shiffman, & Stone, 1999) are run with the help of electronic devices at selected moments during a day or over 1 or more days. Diaries can also involve paper-and-pencil questionnaires (Green, Rafaeli, Bolger, Shrout, & Reis, 2006), telephone interviews (Almeida, Wethington, & Kessler, 2002), and specially designed websites (Schonfeld & Feinman, 2012). The advantage of diary methods is that they help the researcher examine mental states and events occurring at the workplace almost as those events occur in real time, mitigating problems of memory decay. Statistical methods are now available to help minimize subject loss if participants contribute data during some but not all data-collection periods, a circumstance that would be a problem for MLR analyses (Raudenbush & Bryk, 2001; Schonfeld & Rindskopf, 2007).

One particular kind of diary study involves the sampling of representative moments throughout a day or workday in real time. The method is called "ecological momentary assessment" (EMA). The individual reports on momentary states while completing the assessment *in situ*. Typically in EMA, research participants carry electronic devices that signal them, often at randomly[6] generated times, to report their experiences (e.g., affective states, stressors). The accuracy of the characterization of a person depends on having a representative sample of momentary states "much in the way that representative sampling of participants is seen as essential for valid inferences from a sample to a population of people" (Stone & Shiffman, 2002, p. 237).

An innovation in research design involves coordinating EMA and more standard longitudinal designs in which waves of data collection are separated by months. During a 2-year, six-wave longitudinal study of stressors affecting teachers, McIntyre et al. (2016) evaluated the feasibility of teachers completing an iPod-based diary on a single day or on 2 or 3 consecutive days during the fall, winter, and spring. The teachers completed the diaries up to seven times per day, each time after a class period ended. McIntyre et al. found very good compliance, item completion, and user-friendliness. The findings suggest that this kind of research design could be useful in efforts to look closely at stress processes as they play out during the work day as well as provide a look at the longer-term picture. Moreover, the close look can provide clues to identifying transactions that can be improved upon in terms of both reducing teacher stress (or stress in other types of jobs) and improving student achievement.

Natural Experiment

The idea of a natural experiment was introduced in the first chapter, with a description of Parkes's (1982) research on two groups of student nurses who, as part of their training, were randomly rotated through medical and surgical wards in different orders. A natural experiment simulates a true experiment in which participants are randomly assigned to treatment and control conditions. In a natural experiment, "nature" or social conditions outside the investigator's control assign, in an implicitly random manner, individuals to alternative treatments. Without the implicit randomization, a researcher would not be able to draw a causal inference, and the research would reduce to an observational study (DiNardo, 2008). Sometimes, studies are mislabeled natural experiments (e.g., Kompier, Aust, van den Berg, & Siegrist, 2000). For example, they lack a comparison group or, when they have a comparison group, they lack implicit randomization.

Hearst, Newman, and Hulley (1986) described a natural experiment that capitalized on the lottery the U.S. military used to identify men who would be eligible for the draft during the Vietnam War. Compared with men who on account of the lottery were ineligible for the draft, draft-eligible men, over the course of 10 postwar years, were more likely to die by suicide and vehicular accidents, adjusting for wartime deaths. Because about only a quarter of the draft-eligible men served in the military and just 9% of the draft-exempt men served, Hearst et al. (1986) used those figures to calibrate the actual risk associated with military service. The researchers supplemented the analysis with a case-control study that also linked service to subsequent suicide and vehicular death.

---

[6] In the study described next, which involves teachers, participants, for practical reasons, cannot complete an electronic diary at random times during a school day.

Interrupted Time-Series

A time-series involves multiple observations over time. The observations could be of (a) the same individuals or units (e.g., organizational units) or (b) different but similar individuals (e.g., different individuals who come from the same population). What makes a time-series an *interrupted* time-series is that at a point in time within the sequence of observations, a treatment or environmental event occurs. Researchers assess whether the observations obtained after the event differ from the observations obtained before it (Cook & Campbell, 1979).

Many time-series studies extend long enough to encompass more than one environmental event. For example, in an individual-level interrupted time-series study, Eden (1982) followed 39 nursing students for 10 months over five observational periods—three objectively low-stress periods interlarded with two objectively high-stress periods. He found that anxiety, blood pressure, and pulse rate rose during the high-stress periods and fell during the low-stress periods. Although the study was uncontrolled, it is likely that the stressors were causally related to the outcomes. Given that the high-stress periods were sandwiched between the low-stress periods, it is improbable that history and maturational effects, the most likely confounders, could explain the zig and zag of the outcome measures.

Interrupted time-series designs more commonly employ aggregate-level, population-based data. For example, Norström and Grönqvist (2015) assembled data on unemployment rates and suicide rates from 30 countries. The researchers found that, except in Scandinavian countries, male suicide rates over a 52-year period rose or fell with the rise or fall of a country's unemployment rate.[7] In general, the effect of unemployment was stronger in countries with less generous protections for the jobless. A weakness of interrupted time-series studies like Norström and Grönqvist's is that by employing aggregate-level data, one ordinarily cannot discern whether a suicide victim was himself unemployed (see the section of Chapter 3 entitled "Two Pathways for Research on Unemployment"). On the other hand, a country's or region's unemployment rate can serve as a proxy for general economic conditions. Other aggregate-level interrupted time-series studies show that periods of economic recession are associated with elevations in the country's or region's suicide rate (Oyesanya, Lopez-Morinigo, & Dutta, 2015).

Qualitative Research Methods

Qualitative research is not a unitary concept. Qualitative research embraces a variety of methods. Some qualitative OHP researchers interview workers to ask about stressful work experiences and ways in which workers manage or cope with a stressor (e.g., Dewe, 1989; O'Driscoll & Cooper, 1994). Sometimes, workers complete questionnaires in which they freely write responses to open-ended questions about work (e.g., Schonfeld & Santiago, 1994). Other investigators use focus groups (e.g., Kidd, Scharf, & Veazie, 1996), which are group interviews. Some researchers place themselves in locations in which they can observe workers firsthand (Kainan, 1994). Other researchers employ participant observation (Palmer, 1983): the researcher obtains the job he or she intends to study, and learns about the job from the inside.

Glaser and Strauss (1967) propounded a bottom-up approach that has influenced investigators who conduct qualitative research. Glaser and Strauss advanced the

---

[7] Female suicide rates rose or fell with the unemployment rate only in Eastern European countries.

view that researchers should let theoretically interesting categories and hypotheses emerge from qualitative data; it is important *not* to approach qualitative data with preconceptions about what the data should reveal. Content analysis is an empirical methodology that helps organize and make sense of qualitative data. The term "content analysis" refers to a method of analysis, with its own procedures, that helps a researcher obtain insights into textual and symbolic phenomena (e.g., writing, speech, images), including the manifest and latent (shared and unshared) meanings of those phenomena (Krippendorff, 2004).

Although qualitative methods have limitations including the inability to test hypotheses (Schonfeld & Farrell, 2010), they have a number of advantages. For example, qualitative research can help with hypothesis generation, the identifying of as-yet undiscovered stressors and coping strategies, and help with understanding difficult-to-interpret quantitative findings (Schonfeld & Mazzola, 2013). With regard to the latter, Büssing and Glaser (1999) used qualitative data to help understand a paradoxical finding in a quasi-experiment involving nurses. In comparison with control nurses in traditional wards, experimental nurses worked in innovative wards in which job stressors such as time pressure were reduced because they were given greater responsibility but for fewer patients. The experimental nurses, however, experienced higher levels of emotional exhaustion. Qualitative data revealed that compared with nurses in traditional wards who had more piecemeal patient contact, the nurses in the experimental group had less opportunity to withdraw from difficult patients and thus experienced greater interactional stress.

Some OHP investigators collect both quantitative and qualitative data in a single study and integrate them into one set of data analyses.[8] An advantage of this strategy is that researchers can obtain a more complete picture of the stress process (Mazzola, Schonfeld, & Spector, 2011). Elfering et al. (2005) used qualitative methods to identify episodic work and nonwork stressors in workers at a counseling agency. The episodic stressors were assessed every day over the course of a week. Job control and chronically occurring stressors were assessed with standard, quantitatively constructed scales. Compared with chronically occurring stressors, episodically occurring stressors were more idiosyncratic, and therefore more suited to qualitative assessment. Elfering et al. (2005) found that compared with other workers, workers with more job control and lower-intensity chronic stress experienced higher levels of situational well-being in the aftermath of episodic job stressors.

MEASUREMENT

In the previous section, the types of study designs employed in OHP research were outlined. Study designs cannot be implemented in the abstract. Research cannot advance unless researchers effectively measure the factors and conditions they want to study. OHP researchers measure such entities as decision latitude, coworker support, depressive symptoms, and so forth. Before using a specific method of measuring

---

[8] This approach differs from the approach taken by Büssing and Glaser (1999), who also used quantitative and qualitative methods in the same study. Büssing and Glaser used the qualitative data to elucidate an unanticipated finding obtained in the quantitatively organized side of the study rather than combine quantitative and qualitative data in the same analyses.

a factor, OHP researchers, like researchers in other branches of psychology, require evidence that a candidate measure provides a reasonable way to proceed. Researchers can shop around for alternatives. This section briefly covers the measurement aspect of OHP research.

Reliability

Any variable measured should be measured reliably. Reliability reflects the consistency with which researchers measure a given variable. Consider a man's trip to his physician's office. The physician may want to measure the man's weight. Suppose the man steps on the scale, and she measures his weight at 150 lb (68 kg). Then 5 minutes later, the man steps on the scale again, and she measures his weight once more. She now says he weighs 125 lb (57 kg). Then after another 5-minute interval, she weighs him again. But now he weighs 165 lb (75 kg). The scale is not reliable. It does not return consistent measurements from one weighing to the next. Of course, if a year had passed between measurement occasions, it is possible that the scale would return a substantially different weight. The scale could be reliable because people lose and gain weight over time. However, because the measurement occasions in the doctor's office were close in time, the best explanation for the change in weight is that the scale is unreliable. A reliable scale would return the same weight each time the man stepped on it.

In classical test theory, the core of reliability is the "true score." The true score is an unmeasurable, underlying score thought to characterize the person or the condition being assessed. It is thought to be unchanging over short periods of time. Imagine that a sample of workers is administered a five-item job satisfaction scale. Does a worker's score on the scale map exactly onto the worker's true score[9] at that point in time? No. His true score likely contributes to the observed scale score, but a number of other factors may have also contributed to the observed score: if a coworker told him a joke; if he had an argument one morning just before completing the scale; random error.

Suppose a psychologist administers a job satisfaction scale to 100 workers. In addition, an alternate form of the scale (different items that are thought to cover the same ground) is also administered. Each worker is now assigned the mean of his or her scores on the two scales. Is that mean the worker's true score? No it isn't, but it is an improvement. Suppose the psychologist administers 10 alternate forms of the job satisfaction scale, one in the morning and one in the afternoon, every day over the course of a work week. Next each worker is assigned the mean of his or her 10 job satisfaction scores. Is that mean the worker's true score for job satisfaction? The answer is still NO. But that mean is theoretically closer to the true score.

A "reliability coefficient" (its symbol is r_{1t}.), although it looks like a correlation coefficient, is more akin to a coefficient of determination, an r^2. A reliability coefficient is an estimate of the proportion of total scale variance that is true score variance. A reliability estimate of .80 means that 80% of the variance of scale scores is estimated to be true score variance; the remaining 20% of the variance reflects measurement

---

[9] The true score underlying the observed score refers to something largely responsible for the observed score, although reliability alone does not establish what exactly a scale score represents. The section on validity describes what the creators of a scale do to help researchers feel confident that the scale is measuring what the scale is purported to measure.

error or random noise. OHP researchers rarely use scales that have reliability coefficients less than .70. As a reliability coefficient approaches 1.00 (at which point 100% of scale variance is true score variance), more and more scale variance is reflective of true variance. Because true variance is thought to reflect something true about the people responding to scale items, there should be greater consistency from one administration of the scale to the next (at least over short periods of time) and how individuals respond from one scale item to the next. Investigators use a variety of approaches to estimate scale reliability.

Internal Consistency Reliability

The most commonly used reliability coefficient in OHP research is the alpha coefficient, which is also known as "Cronbach's alpha." The strength of the alpha coefficient depends on item-to-item correlations. If you were to open an issue of *Work & Stress* or the *Journal of Occupational Health Psychology*, you would likely find an article in which a scale's coefficient alpha (sometimes seen as the Greek letter α) is reported.

According to classical test theory (Nunnally & Bernstein, 1994), how an individual responds to scale items depends on at least two components, the individual's true score and random error (see Viswanathan [2005] for a discussion of other test score components such as systematic errors). True scores are additive, and sum when the scores on individual items are added to obtain a total score. Item-level random errors, on the other hand, are just that, random. By virtue of their being random, the error components of items are uncorrelated with true scores and each other. Because these errors are essentially random noise, they don't repeat in the same way from item to item. Random errors are not additive; they average out when summing over many items.

One consequence of the randomness of measurement error is that there is a straightforward way to improve the reliability of a scale. Let's suppose that a researcher would like to increase the reliability of a three-item scale designed to measure job satisfaction. Even if the interitem correlations in the original scale are moderate, say around .20 or .30, the researcher can improve the scale's reliability by adding items from the same domain, that is to say, from the domain of items reflecting job satisfaction, that have similar moderate correlations with each other and the original items. The items' true score components will sum, but measurement error associated with the items will not.

Alternate Forms and Test–Retest Reliability

Other kinds of reliability include test–retest reliability and alternate forms reliability (Anastasi & Urbina, 1997). Alternate forms reliability is established by administering two or more forms of the same test or scale within a short time frame, the instruments presumably reflecting similar content but comprising different items. The instruments should be highly correlated with each other. Alternate forms reliability is more likely to be observed in research on psychoeducational tests than in OHP. By contrast, test–retest reliability, which involves correlating the scores obtained in two separate administrations of the same scale, has been employed more often in OHP research. For example, in a measurement study conducted to evaluate the consistency of scales designed to measure the stressfulness of schoolteachers' work environments, Schonfeld (1996) conducted a 2-week test–retest reliability study.

Interrater (Scorer) Reliability: Continuous Measures

Interrater reliability involves having two or more *independent* scorers rate a sample of behavior. Confidence in the measure of behavior depends upon the extent to which the independent ratings are highly correlated. An example of interrater reliability borrowed from a domain outside of OHP would make the idea clear. Two professors of English are independently reading and grading the essays of 100 college students. With a solid scoring rubric and some prior practice, a high correlation between how the two professors rate the 100 essays should obtain.

One could use the Pearson correlation coefficient to assess the reliability of the two sets of ratings. Let's suppose (although this is highly unlikely) that, owing to leniency bias, Professor B awards each student's essay a grade that is exactly 10 points higher than the grade Professor A awards the essay. The Pearson would be perfect, $r = 1.00$, because the corresponding grades awarded by Professors A and B are in exactly the same relative position. This result is to be expected because the Pearson reflects the extent to which the two sets of measurements are linearly related. However, if one is specifically concerned about the exactness with which the two raters agree, that is, the extent to which the raters' ratings are replicates of each other (Bartko, 1991), then it would be helpful to use another statistic, the intraclass correlation coefficient (ICC).[10] The ICC in the essay example would be less than 1.00 because the professors' ratings are not perfect replicates of each other. Of course, applications of the ICC are not limited to professors' ratings of student essays. The ICC can apply to independent observers rating how much complexity there is in job tasks or how much autonomy workers are allowed.

Regardless of whether one is using the Pearson or the ICC in conducting research in which ratings are involved, certain other statistics need to be appreciated and published. With regard to research involving the application of the Pearson correlation coefficient (assuming normality) to evaluate the reliability of raters' ratings, an investigator needs to report in a publication the means and standard deviations (*SD*s) of each rater's ratings. Mean differences could reflect systematic differences (biases) in the raters' ratings. Differences in the *SD*s tell us whether the raters are unequally discriminating. An advantage of the ICC is that, in telling us how closely the corresponding ratings match, the coefficient is affected by rater-related differences in means and *SD*s, although that knowledge may not be obvious to a reader (D. Rindskopf, personal communication, March 14, 2014).

Interrater reliability has been employed in OHP research. Murphy (1991) examined the relation of job characteristics to cardiovascular disease disability. Murphy capitalized on the results of independent research on more than 2,400 U.S. job titles. In that research, job analysts, using observations of job incumbents and interviews of both job incumbents and supervisors, rated 194 work-related activities as specified in the Position Analysis Questionnaire. The interrater reliabilities of the analysts' ratings were satisfactory. The analysts' ratings then became building blocks for the creation of multirating measures of the occupational titles.

---

[10] The intraclass correlation is a family of statistics (Shrout & Fleiss, 1979), but in the interest of making this section relatively nontechnical, the aforementioned example was created.

Interrater Reliability: Categorical Measurement

Some measures used in OHP research are categorical. Examples of categorical measurement include diagnosing a psychiatric disorder. Categorical measurement includes content-analyzing workers' reports about job conditions (e.g., deciding that a worker's written description of a recent interaction with a supervisor reflects whether or not the supervisor was supportive). The coefficient kappa (κ) provides a useful approach to assessing the reliability of procedures employed in categorical measurement (Cohen, 1960).

Suppose, for example, two clinicians independently diagnose 100 workers for a current episode of major depression. For illustrative purposes, the clinicians do something unorthodox. The clinicians believe that the base rate (the normal rate of major depression in the general population) is 10% (it is actually lower), and assign a randomly chosen 10% of the sample a diagnosis of depression. This example is revealing because in earlier times, researchers employed percent agreement as a measure of the reliability of their categorical measurements. Table 2.1 shows what would happen.

Two clinicians assigning a diagnosis to a random 10% of the sample would agree, on average, 82% of the time. They would, on average, agree 81% of the time (0.90×0.90) on which workers are not depressed, and agree about 1% of the time (0.10×0.10) on which workers are depressed. An 82% level of agreement seems impressive; the agreement, however, is largely the result of chance, given the low base rate for the disorder. κ, which adjusts for chance agreement given the base rate (Cohen, 1960), would be .00 for the data in Table 2.1. κ typically ranges from 0, where agreement is purely chance, to 1.00, where there is perfect agreement, as in Table 2.2.[11] An acceptable κ is greater than .40, and κ is considered good when it exceeds .60.

In laying a foundation for the creation of an online diary (Schonfeld & Feinman, 2012), a preliminary study was conducted in which 74 teachers were interviewed for the purpose of identifying job stressors teachers commonly encounter. Two readers *independently* read interview transcripts, content-analyzed the text, and sorted the teachers' descriptions into stressor categories (e.g., episode of student-on-student violence). The median κ was .82 (range: .61 to 1.00). The stressors the 74 teachers identified would become the nucleus of the stressors that would be included in the online diary used in a much larger study.

Final Word on Reliability

Consider an imaginary study in which a researcher measures the height of 25 people in a New York City apartment. The researcher would expect the correlation between height and weight to be moderate, about .60. Let's suppose weight was reliably assessed at another site. What would happen if the measure of height varied in reliability? Suppose the researcher lives near an elevated subway line, with trains passing his window every minute. With subway traffic outside, his hands shake when he measures each person's height. That shaking introduces a little random noise, measurement error, into the height he records next to each person's weight. Some individuals' heights will be slightly lower than they should be, and others', slightly higher. What happens if

---

[11] κ can trend less than 0 when one rater indicates one category, whereas the other rater trends toward indicating the opposite.

TABLE 2.1   Two Clinicians Assigning a Random 10% of a Sample of Workers' Diagnoses of Major Depression

		Clinician 2		
		Not Depressed	Depressed	Row Marginals
Clinician 1	Not Depressed	81	9	90
	Depressed	9	1	10
	Column Marginals	90	10	

TABLE 2.2   Two Clinicians in Perfect Agreement in Assigning Diagnoses of Depression to a Sample of Workers

		Clinician 2		
		Not Depressed	Depressed	Row Marginals
Clinician 1	Not Depressed	90	0	90
	Depressed	0	10	10
	Column Marginals	90	10	

express trains rattle by, causing his hand to shake more, adding even greater variability in the measures of height? The heights he records will contain even more measurement error. Finally, suppose that his hand wobbles so much that the heights he obtains may as well be random numbers. What happens to the correlation between height and weight? As more random error is injected into the recorded heights, the correlation between height and weight weakens (or in statistical language "attenuates"). When the height variable is totally random, that is, 100% of the variability in height represents measurement error, the correlation between height and weight approaches 0. See Cohen, Cohen, West, and Aiken (2003) for a more formal description of the impact of unreliability on correlations. The aforementioned example underlines for the reader that the foundation of all OHP research (in fact, all research in psychology) is the solidity of the measurement properties of the variables being investigated.

Validity

At its most general level, validity concerns establishing that a scale measures what its creators and users profess it to measure. How do we know that a scale purported to measure the stressfulness of a work environment actually measures that construct? How do we know that a scale measuring psychological distress actually measures distress? To establish that a scale measures what the scale's creators claim it measures, three interconnected types of scale validity need to be established: content, criterion-related, and construct validity.

Content Validity

Before looking at scales used in OHP research, it is helpful to turn to psychoeducational testing because (a) it is the arena in which much work on psychometric theory began and (b) an example from that area provides an intuitive way to introduce content validity. In the area of psychoeducational testing, subject area experts establish the content validity of a test by closely examining items to ensure that they are understandable and map onto the content found in curriculum guides and other documents bearing on educational attainment. For example, subject area experts examining an arithmetic test for fourth graders determine whether items map onto the cognitive skills and knowledge that curriculum guides from representative school districts indicate should be taught in the fourth grade.

Content validity in OHP broadly follows the path just described. In creating a scale to assess the extent to which teachers are exposed to workplace stressors, veteran teachers, that is, the experts in the area of stressors confronting teachers, could inspect the items and judge whether they represent stressors teachers ordinarily confront. In creating a depressive symptom scale, experts such as psychiatrists and clinical psychologists inspect the items to judge whether they reflect the symptoms used in clinical settings to diagnose depression.

Criterion-Related Validity

A criterion is something external to the test or scale that the test or scale is expected to predict. Criterion-related validity reflects how well, that is, accurately, the test or scale predicts that external criterion. For illustrative purposes, it is helpful to turn again to the domain of education. Consider the criterion-related validity of a test such as a U.S. college admissions exam (e.g., the ACT) that is administered to upper-level high school students. A college admissions exam's criterion-related validity would depend on how well scores on the exam predict college grades. By the same token, an OHP practitioner would expect scores on a job satisfaction scale to predict workers' contemporaneous intentions to leave their jobs or actual future quitting. A "validity coefficient" is the correlation between the scores on the scale and the behavior the scale is expected to predict. The higher the validity coefficient, the more accurately the scale predicts.

There are two kinds of criterion-related validity. Both apply to the temporal relation of the criterion to the scale in question. Concurrent validity applies to the correlation between the scale and a contemporaneous criterion, for example, the correlation between scores on a job satisfaction scale and current intentions to quit. One would expect the correlation to be positive. Predictive validity applies to the correlation between the scale and a criterion measured at some future time, for example, quitting over the next 2 years.

Construct Validity

When OHP investigators conduct research, they may be interested in such relationships as the influence of decision latitude on psychological distress. But when investigators conduct research, what they do in practice is evaluate the relation of scores on a particular 5-item decision latitude scale to scores on a particular 20-item measure of distress.

OHP researchers also want to draw conclusions at a level of abstraction that goes beyond the particular observables. They would like to draw conclusions about the relation of an abstraction called "decision latitude" to an abstraction called "psychological distress." As mentioned at the beginning of the chapter, abstractions such as decision latitude and psychological distress are constructs. Constructs, not observables, are the constituents of scientific theories (Nunnally & Bernstein, 1994). Construct validation concerns establishing that a particular observable, such as a score on a certain symptom scale, is a reasonable reflection of the construct psychological distress. As in research in other branches of psychology, the construct validity of the measures used in OHP research is of great importance (Hurrell, Nelson, & Simmons, 1998).

Scientific theories generate hypotheses. On the basis of a scientific theory, OHP investigators develop hypotheses that predict how constructs are related to each other. The constructs have to be operationalized in observable measures. Conceptual hypotheses give rise to operational hypotheses (Kleinbaum et al., 1982) that imperfectly mirror the way the constructs will behave (Cronbach & Meehl, 1955). To the extent the observables behave in ways that are consistent with the relevant operational hypotheses, OHP investigators have evidence bearing on the construct validity of their measures.

So far, the discussion of construct validity has been abstract, like a construct itself. Let's bring the discussion down to earth. Schonfeld (2001) developed a measure of the stressfulness of teachers' work environments, the Episodic Stressor Scale (ESS). Teachers indicated how frequently they encountered episodically occurring stressors (e.g., a fight between students). The ESS is supposed to reflect the stressfulness of a teacher's work environment. A hypothesis he tested was that the ESS would correlate with a second measure of workplace stressfulness, the Ongoing Stressor Scale (OSS), which assesses chronically occurring stressors (e.g., low student motivation), because the two scales presumably measure the same construct. This hypothesis reflects Campbell and Fiske's (1959) idea of convergent validity, a component of the construct validation process. Convergent validity requires that two measures of the same construct correlate substantially with each other. The ESS and OSS did, indeed, correlate substantially ($r = .65$).

Every construct in psychology can't be related to every other construct. Construct relationships have borders. A psychological theory often stipulates that a construct central to the theory is unrelated, or weakly related, to another construct. This idea derives from Campbell and Fiske's (1959) concept of discriminant validity, another component of the construct validation process. Schonfeld (2001) hypothesized that the correlation of (a) the ESS administered during the first-year teachers' first fall term with (b) depressive symptoms measured during the summer, preemployment period *before* the women entered the teaching profession would be much weaker than the correlation of the first-term ESS with the first-term OSS. That hypothesis was borne out. The fall-term ESS correlated weakly with preemployment symptoms ($r = -.01$).

It was also expected that compared with the correlation of the fall-term ESS with preemployment symptoms, the fall-term ESS would correlate more strongly with concurrent depressive symptoms and spring-term (measured 4 months later) symptoms because the construct underlying fall-term ESS scores (the extent of chaotic working conditions) would give rise to depressive symptoms. These expectations were also borne out (see Table 2.3). The fall-term ESS scores would *not* be related to preemployment depressive symptoms because the two constructs should be largely

TABLE 2.3 Correlation Matrix

		1	2	3
1	Fall-term Episodic Stressor Scale			
2	Preemployment Depressive Symptoms	−.01		
3	Fall-term Depressive Symptoms	.44*	.47*	
4	Spring-term Depressive Symptoms	.31*	.46*	.55*

*$p < .001$.
Source: Excerpted from Schonfeld (2001).

independent of each other *unless* there was faulty measurement; for example, the fall-term ESS was confounded with prior symptoms/distress.

Schonfeld developed the ESS by populating it with neutrally worded self-report items in reaction to job stress research conducted in an earlier era. In the context of this study, neutral wording refers to items that asked a teacher in unemotional language to indicate how frequently he or she encountered an event such as student fighting. In an earlier research era, job incumbents were often asked how stressed or distressed they were by a work event like student fighting (e.g., Kyriacou & Pratt, 1985). Asking how disturbed a worker is by a working condition (which is fine when done in ordinary conversation) creates an instrument that simultaneously measures at least two constructs: the presumed cause, that is, the job stressors, and the presumed effect, that is, the distress the stressors are hypothesized to provoke. A consequence of this kind of scale construction is that it risks inflating the correlation between the work stressor scale and commonly used dependent variables such as measures of psychological distress. Neutrally worded self-report items, by contrast, minimize emotional language, and concentrate on pinning down how frequently each work event occurred (Frese & Zapf, 1988; Kasl, 1987; Schonfeld, 1996).

RESEARCH ETHICS

Like all professionals, OHP investigators must adhere to ethical standards. The American Psychological Association (APA), the British Psychological Society, the National Institutes of Health, and other prominent organizations have promulgated ethical standards (APA, 2010; Ethics Committee of the British Psychological Society, 2009; National Institutes of Health, 2011). Some major ethical requirements advanced by the APA are highlighted, along with the observation that the APA's ethical standards are generally consistent with those of other, comparable organizations.

The APA's ethical standards follow from a set of general principles the APA has advanced. An example of an ethical principle is the principle of beneficence and nonmaleficence. This principle requires the researcher to do no harm and safeguard the research participant's "welfare and rights." Another principle is that of respect for the rights and dignity of individuals. The principle holds that individuals have the right to "privacy, confidentiality, and self-determination."

More specific standards of conduct are derived from the principles. For example, all proposed empirical research requires approval from the researcher's home institution. The APA requires researchers to provide accurate information to their home institution's institutional review board (IRB). The IRB has the power to approve the research's launch. In the formal application to the IRB, the investigator, in describing the study's procedures, also describes the study's risks and benefits, and the steps the investigator has taken to minimize risk or harm to participants. For example, the investigator describes how he or she will safeguard the privacy of the participants.

For empirical research with human subjects, the investigator must obtain informed consent from each participant. Informed consent is often framed in a letter to the participant (one to be signed and given to the investigator and an identical copy kept by the participant). The investigator, using language that is clearly understandable to participants, explains the purpose of the research, the risks and benefits of the research, and what the investigator has done to minimize risk (e.g., how the participant's privacy will be safeguarded). The letter (in some research projects informed consent can be communicated orally) explains that participation in the research is voluntary and that the individual can stop participating at any time with no penalty.

In some circumstances, informed consent is not needed. When an investigator uses an anonymous questionnaire that his or her IRB has approved and judged not to cause harm, informed consent can sometimes be waived. When conducting research based on archival data, informed consent is not required.

The APA has ethical standards regarding publication credit once a research effort has concluded and a group of investigators has decided to write a paper about its findings. The APA standards indicate that who becomes the first author, the second author, and so forth depends on the extent of the individual's scientific and professional contribution to the paper. The standards make it clear that having senior status (e.g., an individual who is a department chairperson) does not entitle an individual to author status. Author status depends on the individual's contribution to the project.

SUMMARY

This chapter sketches the principal designs used in OHP research. Research is often guided by theory-generated hypotheses that investigators plan to test. Sometimes, however, research is guided by the accumulation of past findings. Much research is motivated by a combination of both. It should be borne in mind that the designs found in OHP research are commonly used in other branches of psychology and in medicine. The chapter emphasizes the value of the random allocation of research participants to experimental and control conditions in research evaluating the efficacy of workplace interventions. Random assignment of participants to treatment and control groups distinguishes the experiment from the quasi-experiment.

Researchers cannot ethically conduct experiments in which they deliberately expose participants to risk factors for health-related problems. Investigators can, however, conduct longitudinal studies in which they can statistically adjust for measured confounding factors such as baseline levels of the dependent variable, the variable that is expected to be affected by the work-related exposures. A diary study is a special kind of longitudinal study, the duration of which is usually brief, but captures events at work in, or close to, real time. Investigators conduct another special kind of longitudinal study called the prospective study, a study that is limited to participants who at the time 1 baseline are free of the disorder hypothesized to emerge later as a result of work-related exposures. A natural experiment, a kind of accident of the social, if not the natural, world, mimics a true experiment. An interrupted time-series study also takes advantage of events occurring in the world provided there are a sufficient number of assessments, either at the level of the individual or at the aggregate level, before and after the occurrence of the event in question.

Other types of research designs include the cross-sectional study and the case-control study. In cross-sectional studies, variables are assessed at a single point in time. Case-control studies involve individuals with and without a disorder. Investigators obtain data on the participants' life histories in order to learn whether the cases and controls were subject to different exposures over time. Both of these designs are useful for assessing whether an exposure and a health problem are related, but are usually unsuited to drawing cause–effect conclusions. One- and two-stage meta-analyses pool data at the participant or study level. Meta-analyses provide a basis for obtaining broad summary findings across multiple studies. Qualitative methods help us understand the work lives of individuals at a highly descriptive level. Although not an effective vehicle for hypothesis testing, qualitative methods help investigators in the context of discovery and hypothesis generation.

Measurement is an important part of OHP research. We cannot study what we cannot adequately measure. OHP researchers want to employ reliable and valid measures of the variables they investigate. Investigators want evidence that they are reliably measuring every factor pertinent to their research. In other words, researchers want evidence that a factor (e.g., decision latitude) will remain largely unchanged if measured today and tomorrow. Of course, investigators want evidence that the instruments they use are valid. In other words, researchers want evidence that an instrument they use to measure a factor (e.g., depression) is truly assessing that factor.

Research must be conducted ethically. Research should do no harm. Those who participate in a study should do so voluntarily; they must give their informed consent in order to participate in a study. Coercion is unacceptable. Participants can withdraw from a study at any time and for any reason. When publishing a paper, researchers must allocate credit fairly.

REFERENCES

Almeida, D. M., Wethington, E., & Kessler, R. C. (2002). The daily inventory of stressful events: An interview-based approach for measuring daily stressors. *Assessment, 9*, 41–55. doi:10.1177/1073191102009001006

American Psychological Association. (2010). *Ethical principles of psychologists and code of conduct.* Retrieved from www.apa.org/ethics/code/index.aspx

Anastasi, A., & Urbina, S. (1997). *Psychological testing* (7th ed.). Upper Saddle River, NJ: Prentice Hall.

Bartko, J. J. (1991). Measurement and reliability: Statistical thinking considerations. *Schizophrenia Bulletin, 17*(3), 483–489.

Bond, F. W., & Bunce, D. (2001). Job control mediates change in a work reorganization intervention for stress reduction. *Journal of Occupational Health Psychology, 6*, 290–302. doi:10.1037/1076-8998.6.4.290

Borenstein, M., Hedges, L., & Rothstein, H. (2007). *Meta-analysis: Fixed effect vs. random effects.* Retrieved from www.meta-analysis.com/downloads/Meta%20Analysis%20Fixed%20vs%20Random%20effects.pdf

Burke, R. J., & Greenglass, E. (1995). A longitudinal study of psychological burnout. *Human Relations, 48*, 187–202. doi:10.1177/001872679504800205

Büssing, A., & Glaser, J. (1999). Work stressors in nursing in the course of redesign: Implications for burnout and interactional stress. *European Journal of Work and Organizational Psychology, 8*, 401–426. doi:10.1080/135943299398249

Campbell, D. T., & Fiske, E. W. (1959). Convergent and discriminant validation by the multitrait-multimethod matrix. *Psychological Bulletin, 56*, 81–105. doi:10.1037/h0046016

Case, R. A., Hosker, M. E., Mcdonald, D. B., & Pearson, J. T. (1954). Tumours of the urinary bladder in workmen engaged in the manufacture and use of certain dyestuff intermediates in the British chemical industry. Part I. The role of aniline, benzidine, alpha-naphthylamine, and beta-naphthylamine. *British Journal of Industrial Medicine, 11*(2), 75–104.

Cohen, J. (1960). A coefficient of agreement for nominal scales. *Educational and Psychological Measurement, 20*, 37–46. doi:10.1177/001316446002000104

Cohen, J. (1992). A power primer. *Psychological Bulletin, 112*, 155–159. doi:10.1037/0033-2909.112.1.155

Cohen, J., Cohen, P., West, W. G., & Aiken, L. S. (2003). *Applied multiple regression/correlation analysis for the behavior sciences* (3rd ed.). Hillsdale, NJ: Erlbaum.

Cook, T. D., & Campbell, D. T. (1979). *Quasi-experimentation: Design and analysis issues in field settings.* Boston, MA: Houghton Mifflin.

Cronbach, L., & Meehl, P. (1955). Construct validity in psychological tests. *Psychological Bulletin, 56*, 81–105. doi:10.1037/h0040957

Dewe, P. J. (1989). Examining the nature of work stress: Individual evaluations of stressful experiences and coping. *Human Relations, 42*, 993–1013. doi:10.1177/001872678904201103

DiNardo, J. (2008). Natural experiments and quasi-natural experiments. In S. N. Durlaur & L. E. Blume (Eds.), *The new Palgrave dictionary of economics* (2nd ed.). New York, NY: Palgrave Macmillan. doi:10.1057/9780230226203.1162

Eden, D. (1982). Critical job events, acute stress, and strain: A multiple interrupted time series. *Organizational Behavior & Human Performance, 30,* 312–329. doi:10.1016/0030-5073(82)90223-9

Elfering, A., Grebner, S., Semmer, N. K., Kaiser-Freiburghaus, D., Lauper-Del Ponte, S., & Witschi, I. (2005). Chronic job stressors and job control: Effects on event-related coping success and well-being. *Journal of Occupational and Organizational Psychology, 78,* 237–252. doi:10.1348/096317905X40088

Ethics Committee of the British Psychological Society. (2009). *Code of ethics and conduct.* Retrieved from www.bps.org.uk/sites/default/files/documents/code_of_ethics_and_conduct.pdf

Flaxman, P. E., & Bond, F. W. (2010). Worksite stress management training: Moderated effects and clinical significance. *Journal of Occupational Health Psychology, 15,* 347–358. doi:10.1037/a0020522

Fransson, E., Heikkilä, K., Nyberg, S., Zins, M., Westerlund, H., Westerholm, P., & Kivimäki, M. (2012). Job strain as a risk factor for leisure-time physical inactivity: An individual-participant meta-analysis of up to 170,000 men and women: The IPD-Work Consortium. *American Journal of Epidemiology, 176,* 1078–1089. doi:10.1093/aje/kws336

Frese, M., & Zapf, D. (1988). Methodological issues in the study of work stress: Objective vs subjective measurement of work stress and the question of longitudinal studies. In C. L. Cooper & R. Payne (Eds.), *Causes, coping and consequences of stress at work* (pp. 375–411). Oxford, England: Wiley.

Glaser, B., & Strauss, A. (1967). *The discovery of grounded theory: Strategies for qualitative research.* Chicago, IL: Aldine.

Green, A. S., Rafaeli. E., Bolger, N., Shrout, P. E., & Reis, H. T. (2006). Paper or plastic? Data equivalence in paper and electronic diaries. *Psychological Methods, 11,* 87–105. doi:10.1037/1082-989X.11.1.87

Hearst, N., Newman, T. B., & Hulley, S. B. (1986). Delayed effects of the military draft on mortality: A randomized natural experiment. *New England Journal of Medicine, 314,* 620–624. doi:10.1056/NEJM198603063141005

Hurrell, J. J., Jr., Nelson, D. L., & Simmons, B. L. (1998). Measuring job stressors and strains: Where we have been, where we are, and where we need to go. *Journal of Occupational Health Psychology, 3,* 368–389. doi:10.1037/1076-8998.3.4.368

Kainan, A. (1994). Staffroom grumblings as expressed teachers' vocation. *Teaching and Teachers Education, 10,* 281–290. doi:10.1016/0742-051X(95)97310-1

Karasek, R. A. (1979). Job demands, job decision latitude, and mental strain: Implications for job redesign. *Administrative Science Quarterly, 24*(2), 285–308.

Kasl, S. V. (1983) Pursuing the link between stressful life experiences and disease: A time for reappraisal. In C. L. Cooper (Ed.), *Stress research* (pp. 79–102). Chichester, England: UK: Wiley.

Kasl, S. V. (1987). Methodologies in stress and health: Past difficulties, present dilemmas, future directions. In S. V. Kasl & C. L. Cooper (Eds.), *Stress and health: Issues in research methodology* (pp. 307–318). Chichester, England: UK: Wiley.

Kelloway, E. K., & Francis, L. (2013). Longitudinal research and data analysis. In R. R. Sinclair, M. Wang, & L. E. Tetrick (Eds.), *Research methods in occupational health psychology: Measurement, design, and data analysis* (pp. 374–394). New York, NY: Routledge.

Kidd, P., Scharf, T., & Veazie, M. (1996) Linking stress and injury in the farming environment: A secondary analysis. *Health Education Quarterly, 23,* 224–237. doi:10.1177/109019819602300207

Kivimäki, M., Elovainio, M., Vahtera, J., & Ferrie, J. E. (2003). Organisational justice and health of employees: Prospective cohort study. *Occupational and Environmental Medicine, 60*(1), 27–34.

Kleinbaum, D. G., Kupper, L. L., & Morgenstern, H. (1982). *Epidemiologic research: Principles and quantitative methods.* Belmont, CA: Lifetime Learning.

Kompier, M. J., Aust, B., van den Berg, A., & Siegrist, J. (2000). Stress prevention in bus drivers: Evaluation of 13 natural experiments. *Journal of Occupational Health Psychology, 5,* 11–31. doi:10.1037/1076-8998.5.1.11

Krippendorff, K. (2004). *Content analysis: An introduction to its methodology* (2nd ed.). Thousand Oaks Hills, CA: Sage.

Kuper, H., & Marmot, M. (2003). Job strain, job demands, decision latitude, and risk of coronary heart disease within the Whitehall II study. *Journal of Epidemiology and Community Health, 57*(2), 147–153.

Kyriacou, C., & Pratt, J. (1985). Teacher stress and psychoneurotic symptoms. *British Journal of Educational Psychology, 55,* 61–64. doi:10.1111/j.2044-8279.1985.tb02607.x

LeLorier, J., Grégoire, G., Benhaddad, A., Lapierre, J., & Derderian, F. (1997). Discrepancies between meta-analyses and subsequent large randomized, controlled trials. *New England Journal of Medicine, 337*(8), 536–542.

Link, B. G., Dohrenwend, B. P., & Skodol, A. E. (1986). Socio-economic status and schizophrenia: Noisome occupational characteristics as a risk factor. *American Sociological Review, 51*, 242–258. doi:10.2307/2095519

MacMahon, B., & Pugh, T. R. (1970). *Epidemiology: Principles and methods.* Boston, MA: Little, Brown.

Marco, C. A., Neale, J. M., Schwartz, J. E., Shiffman, S., & Stone, A. A. (1999). Coping with daily events and short-term mood changes: An unexpected failure to observe effects of coping. *Journal of Consulting and Clinical Psychology, 67*, 755–764. doi:10.1037/0022-006X.67.5.755

Mazzola, J. J., Schonfeld, I. S., & Spector, P. E. (2011). What qualitative research has taught us about occupational stress. *Stress and Health, 27*, 93–110. doi:10.1002/smi.1386

McIntyre, T. M., McIntyre, S. E., Barr, C. D., Woodward, P. S., Francis, D. J., Durand, A. C., & Kamarck, T. W. (2016). Longitudinal study of the feasibility of using ecological momentary assessment to study teacher stress: Objective and self-reported measures. *Journal of Occupational Health Psychology, 21*, 403–414. doi:10.1037/a0039966

Murphy, L. R. (1991). Job dimensions associated with severe disability due to cardiovascular disease. *Journal of Clinical Epidemiology, 44*(2), 151–166.

National Institutes of Health. (2011). *NIH research ethics.* Retrieved from http://researchethics.od.nih.gov/CourseIndex.aspx

Ng, S. (1991). Does epidemiology need a new philosophy? A case study of logical inquiry in the acquired immunodeficiency syndrome epidemic. *American Journal of Epidemiology, 133*(11), 1073–1077.

Norström, T., & Grönqvist, H. (2015). The Great Recession, unemployment and suicide. *Journal of Epidemiology and Community Health, 69*, 110–116. doi:10.1136/jech-2014-204602

Nunnally, J. C., & Bernstein, I. H. (1994). *Psychometric theory.* New York, NY: McGraw-Hill.

O'Driscoll, M. P., & Cooper, C. L. (1994). Coping with work-related stress: A critique of existing measures and proposal for an alternative methodology. *Journal of Occupational and Organizational Psychology, 67*, 343–354. doi:10.1111/j.2044-8325.1994.tb00572.x

Oyesanya, M., Lopez-Morinigo, J., & Dutta, R. (2015). Systematic review of suicide in economic recession. *World Journal of Psychiatry, 5*, 243–254. doi:10.5498/wjp.v5.i2.243

Palmer, C. E. (1983). A note about paramedics' strategies for dealing with death and dying. *Journal of Occupational Psychology, 56*, 83–86. doi:10.1111/j.2044-8325.1983.tb00114.x

Parkes, K. R. (1982). Occupational stress among student nurses: A natural experiment. *Journal of Applied Psychology, 67*, 784–796. doi:10.1037/0021-9010.67.6.784

Platt, J. R. (1964). Strong inference: Certain systematic methods of scientific thinking may produce much more rapid progress than others. *Science, 146*(3642), 347–353.

Popper, K. (1963). *Conjectures and refutations: The growth of scientific knowledge.* New York, NY: Basic Books.

Raudenbush, S. W., & Bryk, A. S. (2001). *Hierarchical linear models: Applications and data analysis methods* (2nd ed.). Newbury Park, CA: Sage.

Richardson, K. M., & Rothstein, H. R. (2008). Effects of occupational stress management intervention programs: A meta-analysis. *Journal of Occupational Health Psychology, 13*, 69–93. doi:10.1037/1076-8998.13.1.69

Rosnow, R. L., & Rosenthal, R. (1989). Statistical procedures and the justification of knowledge in psychological science. *American Psychologist, 44*, 1276–1284. doi:10.1037/0003-066X.44.10.1276

Schonfeld, I. S. (1990). Coping with job-related stress: The case of teachers. *Journal of Occupational Psychology, 63*, 141–149. doi:10.1111/j.2044-8325.1990.tb00516.x

Schonfeld, I. S. (1996). Relation of negative affectivity to self-reports of job stressors and psychological outcomes. *Journal of Occupational Health Psychology, 1*, 397–412. doi:10.1037/1076-8998.1.4.397

Schonfeld, I. S. (2001). Stress in 1st-year women teachers: The context of social support and coping. *Genetic, Social, and General Psychology Monographs, 127*(2), 133–168.

Schonfeld, I. S., & Farrell, E. (2010). Qualitative methods can enrich quantitative research on occupational stress: An example from one occupational group. In D. C. Ganster & P. L. Perrewé (Eds.), *Research in Occupational Stress and Well Being Series: New developments in theoretical and conceptual approaches to job stress* (Vol. 8, pp. 137–197). Bingley, England: Emerald.

Schonfeld, I. S., & Feinman, S. J. (2012). Difficulties of alternatively certified teachers. *Education and Urban Society, 44*, 215–246. doi:10.1177/0013124510392570.

Schonfeld, I. S., & Mazzola, J. J. (2013). Strengths and limitations of qualitative approaches to research in occupational health psychology. In R. R. Sinclair, M. Wang, & L. E. Tetrick (Eds.), *Research methods in occupational health psychology: State of the art in measurement, design, and data analysis* (pp. 268–289). New York, NY: Routledge.

Schonfeld, I. S., & Rindskopf, D. (2007). Hierarchical linear modeling in organizational research: Longitudinal data outside the context of growth modeling. *Organizational Research Methods, 18*, 417–429. doi:10.1177/1094428107300229

Schonfeld, I. S., & Santiago, E. A. (1994). Working conditions and psychological distress in first-year women teachers: Qualitative findings. In L. C. Blackman (Ed.), *What works? Synthesizing effective biomedical and psychosocial strategies for healthy families in the 21st century* (pp. 114–121). Indianapolis: University of Indiana Press.

Shrout, P. E., & Fleiss, J. L. (1979). Intraclass correlations: Uses in assessing rater reliability. *Psychological Bulletin, 86*, 420–428. doi:10.1037/0033-2909.86.2.420

Siegel, J. M., Prelip, M. L., Erausquin, J. T., & Kim, S. A. (2010). A worksite obesity intervention: Results from a group-randomized trial. *American Journal of Public Health, 100*, 327–333. doi:10.2105/AJPH.2008.154153

Spector, P. E., & Zhou, Z. E. (2014). The moderating role of gender in relationships of stressors and personality with counterproductive work behavior. *Journal of Business and Psychology, 29*, 669–681. doi:10.1007/s10869-013-9307-8

Stansfeld, S., & Candy, B. (2006). Psychosocial work environment and mental health: A meta-analytic review. *Scandinavian Journal of Work, Environment & Health, 32*(Special Issue 6), 443–462.

Stewart, G., Altman, D., Askie, L., Duley, L., Simmonds, M., & Stewart, L. (2012). Statistical analysis of individual participant data meta-analyses: A comparison of methods and recommendations for practice. *PLOS ONE, 7*(10), e46042. doi:10.1371/journal.pone.0046042

Stone, A. A., & Shiffman, S. (2002). Capturing momentary, self-report data: A proposal for reporting guidelines. *Annals of Behavioral Medicine, 24*, 236–243. doi:10.1207/S15324796ABM2403_09

Susser, M. (1979). *Causal thinking in the health sciences.* New York, NY: Oxford University Press.

Tennant, C., Bebbington, P., & Hurry, J. (1981). The role of life events in depressive illness: Is there a substantial causal relation? *Psychological Medicine, 11*, 379–389. doi:10.1017/S0033291700052193

Viswanathan, M. (2005). *Measurement error and research design.* Thousand Oaks, CA: Sage.

THREE

The Impact of Psychosocial Working Conditions on Mental Health

KEY CONCEPTS AND FINDINGS COVERED IN CHAPTER 3

Many types of workplace hazards can compromise a worker's health. For example, physical hazards such as extreme temperatures or excessive noise can adversely affect a worker's health. Chemical hazards such as benzene and insecticides can harm a worker's health. The central aim of this book, however, is to examine the impact of a different category of workplace hazards, namely, psychosocial hazards. This chapter examines the impact of the psychosocial work environment on the mental health of people who work. Although it is widely recognized that the causes of mental health problems such as depression are multifactorial (e.g., genetic, stressful life events occurring outside of work), psychosocial working conditions are also part of that "multifactorial" set of causes. This chapter is largely confined to depression and elevated levels of depressive symptoms, although some research that the chapter examines involves suicide, excessive alcohol use, psychosomatic symptoms (headaches, backaches, stomachaches, etc.), and burnout. Sometimes, researchers label these mental health outcomes as "psychological strains."

It is important to examine mental health for two reasons. The first, and most important, reason is that a great deal of suffering is associated with mental health problems such as depression. Depression increases the risk of suicide (Miret, Ayuso-Mateos, Sanchez-Moreno, & Vieta, 2013; Rihmer, 2001). Research on the global burden of disease indicates that depression is a gateway to poor physical health, disability, and premature death from a variety of causes (Baxter, Charlson, Somerville, & Whiteford, 2011; Bruce, Leaf, Rozal, & Florio, 1994). Prospective studies have linked depression to increased risk of cardiovascular disease (e.g., Pratt et al., 1996), although the prospective evidence is not unambiguous (Nicholson, Kuper, & Hemingway, 2006). The World Health Organization (WHO) considers depression to be "the most burdensome disease in the world" in terms of total disability affecting people at midlife (Gotlib & Hammen, 2009, p. 1). The second reason for a chapter on mental health is that workers' mental health affects the smooth and safe running of businesses and other organizations. Workers suffering from mental health problems such as depression have more absences and show reduced performance while at work ("presenteeism"). They constitute an economic burden for employers, and compromise safety (Ford, Cerasoli, Higgins, & Decesare, 2011; Goetzel, Ozminkowski, Sederer, & Mark, 2002; Kessler et al., 2006; Laitinen-Krispijn, & Bijl, 2000; McTernan, Dollard, & LaMontagne, 2013). Other research indicates that depression is related to reduced performance on work-related interpersonal tasks, time management, and timely handling of workload (D. A. Adler et al., 2006). If we can identify workplace factors that increase the risk of depression, then we can target those factors in planning to create healthier workplaces.

In examining the research bearing on the impact of psychosocial working conditions on mental health, the chapter is largely confined to higher quality longitudinal studies, many of which have been population based, and have controlled for workers' psychological functioning at the first wave of data collection (at baseline). With some exceptions, the chapter largely excludes cross-sectional studies because they are unable to determine the temporal ordering of the putative causes (e.g., a factor

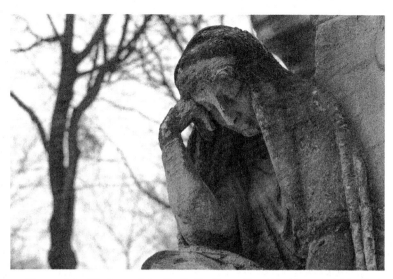

Depression. (Photograph by Kerttu Jaatinen. Reprinted by permission.)

in the psychosocial work environment) and effects (e.g., depression). In addition, four types of longitudinal studies are also excluded. First, longitudinal studies in which the lag between measurement periods is exceedingly long (e.g., >20 years) are excluded. Such studies do not allow us to draw reasonable conclusions about the impact of baseline psychosocial features on outcomes (e.g., Michélsen & Bildt, 2003). Second, longitudinal studies are excluded in which working conditions that were linked to mental health were limited to measures that were obtained contemporaneously with the assessments of mental health (e.g., Parkes, Mendham, & von Rabenau, 1994; Schonfeld, 1996). These studies make it difficult to get the causal ordering right despite their longitudinal design. Third, longitudinal studies that do not control for mental health at time 1 (e.g., Olstad, Sexton, & Søgaard, 2001) are excluded. When assessing the impact of time 1 work stressors on time 2 mental health outcomes, investigators should control for time 1 mental health (see the explanation in Chapter 2). Finally, with a few exceptions, longitudinal studies in which changes in working conditions between time 1 and time 2 are used to predict time-1-to-time-2 changes (e.g., Barnett & Brennan, 1997) in mental health are excluded. These change–change studies are problematic because they prevent us from ascertaining which change had temporal priority.

ASSESSING MENTAL HEALTH IN OHP RESEARCH

Occupational health psychology (OHP)–related research on mental health has focused largely on the relation of psychosocial working conditions to three types of outcomes. One is psychological distress. The second is depression. The third is burnout.

Psychological Distress and Depression

In much of the research that is described in this chapter, mental health is often measured with well-known, reliable, and valid symptom scales and rarely through ascertaining the presence of a mental disorder diagnosed by clinical interview (e.g., Plaisier et al., 2007). The most prominent symptom scales are the General Health Questionnaire (GHQ; Goldberg, 1972), the Center for Epidemiologic Studies Depression Scale (CES-D; Radloff, 1977), the Symptom Checklist-90 (SCL-90[-R]; Derogatis, 1977, 1983), the Beck Depression Inventory (BDI; Beck, Ward, Mendelson, Mock, & Erbaugh, 1961), and the Self-Rating Depression Scale (Zung, 1965, commonly called the "Zung scale"). High scores on any of these scales are not equivalent to a diagnosis of mental disorder. However, a considerable amount of research shows that a score above a predetermined threshold indicates that an individual is at high risk for meeting criteria for a mental disorder (Goldberg, Oldehinkel, & Ormel, 1998; Schonfeld, 1990). It is also possible to obtain a high score on one of the aforementioned scales, yet not meet criteria for a diagnosable mental disorder. Such an individual is *not* free of suffering. Ordinarily, a high score on a symptom scale without meeting diagnostic criteria indicates that an individual is experiencing considerable nonspecific psychological distress or demoralization (Dohrenwend, Shrout, Egri, & Mendelsohn, 1980).

The GHQ is a screening instrument reflecting "psychiatric distress covering symptoms of anxiety and depression, social dysfunction and loss of confidence" (Aalto, Elovainio, Kivimäki, Uutela, & Pirkola, 2012, p. 164). GHQ items refer to such symptoms as loss of sleep, lost concentration, feeling happy (reverse scored), and so on. The SCL-90 (Derogatis, 1977, 1983), but not the other symptom scales mentioned in this section, contains subscales comprising different combinations of its 90 items. Each subscale is devoted to a particular set of psychiatric symptoms (e.g., depression, phobic anxiety). Depression items on the SCL-90 cover symptoms such as "feeling lonely" and "feelings of worthlessness." The SCL-90 also includes a Global Severity Index (GSI), a measure that combines the number of symptoms and symptom severity. The items on the CES-D reflect depressive symptoms (Radloff, 1977). CES-D items refer to feeling depressed, having trouble concentrating, and feeling hopeful about the future (reverse scored). BDI items reflect behavioral, affective, and somatic symptoms (Beck et al., 1961). Items on the Zung scale cover feeling "down-hearted and blue" and not experiencing sexual pleasure (Zung, 1965).

The studies described in this chapter rarely ascertained the presence of a mental disorder such as depression. One study (Ylipaavalniemi et al., 2005) relied on worker reports of a doctor-confirmed diagnosis of "clinical depression." Some studies (Bromet, Dew, Parkinson, & Schulberg, 1988; Plaisier et al., 2007; Muntaner, Tien, Eaton, & Garrison, 1991) employed diagnostic interviews at two points in time. It is not surprising that so few longitudinal studies ascertained the presence of diagnosable mental disorders and that most of the research in this area relied largely on symptom scales. The studies covered in these chapters tended to have large numbers of participants. It would have been impractical and extremely costly to organize clinician-administered diagnostic interviews at multiple points in time. In the studies by Plaisier et al. (2007) and Mutaner et al. (1991), costs of diagnostic interviews were somewhat controlled because the interviews were highly structured and administered by lay interviewers (not clinicians, who are more expensive), with algorithmically generated diagnoses.

Burnout

A number of studies examined the impact of job stressors on burnout, a concept first identified by Herbert J. Freudenberger (1974), based on his qualitative observations of volunteers (including himself) working in a free clinic for drug abusers. The concept was soon extended to embrace other helping professionals, including teachers, nurses, and social workers. According to Freudenberger, burnout is a syndrome, the core of which is exhaustion and fatigue. He also noted concomitant symptoms, including frustration and quickness to anger. He observed that a burned-out individual "looks, acts and seems depressed" (p. 161). A number of scales have been developed to measure burnout. One, the Maslach Burnout Inventory (MBI; Maslach & Jackson, 1986), which comprises three dimensions: emotional exhaustion, depersonalization (viewing in a cynical manner the clients the individual is supposed to help), and lack of a sense of personal accomplishment on the job. Shirom (1989), however, adduced evidence for the view that exhaustion, in the form of "physical fatigue, emotional exhaustion, and cognitive weariness" (p. 33), is the core of burnout, and that the other components are reflections of coping efforts (depersonalization) or self-esteem problems (lack of personal accomplishment). The later-developed MBI-General Survey (MBI-GS; Schaufeli, Leiter, Maslach, & Jackson, 1996), a revision of the original MBI, also contains three dimensions, now named "exhaustion" (e.g., feeling emotionally drained by one's work; feeling used up at the end of the workday), "cynicism" (e.g., having become less enthusiastic about one's job), and "professional efficacy" (believing that one is competent at one's job).

Although the MBI was originally applied to the helping professions, the MBI-GS applies to almost any occupation. An alternative instrument, the Oldenburg Burnout Inventory (OLBI), comprises two dimensions, exhaustion (e.g., feeling worn out and weary after work) and disengagement from the job (e.g., talking about work in a derogatory way), and can be used with almost all occupations (Demerouti, Bakker, Nachreiner, & Schaufeli, 2001). The Shirom-Melamed Burnout Inventory (Shirom & Melamed, 2006) applies to all occupations and reflects "physical, emotional, and cognitive exhaustion" (p. 194). Other burnout instruments also apply to all occupations *and* to stressful circumstances outside of work (Kristensen, Borritz, Villadsen, & Christensen, 2005; Malach-Pines, 2005).

Although Freudenberg (1974) observed that burned-out volunteer mental health workers appeared depressed, he considered burnout a separate syndrome. Other investigators (Bianchi, Schonfeld, & Laurent, 2014; Meier, 1984; Schonfeld & Bianchi, 2016a) advanced the idea that burnout, as measured on burnout scales, overlaps depressive symptoms and that clinical burnout reflects a depressive disorder that originates with very bad working conditions. By contrast, Frone and Tidwell (2015) observed a great deal of overlap between burnout and work-related fatigue.

THE IMPACT OF JOB LOSS ON MENTAL HEALTH

Sigmund Freud rarely discussed the role of work in his vast writings. However, in a footnote in one of his books, he wrote that "no other technique for the conduct of life attaches the individual so firmly to reality as laying emphasis on work; for his work at least gives him a secure place in a portion of reality, in the human community" (Freud, 1962/1930, p. 27). Losing one's job can mean losing one's moorings. The Marienthal study described in Chapter 1 painted a troubled picture of unemployed people living in a community bearing the weight of the Great Depression (Jahoda, Lazarsfeld, & Zeisel, 1971/1933). Many years after the Marienthal study was published,

Jahoda (1981), taking a cue from Robert Merton *and* Sigmund Freud, developed a theory of the latent functions of work—the manifest functions, such as earnings and prestige, are more easily observed. The latent functions of work include the establishment of a time structure for activities conducted during the day, the sharing of experiences and contacts with people outside one's nuclear family, and the provision of opportunities to work with others toward common goals. Other latent functions include helping to define the individual's identity and ensuring that an individual remains active. Unemployment robs individuals of these manifest and latent functions. A corollary is that unemployment has adverse psychological effects on the individual. Warr (1987, 1994) advanced the view that work provides a number of psychological benefits that are analogous to vitamins' benefits vis-à-vis physical health. Work's benefits include opportunities for control and skill use, earnings, physical security, opportunities for contact with others, and so on. He advanced the view that these factors are important to mental health.[1] Unemployment, because it largely deprives the individual of these benefits (although Warr allows for exceptions), has an adverse effect on psychological well-being.

The first author of this book suffered job loss twice in his life. The first time was when he was a student at a commuter college, and living at home with his parents in a New York City housing project. At the end of his freshman year, he obtained a job as a tool and die operator in a factory that manufactured ladies' slippers. Every weekday, he commuted by bus and subway to a factory located in an upper floor of an industrial building on the Brooklyn waterfront. It was the summer, and between the heat, dust, and humidity, it felt to him as if it were 120 degrees on the shop floor. If he made a mistake operating the machinery needed to cut sole-shaped silhouettes out of the giant rolls of fabric, leather, and rubber he was assigned, he could have crushed his hand. He was surprised when he was called into the factory-owner's office and told that, because business had slowed, he was laid off. Despite the job being hazardous, repetitive, and ill-paying, he still felt upset about losing it. Later in life, he was a new PhD holding the position of research associate at New York State Psychiatric Institute, an institution that was essentially the Department of Psychiatry for Columbia University. It was his dream job. He was part of a team conducting exciting research on the origins of mental disorder in youth. A newly elected governor took office, and cut the state budget substantially. Everyone with the job title "research associate" lost his or her position. What made the termination particularly distressing was that his wife was four months pregnant with their first child.

Two Pathways for Research on Unemployment

Research on job loss and unemployment has generally followed two paths, one at the aggregate level, and the other at the individual level. At the aggregate level, unemployment rates come into play. An example of aggregate-level research would be a study of the correlation between the unemployment rates in different U.S. states, on the one hand, and the rate of admissions to psychiatric hospitals (or the suicide rate) in each state, on the other. This type of group-level correlation is called an

---

[1] Warr also advanced the view that beyond some threshold, increments in the factor do not further mental health and that beyond some critical point, increments (like the impact of very large doses of vitamins on physical health) adversely affect mental health.

"ecological correlation." A limitation of such aggregate findings is that they do not show what is occurring at the individual level (Robinson, 1950). Based on a group-level correlation between unemployment rates and psychiatric admission rates, one does not know whether unemployed individuals, compared with individuals with jobs, are more likely to be admitted to psychiatric hospitals.[2] It is possible that working individuals, not the unemployed, are entering the hospital at higher rates given the group-level correlation. To find out what is happening to individuals, an investigator needs to focus on data collected at the level of the individual.

Studying the individual psychological consequences of job loss is challenging.[3] Complicating research efforts on the impact of unemployment is the fact that workers suffering from poor health, including poor mental health, are at risk for job loss (Dooley, Fielding, & Levi, 1996). The extensiveness of the safety net (e.g., government unemployment benefits, programs to ensure health care) for the unemployed varies from country to country, further complicating research on the impact of job loss (Dooley et al. 1996). Another difficulty is that of distinguishing a job loss that is outside a worker's control from a job loss to which a worker contributed. There is also the difficulty of planning a longitudinal study (a) having appropriate controls for baseline measures of key health outcomes with (b) the baseline wave of data collection strategically timed such that it not only antedates the job loss in question but also antedates workers' anticipation of job loss (c.f. Kessler, House, & Turner, 1987). Anticipation alone could exert effects. Of course, such a study would require comparable workers who do not experience or anticipate job loss. Many studies do not address all of these challenges.

What the Research on Unemployment Has to Tell Us

There has been more research on unemployment than any other work-related psychosocial condition. Unemployment is of interest not only to psychologists. Epidemiologists, sociologists, and economists have also been concerned with the psychological impact of unemployment. Thus, a vast literature on the impact of unemployment on mental health has developed. Cross-sectional research shows that workers who lost their jobs "through no fault of their own" (e.g., factory closings) experienced higher levels of psychological symptoms than stably employed workers (e.g., Kessler et al., 1987). Longitudinal research shows that involuntary job loss in the form of plant closings and layoffs is related to elevations in psychological symptoms (e.g., Brand, Levy, and Gallo, 2008), a pattern that runs through the literature (Paul & Moser, 2009). Other research suggests that business closings lead to increased alcohol consumption in individuals whose consumption already tends toward unhealthful levels (Deb, Gallo, Ayyagari, Fletcher, & Sindelar, 2011).

Two two-stage meta-analyses help order some of the literature. The meta-analysis conducted by McKee-Ryan, Song, Wanberg, and Kinicki (2005) comprised 52 cross-sectional studies cumulatively involving more than 22,000 individuals and

---

[2] The idea that group-level correlations inform us of the nature of relationships at the individual level, that is to say, at the level of the members of the groups, is called the "ecological fallacy" (Selvin, 1958).

[3] An orientation not taken here is research on the impact of underemployment (holding a part-time job when wanting or needing full-time employment), a fertile field for study.

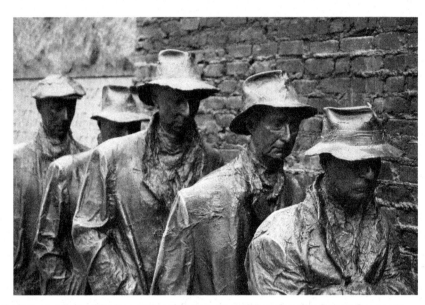

George Segal's sculpture of jobless men waiting on a bread line, Franklin Delano Roosevelt Memorial, Washington, DC. (Photo in the public domain.)

15 longitudinal studies involving more than 1,900 individuals. The cross-sectional findings suggest that the effect of unemployment on mental health is moderate, Cohen's $d = 0.57$,[4] corrected for measurement error. In other words, on average, unemployed individuals, compared with employed individuals, are disadvantaged by a little more than half a standard deviation in terms of scores on psychological symptom scales (e.g., GHQ, CES-D), bearing in mind caveats such as the fact that cross-sectional findings are consistent with the possibility that psychological problems precipitated unemployment as well as the reverse. Assume for a moment that the "true" effect size for unemployment is 0.57. Consider McKee-Ryan et al.'s finding, based on longitudinal studies, bearing on the impact of reemployment. These findings indicate that, on average, Cohen's $d = -0.89$, corrected for measurement error. The pair of findings suggest that a person who loses his or her job, spends time unemployed, and then regains employment is, in sum, better off (shows greater psychological growth) than a person who remains stably employed over the same period of time. Taken together, the findings are puzzling because they suggest, incorrectly, that working, losing a job, and regaining a job is, somehow, "therapeutic" (Paul & Moser, 2009).

Paul and Moser's more comprehensive meta-analysis suggests why the foregoing interpretation is wrong. First, they recognized that individuals subjected to repeated assessments with instruments such as the GHQ tend to manifest small improvements over time (a repeated testing effect). Second, they highlighted studies that compared workers who remained employed with workers who lost their jobs through factory closings and other mass layoffs because such studies reflect natural experiments that occurred independently of the personalities of the workers, and therefore better justify causal conclusions about the impact of job loss. Cumulating the results of 86 longitudinal studies ($n > 50,000$; K. Paul, personal communication, February 19, 2014),

---

[4] Chapter 2 contains a discussion of Cohen's d.

analyses indicated that the mental health of an individual who lost his or her job was, on average, about half a standard deviation worse off than that of a stably employed individual, a moderate effect. The impact of unemployment was weaker in countries that had greater income equality and more unemployment protections; the impact was stronger in countries with greater inequality and fewer unemployment protections. In addition, Paul and Moser, capitalizing on the longitudinal data, found evidence that poorer mental health had a small but significant effect on risk of future unemployment and that reemployment has beneficial effects on mental health. However, they found no evidence for the hypothesis that unemployment followed by reemployment leads to psychological growth when controlling for measurement error and retesting effects. They also found a comparatively weak trend for unemployment to have a greater adverse effect on the mental health of cultural and ethnic minorities; however, too few studies pertinent to this issue were available to draw a firm conclusion. Overall, male blue-collar workers were the group most at risk for adverse mental health effects in the face of job loss.

Job Loss and Suicide

It is a corollary to the aforementioned findings that if job loss precipitates ill effects on mental health, and mental health problems such as depression contribute to suicide (Berman, 2009), then we should expect higher rates of suicide among individuals who lose their jobs. A small number of longitudinal studies bear out the connection between job loss and suicide; the studies, however, are structured such that it is almost impossible to assess an intervening variable such as mental disorder or psychological distress, although one could argue that suicide itself reflects a substantial degree of despair.

Research linking job loss to suicide is difficult to conduct because of the large sample sizes required for statistical purposes. To illustrate this point, consider that according to the World Health Organization (2013), the rate of suicide in Swedish males in 2008 was 18.7 per 100,000. A study conducted on 100,000 Swedish men would likely yield too few suicides to provide a statistically clear picture of the relation of risk factors to that terrible outcome. Assuming the rate remains somewhat stable over time, a research effort would need to follow 1,000,000 men over 1 year or 100,000 men over 10 years to assemble a sample that included an estimated 187 suicides to study in detail. The studies described next are large and have been conducted in countries in which researchers have access to records that antedate the suicides; privacy regulations in other countries (e.g., the United States) would make such research extremely difficult to conduct in those countries.

In a large ($n \approx 80,000$) Danish study, Mortensen, Agerbo, Erikson, Qin, and Westergaard-Nielsen (2000)[5] found that unemployment, controlling for income, past psychiatric hospitalization, family structure, and so forth, predicted suicide in males and females, although the effect size was larger in males. Given limitations in the records used, the investigators could not control for two other risk factors—(a) mental disorders that did not lead to hospitalization or (b) previous suicide attempts. In a larger ($n \approx 421,000$) Danish study,[6] Qin, Agerbo, and Mortensen (2003) found that

---

[5] Mortensen et al. conducted what is known as a "nested case-control design," a study that despite its "case-control" label, is similar to the retrospective cohort study described in Chapter 2.
[6] This study also had a nested case-control design.

unemployment predicted suicide controlling for income, past psychiatric hospitalization, and family history (first-degree relatives, i.e., mother, father, sister, brother, son, daughter) of both suicide attempts and psychiatric hospitalization. Unemployment *and* low income exerted larger effects in males than females.

Mäki and Martikainen (2012), capitalizing on the changing macroeconomic conditions in the Finnish economy over a 16-year period ($n > 1,000,000$), found that, consistent with a social selection explanation, 1-year suicide risk among *un*stably employed men and women (they experienced both employment and spells of unemployment the same year) was higher during periods of low national unemployment than during periods of high unemployment. During periods of high unemployment, less impaired individuals presumably joined the ranks of the unstably employed. Consistent with a social causation explanation, suicide risk was high in long-term unemployed men during either period compared with the risk in their stably employed counterparts. In women who were long-term unemployed, the risks were less consistent from year to year, perhaps owing to smaller numbers of suicides.

Although there was a negative finding in a large ($n > 770,000$) Swedish study (Lundin, Lundberg, Allebeck, and Hemmingsson (2012), a larger ($n > 3.3$ million) Swedish study (Garcy & Vågerö, 2012) found that the duration of unemployment predicted suicide in men but not in women during the ensuing 6 years, adjusting for confounding factors (e.g., income, prior self-injuries, alcohol-related hospitalization). Garcy and Vågerö ruled out a selection-based explanation by documenting each Swede's unemployment experience during a period of mass layoffs, and excluding individuals who were unemployed at the beginning of the period. In a third Swedish study ($n > 37,000$ men), one that capitalized on records dating back to childhood, Lundin, Lundberg, Hallsten, Ottosson, and Hemmingsson (2010) found that long spells of unemployment (>89 days) occurring during a recession predicted suicide during the first 4 years postrecession but not during the next 4 years, controlling for social circumstances during childhood, smoking, psychiatric hospitalization, and so forth. Although longer-term, compared with short-term, unemployment is related to higher suicide risk, Milner, Page, and LaMontagne (2013) found suggestive evidence that the impact of longer-term unemployment on suicide risk is greatest earlier in the period of unemployment with the risk attenuating over time.

Economic recession itself is related to suicidal behavior, particularly in men (Haw, Hawton, Gunnell, & Platt, 2015). Although there are a number of pathways from recession to suicide, two are underlined. First, recessions give rise to unemployment, which paves the way for depression (Paul & Moser, 2009) and binge drinking (Dee, 2001), factors that increase suicide risk. Second, economic stress sets the stage for impulsive behavior, including suicidality. A case-control, psychological autopsy study ($n > 560$; ⅔ male) conducted in India found that sudden bankruptcy was related to completed suicide (Gururaj, Isaac, Subbakrishna, & Ranjani, 2004). An English study (Coope et al., 2015) of a consecutive series of coroners' records linked recession-related problems to suicide in people with no previously recorded evidence of psychiatric disorder or self-harm. Given the health effects of recession and unemployment, it behooves policy makers to (a) develop measures to combat economic turmoil, (b) create programs to train for alternative types of work for individuals who lose their jobs, and (c) enhance the safety net for the victims of recessions, including the provision of unemployment insurance programs and psychological services.

THE DEMAND–CONTROL(–SUPPORT) MODEL

Robert Karasek (1979) advanced the view that our understanding of the mental health consequences of working conditions can be improved if we consider two dimensions of the work role: (a) the extensiveness of the demands, that is, workload, placed on the worker and (b) the amount of decision latitude the worker possesses in determining how to meet those demands. The job demands Karasek investigated in his original article were psychological demands rather than physical demands (e.g., heavy lifting). Examples of psychological demands include task complexity, pace, and so on. Decision latitude, according to Karasek (1985), comprises two components. One is decision authority, which refers to having control over meaningful job-related decisions. The second component is skill discretion, which denotes the variety of job-related skills a worker can exercise as well as the learning of new skills. Some investigators (e.g., Mausner-Dorsch & Eaton, 2000), however, have suggested that decision authority is more important than skill discretion in terms of mental health consequences.

According to Karasek's (1979) model, workload demands "place the individual in a motivated or energized state of 'stress'" that has the potential to become a psychologically disagreeable state (p. 287). Job-related decision latitude "modulates the release or transformation" of that energy into "the energy of action" (p. 287). In Karasek's terminology, when a worker experiences high levels of job demands but has little decision latitude, he or she would experience "job strain." Karasek labeled such jobs "high strain" jobs. Put another way, the model proposes that in high-strain jobs, biologically wired arousal—arousal resulting from high levels of psychological demands (psychological workload)—"is transformed into damaging, unused residual strain" because the lack of decision latitude is a "constraint on the person's optimal response" to the conditions in which the individual works (p. 33; Karasek & Theorell, 1990). Karasek's idea is consistent with a biological view of depression. Psychosocial stressors exert effects through the central and autonomic nervous systems. Stressors are interpreted by the hippocampus and amygdala and, when chronically occurring (as in high-strain jobs), can create an imbalance in allostatic (i.e., adaptive) systems such as the hypothalamic–pituitary–adrenal, or stress, axis (Hintsa et al., in press; McEwen, 2004). Excessive allostatic load can also give rise to cardiovascular disease (allostatic load is discussed in more detail in Chapter 4), although biomarkers of allostatic load appear in depression as well (McEwen, 2004).

Decision latitude is thought to interact with work-related demands to buffer the impact of those demands on psychological health. Strain is measured with scales that assess psychological distress, depressive symptoms, job dissatisfaction, psychosomatic symptoms, and so forth. Karasek suggested that the traditional multiplicative type of interaction commonly assessed in analyses such as those seen with multiple linear regression may not be reflective of the interaction he had in mind because he also believed that "passive jobs" are harmful to workers. Passive jobs combine low latitude with low demands or workload and, according to the model, promote job dissatisfaction and learned helplessness.

Individuals who experience high levels of demands but have a great deal of latitude in meeting the demands have what Karasek called "active jobs" (see Table 3.1). Because active jobs help workers realize accomplishment after accomplishment, such jobs are personally satisfying. Incumbents in active jobs are expected to experience

TABLE 3.1 Karasek's Job Strain Model			
		Job Demands	
		Low	**High**
Decision Latitude or Control	Low	Passive jobs	High-strain jobs
	High	Low-strain jobs	Active jobs

low levels of strain and high levels of job satisfaction. The combination of low work-load and high latitude makes for a "low strain job."

The question of whether job demands and control exert effects on mental health additively or whether control buffers the impact of demands is more than academic. If there is buffering, affording workers high levels of control would be expected to reduce the impact of an organization's increasing its demands on workers. However, if the impact of demands and control is additive, increasing demands are likely to adversely affect mental health independently of control (Häusser, Mojzisch, Niesel, & Schulz-Hardt, 2010). This section of the chapter is concerned with both the individual effects of each factor and their potential for interactive effects, preferring to underline the fact that there are two important factors that separately *or* in combination bear on the relation of work to mental health.

Social Support Becomes Part of the Model

Karasek and his colleagues (1981) extended the Demand–Control (DC) model to apply to the development of cardiovascular disease (CVD; see Chapter 4), which in turn paved the way for an examination of an additional psychosocial risk factor relevant to both CVD *and* mental health. Johnson, Hall, and Theorell (1989), in their research on CVD, expanded the DC model by bringing into the picture social isolation or its opposite, social support from coworkers, giving birth to the "iso-strain" or Demand–Control–Support (DCS) model. The expanded model would influence future research.

Social support fits well with research concerning the relation of psychosocial workplace factors to mental health because coworker and supervisor support *are* psychosocial workplace factors. Research on the relation of support at work to mental health did not develop quickly. Research interest in social support has roots that date back to Émile Durkheim. Durkheim (1951/1912), in addition to his work on suicide and the business cycle, also found that social ties in the form of marriage and children are "preservative," that is, protect individuals from suicide by way of integrating the individual into a larger social unit. According to Durkheim, within the collectivity of spouses and children, a certain emotional intensity is reflected back and forth, serving as a kind of life-preserving bond. Durkheim's work was a stimulus for the growth of research on the impact of social connections. If family ties are protective, what about other types of social ties? Research had begun to show that social ties in general (Berkman & Syme, 1979) and social support are related to health and longevity (House, Landis, & Umberson, 1988). By the mid-1980s, research on the relation of social support—the research largely concerned support from family and friends—to psychological distress had grown substantially (Cohen & Wills, 1985). Explanations of why social support may exert a positive effect on mental health include at least two theoretical ideas: (a) supportive social relationships encourage an individual, either explicitly or tacitly, to engage in adaptive behavior and

(b) supportive social relationships, perhaps from an evolutionary standpoint, may have a healthful influence on the neuroendocrine axis that underlies stress responding. Of course, social ties are not limited to family and friends. Because work constitutes a major part of an individual's life, relationships with coworkers and managers are likely to be important in the context of the stress process as it plays out in workplaces. That Johnson et al. (1989) brought social connectivity into the DC model is thus an important milestone. Meta-analytic research has emphasized that coworker and supervisor support can be differentiated, and have independent effects on burnout (Luchman & González-Morales, 2013).

Measuring DCS Factors

Two different frameworks, epidemiological and cognitive appraisal frameworks, underlie different approaches to measuring psychosocial factors such as workplace demands (Kain & Jex, 2010). The cognitive appraisal approach is embodied in an instrument Karasek (1985, 2006) assembled, the Job Content Questionnaire (JCQ), which came to be widely used in OHP research. A worker responds to each item. An item assesses some elements of the worker's psychosocial work environment. The U.S. Department of Labor's *Quality of Employment Surveys* (Quinn & Staines, 1979) were a source of many of the JCQ's core items. The JCQ comprises scales reflecting psychological workload, decision latitude, coworker support, supervisor support, and other factors. In the JCQ, the decision latitude scale comprises the sum of the scores on two subscales, the decision authority and skill discretion subscales. The scores the worker obtains on the JCQ or an instrument like it reflect the worker's psychosocial working conditions.[7] A limitation of cognitively appraised items is that the psychological functioning of a worker can bias the worker's responding in one direction (indicating that the job allows for more control than it actually does) or another (e.g., the job allows less control).

The epidemiological framework favors linking "objective" job-related exposures to health outcomes (Kristensen, 1995). For example, exposures to high and low workload can be assessed using average JCQ workload scale values from a group of study participants having the same job title, thus averaging out idiosyncratic tendencies that may affect any one individual's scale score. An alternative procedure would be to impute scale values for study participants based on average values obtained from workers who are not study participants, but who have the same job titles as study participants. A third alternative procedure is to use expert ratings based on observations and interviews of nonparticipating workers having the same job titles but studied independently, and then imputing the rater-derived values to characterize the jobs of study participants. Other epidemiological approaches include using "objective" measures such as the density of traffic patterns engaging air traffic controllers or "cycle time" in repetitive factory or clerical work (Kristensen). A limitation of objective measures is that they do not exactly characterize the immediate environment

---

[7] de Jonge, van Vegchel, Shimazu, Schaufeli, and Dormann (2010) suggested a theoretical refinement of the DC model, advancing the view that high levels of skill discretion should be conceptualized as a demand rather than as a component of decision latitude. They argued that a test of the DC model should use the decision authority subscale alone to index decision latitude. They also advanced the view that workload should be treated as three separate dimensions, mental, emotional, and physical demands, of a job.

of each particular worker, and minimize within-occupational variation. In research on teachers, Schonfeld (2001) found considerable within-occupation variation in the stressfulness of the job.

Methodological Concerns

Many of the studies of the impact of psychosocial job factors on mental health covered in this chapter, although superior in some respects (e.g., they are prospective), are biased toward the null hypothesis, suggesting that the studies underestimate the true impact of those job factors. In many studies, factors such as job control, although measured as a continuous variable on instruments like the JCQ, are treated as dichotomous factors based on whether a worker's score is above or below a particular cutoff (there are exceptions such as the study by Bromet et al. [1988]). By dichotomizing continuous, dimensional factors, information is lost, reducing estimates of effect sizes.

For example, suppose Worker A has a score on a job control scale that is just barely above the cutoff used to categorize workers as having high control. Further, suppose Worker B has a score that is many units above the cutoff on the control scale. Workers A and B are considered to have the same high level of control although the amount of control they have is different. Finally, suppose Worker C has a score just below the cutoff and only a couple of ticks below the score of Worker A, Worker C is categorized as having low control. Thus Workers A and C are more similar in terms of job control, but Worker A, like Worker B, is considered to have high control. This kind of problem happens when dimensional measures are dichotomized. In some studies, the dependent variable, although measured on a continuous scale like the GHQ, is treated dichotomously. Again information is lost, and estimates of effect sizes are reduced.

The Evidence Bearing on the Relation of the Demand–Control(–Support) Model to Depression and Distress

The evidence for the influence of decision latitude, psychological workload, and support on mental health comes from a variety of longitudinal studies. The studies were conducted in several different countries including Belgium (Clays et al., 2007), Canada (Marchand, Demers, & Durand, 2005; Shields, 2006; Wang, 2004), Denmark (Rugulies, Bültmann, Aust, & Burr, 2006), Finland (Kivimäki, Elovainio, Vahtera, & Ferrie, 2003; Virtanen et al., 2007), France (Niedhammer, Goldberg, Leclerc, Bugel, & David, 1998; Niedhammer, Malard, & Chastang, 2015; Paterniti, Niedhammer, Lang, & Consoli, 2002), Japan (Kawakami, Haratani, & Araki, 2002; Mino, Shigemi, Tsuda, Yasuda, & Bebbington, 1999), The Netherlands (Bültmann, Kant, Van den Brandt, & Kasl, 2002; Plaisier et al., 2007; de Jonge et al., 2010; de Lange, Taris, Kompier, Houtman, & Bongers, 2004), Sweden (Fandiño-Losada, Forsell, & Lundberg, 2013), the United Kingdom (Stansfeld, Fuhrer, Shipley, & Marmot, 1999), and the United States. (Bromet et al., 1988). Table 3.2 summarizes a number of studies that assess the impact of the DCS factors. Many are at least partially supportive, but there are negative findings too (e.g., Fandiño-Losada et al., 2013). Overall, the longitudinal evidence is more supportive of an additive model than a model that holds that control buffers the impact of demands. Additional evidence not shown in the table suggests that the repeated exposure to high demands and low control over time increases the risk of incident cases of major depression in workers who had not previously had the disorder (Stansfeld, Shipley, Head, & Fuhrer, 2012; Wang, Schmitz, Dewa, & Stansfeld, 2009). A narrative review and two-stage meta-analysis (Theorell et al., 2015) that involved studies with the highest scientific quality revealed that there is "moderately strong evidence" that job strain and low decision latitude have a significant impact on depressive symptoms.

The DCS Factors and Excessive Alcohol Consumption

The studies identified in Table 3.2 implicate the DCS variables with the development of depression, anxiety, and psychological distress. Although there have not been as many longitudinal studies implicating the DCS variables in the onset of excessive alcohol use, in order to round out the picture, it should be noted that there is some longitudinal research on excessive alcohol consumption. Excessive alcohol consumption can be disastrous for the individual because of its implications for general functioning, dependence, accident risk, comorbid psychiatric disorders, and liver disease. Although genetic and personality factors contribute to the onset of alcohol problems, one general but unevenly supported hypothesis has been that alcohol provides a way of coping with distress and tension that build as a result of exposure to environmental stressors (Cooper, Russell, & Frone, 1990). Thus, there is some potential for linking the DCS factors to excessive alcohol consumption. Three longitudinal North American studies (Bromet et al., 1988; Crum, Muntaner, Eaton, & Anthony, 1995; Marchand & Blanc, 2011), two Swedish studies (Hemmingsson & Lundberg, 1998; Romelsjö et al., 1992), one British study (Head, Stansfeld, & Siegrist, 2004), and a large European, one-stage meta-analysis (Heikkilä et al., 2012) are relevant, and are described in Table 3.3. The evidence is mixed, especially given the size of the meta-analysis. No firm conclusions can be drawn.

Workplace Support

Threaded though the DCS section are findings concerning the impact of workplace support. On balance, the evidence indicates that higher levels of support are related to lower risk of distress and depression (research on alcohol use is sketchier). The evidence comes from the earlier-mentioned studies conducted in Belgium (for iso-strain; Clays et al., 2007), Canada (Wang, 2004), Denmark (Rugulies et al., 2006), Finland (Kivimäki et al., 2003), France (Niedhammer et al., 1998; Paterniti et al., 2002), The Netherlands (Bültmann et al., 2002; de Lange et al., 2004; Plaisier et al., 2007), and the U.K. (Stansfeld et al., 1999). An alternate analysis (Ylipaavalniemi et al., 2005) of the data from the same Finnish hospital worker sample examined by Kivimäki et al. (2003) found that team climate, a construct representing how supportive the people in the worker's immediate work environment have been, was related to lower incidence of doctor-diagnosed depression over the next 2 years. By contrast, evidence from the earlier-mentioned U.S. study (Bromet et al., 1988) was more mixed. Research covered in Chapter 5 on workplace bullying, which is different from nonsupport—it is more reflective of a torment-laden interpersonal environment—underscores the impact of bullying on psychological distress.

The Impact of DCS Factors

Sometimes, studies reveal null results. For example, a small longitudinal study ($n = 61$) of London department store employees found no effects of workload and

TABLE 3.2 Longitudinal Studies That Bear on the Relationship of DCS Workplace Factors to Depression, Anxiety, and Psychological Distress

Study Team	Country	Sample	Time Lag	Control Variables	Major Findings	Comments
Bromet et al. (1988)	U.S.	325 ♂s working in power plant	1 y	Baseline disorder	ΨWL but not DL → affective disorder and SCL-90; Unanticipated ΨWL × DL interaction	Used the GSI score from the SCL-90. Workers with less DL & greater ΨWL, surprisingly, had fewer symptoms than workers with "active jobs." IVs treated as continuous variables.
Bültmann et al., 2002	Netherlands	>8,800 individuals (26% ♀)	1 y	Age, education, marital status, GHQ	In ♂s, high ΨWL & emotional demands, low supervisor and coworker support, & high conflict with coworkers → ↑ GHQ but DL not sig.; In ♀s, high ΨWL & emotional demands → ↑ GHQ but DL not sig.	Dichotomized GHQ. Trichotomized ΨWL, demands, DL. Dichotomized support.
Clays et al. (2007)	Belgium	>2,800 workers in variety of sectors (69% ♂)	6½ y	Baseline CES-D	Combination of high ΨWL, low DL, & low support → incidence of ↑ CES-D scores in ♂s ΨWL, DL, & low support do not → CES-D scores in ♂s	Long follow-up likely attenuated effects. CES-D treated dichotomously. But individuals above CES-D cutoff at baseline were excluded from analyses.
de Jonge et al. (2010)	Netherlands	260 nursing home workers (90% ♂)	2 y	Sociodemo., baseline DVs	Classic ΨWL × Control interaction → Ψsomatic symptom & job satisfaction; Classic interaction for emotional demands × Control interaction → symptoms, job satisfaction, & sickness absence	Predictor variables and DVs were treated as continuous factors.
de Lange et al. (2004)	Netherlands	668 workers (69% ♂) The SMASH study	4 waves of data collection of 4 y	Age, gender, and DV assessed the previous wave	ΨWL affected → ↑ CES-D & EE (MBI); Control → ↑ job satisfaction; Supervisor support → ↓ EE Job satisfaction → ↑ supervisor support EE → ↓ supervisor support EE → ↑ ΨWL	Predictor variables and DVs were treated as continuous factors. Used structural equation modeling that controlled for measurement error. Also found sig. but weaker reverse causal effects.

Study	Country	Sample	Duration	Controls	Findings	Comments
Fandiño-Losada et al. (2013)	Sweden	4,427 workers (55% ♀) The PART Study	3 y	Sociodemo., time 1 depressive symptoms	Prospective study: excluded workers with time 1 depressive dx. Poor work support → ↑ depression in ♀s ΨWL, SkD, DA → depression in ♀s DA → depression in ♂s ΨWL, low SkD → ↓ depression in ♂s	Dx was probable depression based on standardized questionnaire. In ♂s, finding that high ΨWL & low SkD → lower depression risk was unexpected. Among ♂s, number of cases at time 2 was low (n = 31; 1.5% of ♂s).
Kawakami et al. (2002)	Japan	460 ♂, blue-collar workers	4 times over 4 y	Sociodemo., medical, Zung	Low control & problematic interpersonal relations → ↑ Zung. High ΨWL not sig.	Job's incompatibility with worker's skills → ↑ Zung. Zung scale was dichotomized.
Kivimäki et al. (2003)	Finland	>5,600 mostly ♀ employees of 10 hospitals	2 y	Sociodemo., health behaviors	High ΨWL & low DA → ↑ GHQ scores Relational justice → low GHQ scores	Trichotomized continuous IVs. Dichotomized GHQ.
Marchand et al. (2005)	Canada	National sample of >6,000 workers (46% ♀) NHPS study	4 time points over 6 y	Sociodemo.	Low DA → severe distress (6-item scale); ΨWL and support were not sig.	Dichotomized continuous DV. Survival analysis to the first episode of severe distress. IVs had low reliability (e.g., ΨWL, support) and were dichotomized.
Mino et al. (1999)	Japan	310 machine workers (53% ♀)	2 y	Sociodemo., excluded those with elevated baseline GHQ	ΨWL → ↑ GHQ	Used single items to assess varieties of workload.
Niedhammer et al. (1998)	France	>11,500 workers (27% ♀) at national gas co.; The GAZEL study	1 y	Absenteeism owing to MH problems but not CES-D	High ΨWL, low DL & low work-related support → ↑ CES-D	Did not control for depression at baseline. Dichotomized CES-D.
Niedhammer et al. (2015)	France	National sample 4,717 workers (≈ 50% ♂)	4 y	Sociodemo., nonwork support & adversity, childhood adversity	ΨWL → GAD not MDD Emotional demands → GAD Control GAD or MDD	Prospective study. One of few studies to look at GAD dx.

(continued)

TABLE 3.2 Longitudinal Studies That Bear on the Relationship of DCS Workplace Factors to Depression, Anxiety, and Psychological Distress *(continued)*

Study Team	Country	Sample	Time Lag	Control Variables	Major Findings	Comments
Paterniti et al. (2002)	France	>8,000 workers (75% ♂) GAZEL study	3 y	Occupational grade, hostility, Type A behavior	DL, ΨWL → ↑ CES-D in ♂s ΨWL → ↑ CES-D in ♀s Work support → ↓ CES-D	IVs were measured during year 2. DV in regression was time-1-time-2 CES-D change score. Better to treat baseline CES-D as IV & time 2 CES-D as the DV.
Plaisier et al. (2007)	Netherlands	>2,600 workers (42% ♂) The NEMESIS study	2 y	Sociodemo., physical health	Prospective study, excluded workers with disorder at baseline. ΨWL but not DL → ↑ depressive & anxiety disorders; No effect for job security. Combined work & nonwork support → ↓ depressive disorders	Incidence study. Used diagnostic instrument CIDI (Robins et al., 1988) to detect disorders. ΨWL, DL, and support were continuous scales (I. Plaisier, personal communication, November 11, 2014).
Rugulies et al. (2006)	Denmark	>4,100 workers (½ ♂) The DWECS study	5 y	Sociodemo., health behaviors; job changing	Low supervisor support & low influence (akin to control) → ↑ depressive symptom levels in ♀s but not ♂s No effect for ΨWL	Long follow-up likely attenuated effects (although there were statistical controls for job changes). Controlled concurrent alcohol abuse, often a comorbid disorder, potentially weakening effects of IVs. DV was dichotomous. Predictors either dichotomous and/or based on single item.
Shields (2006)	Canada	>12,000 (≈50% ♂) NHPS study	2 y	Age, SES, personal stress, mastery	Strain → ↑ depression in ♂s Low coworker support → ↑ depression in ♀s	Incidence study. Depression dx by CIDI module.

Stansfeld et al. (1999)	U.K.	>7,900 civil servants (2/3 ♂) Whitehall II	5 y	Sociodemo., NA, hostility, baseline GHQ or excluded those with elevated baseline GHQ	ΨWL → ↑ GHQ Low DA → ↑ GHQ Low colleague support → ↑ GHQ Low info from supervisor → ↑ GHQ SkD ↛ GHQ	Findings held when controlling for baseline GHQ or excluding those with high baseline GHQ.
Virtanen et al. (2007)	Finland	>3,300 working adults (50% ♀)	3 y	History of psychopathology	High ΨWL & high ΨWL × low control → affective disorder as reflected antidepressant meds. prescriptions	Depression assessed by prescription for antidepressant meds. Many depressed do not take meds., & individuals with anxiety disorders sometimes take antidepressant meds.
Wang (2004)	Canada	Same sample as Marchand et al. (2005)	4 time points over 6 y	Physical health; childhood trauma; stressful life events	Low SkD, high ΨWL, low support → newly incident episode of depression	Survival model to first incidence of diagnosed depression. IVs had low reliability (e.g., ΨWL, support) and were dichotomized. Controlled contemporaneous physical health with depressive episode, likely attenuating IV-DV relation.

♂, male; ♀, female; ΨWL, psychologicial workload or psychological demands; Baseline DVs, baseline versions of the dependent variables; CES-D, Center for Epidemiologic Studies Depression Scale; DA, decision authority; DL, decision latitude; dx, diagnosis; EE, emotional exhaustion; GAD, generalized anxiety disorder; IVs, principal independent variables; MDD, major depressive disorder; meds., medications; MH, mental health; NA, negative affectivity; sig., significant; SkD, skill discretion; Sociodemo., sociodemographic variables.

TABLE 3.3 Longitudinal Studies That Bear on the Relationship of DCS Workplace Factors to Alcohol Problems

Study Team	Country	Sample	Time Lag	Control Variables	Major Findings	Comments
Bromet et al. (1988)	U.S.	325 ♂s working in power plant	1 y	Baseline disorder	DL but not ΨWL→↑ self-reported alcohol problems controlling for baseline alcohol problems	Alcohol problems treated dichotomously. IVs treated as continuous variables.
Crum et al. (1995)	U.S.	500 individuals (45% ♂)	1 y	Sociodemo., age at first alcohol use	Combination of low DL & either high psychological or physical ΨWL → DMS-III alcohol abuse or dependence in ♂s. No effect in ♀s	Used dichotomized imputed values of IVs (high strain = 1 vs. 0). Excluded those with alcohol-related diagnoses at baseline.
Head et al. (2004)	U.K.	>7,300 civil servants (2/3 ♂) Whitehall II	5 y	Sociodemo., health behaviors, support outside work, life events	DCS factors were not related to the onset of alcohol dependence	Trichotomized continuous IVs. Dichotomized continuous DV.
Heikkilä et al. (2012)	Belgium, Finland, U.K.	>48,000 (≈50% ♂)	Av. 4 y	Sociodemo., alcohol at baseline	Strain→excessive alcohol consumption	1-stage meta-analysis (see Chap. 4). No relation between strain & alcohol in the x-sectional part of study too.
Hemmingsson & Lundberg (1998)	Sweden	>42,000 ♂s	8 y	Excluded ♂s with past alcohol problems, controlled childhood factors (e.g., SES, from census)	Low control & low work support →↑ alcohol-related dx. Passive jobs (low control + low demands) →↑ alcohol-related dx	IVs were imputed based on census data 5 y after military service & treated as quartiles. Used military records (conscription near-universal in Sweden) to exclude men with past alcohol problems. Alcohol problems based on national hospital records. Those with alcohol problems that did not lead to hospitalization thus not missed.
Marchand & Blanc (2011)	Canada	NPHS sample described in Table 3.2 >6,000 workers	5 time points over 8 y	Sociodemo.	Low SkU but not DA & ΨWL →↑ alcohol misuse. Coworker support →↓ alcohol misuse. Low SkU, low DA →↑ recurrent misuse. Coworker support →↓ recurrent misuse.	Findings were concurrent, not lagged. DV was dichotomous. IVs treated as continuous variables.
Romelsjö et al. (1992)	Sweden	>1,300 ♂s	6 y	Sociodemo.	Low control & ΨWL →↑ hospitalization for severely high levels alcohol consumption	Based on hospital records; alcohol problems that did not lead to hospitalization were missed. Dichotomized IVs.

♂, male; ♀, female; ΨWL, psychological workload or psychological demands; Baseline DVs, baseline versions of the dependent variables; DA, decision authority; DL, decision latitude; dx, diagnosis; IVs, principal independent variables; SkU, skill utilization; Sociodemo., sociodemographic variables.

support (control was not assessed) on the GHQ (Steptoe et al., 1998). Moreover, not every large study showed that both high levels of demands and low control adversely affected mental health. The balance of longitudinal evidence from studies with large samples, however, suggests that each factor contributes to distress or psychological disorder although there is not perfect consistency—and perfect consistency should not be expected—from study to study. However, evidence that demands and control interact has been relatively rare. In other words, evidence for the view that workers who specifically experience high levels of demands and low levels of control manifest more distress (or higher rates of mental disorder) than would be expected from the additive effects of each factor has not been compelling.

Additional evidence bears on the importance of the DCS factors. Häusser et al. (2010) reviewed DC- and DCS-related cross-sectional and longitudinal research published between 1998 and 2008. Although many of the findings are biased toward the null (e.g., continuous measures of the independent and dependent variables were dichotomized), the authors found that the balance of evidence from 19 longitudinal studies was consistent with the view that high levels of demands and low levels of control had adverse effects on depressive symptoms, distress, and emotional exhaustion. A limitation of the review was the inclusion of weaker change–change studies (e.g., Bourbonnais, Comeau, & Vezina, 1999; Gelsema et al., 2006) with stronger longitudinal studies. As mentioned earlier, longitudinal, change–change studies cannot establish the temporal priority of the DCS factors over putative outcomes such as emotional exhaustion. Häusser et al. (2010) found no systematic gender differences. Five of 11 longitudinal studies that measured all three factors indicated that the DCS model was consistent with expectation regarding psychological distress (results were slightly weaker for emotional exhaustion). Although Häusser et al. found DC buffering-type interactions in about 40% of the studies (which is higher than the Type I error rate), the findings were based mainly on cross-sectional research; relevant reports on longitudinal studies were few.

THE JOB DEMANDS–RESOURCES (JD–R) MODEL AND CONSERVATION OF RESOURCES MODEL

The Job Demands–Resources (JD–R) model is a broader theoretical model than the DC or DCS models, and can be thought of as subsuming those models. Job demands are common to the JD–R and DCS models and can be organizational (e.g., an abusive organizational leader), physical (e.g., exposure to loud noise), or psychological (e.g., worker having to deal with a series of argumentative customers) in nature. According to Demerouti et al. (2001), sustained efforts to meet job demands have "physiological and psychological costs" such as exhaustion. Job resources include "physical, psychological, social, or organizational aspects of the job that may do any of the following: (a) be functional in achieving work goals; (b) reduce job demands [and] the associated physiological and psychological costs; (c) stimulate personal growth and development" (Demerouti et al., 2001, p. 501). Organizational resources include job control, participation in decision-making, and task variety. Job-related social resources include supportive supervisors and coworkers. Physical resources can include things like equipment to help lift loads.

Control and support, as per the DCS model, are elements subsumed under the broader concept of resources. Control itself could represent several different resources. Kain and

Jex (2010) pointed out that control is manifest in several different ways, acknowledging that workers "may have a great deal of control over some aspects of their job and very little over other aspects" (p. 250). Moreover, there are several kinds of support (tangible, informational, etc.). The JD–R model also allows for social resources outside the job context, including supportive friends and family members (Demerouti et al., 2001).

The role of resources in the JD–R model builds upon another theory. The importance of resources is central to Hobfoll's (1989; Halbesleben, Neveu, Paustian-Underdahl, & Westman, 2014) conservation of resources (COR) theory. Resources help pave the way to lower levels of strain, positive affective states, and greater work engagement; work engagement earns positive feedback for the worker and thus broadens the worker's resource base (Bakker & Demerouti, 2014). According to the COR theory (Hobfoll & Shirom, 2001), people are motivated to "obtain, retain, and protect" their resources, which include important objects (e.g., home, car), significant relationships (e.g., job, connections with supportive others), and certain personal characteristics (e.g., self-esteem). Resources are defined as things individuals value.[8] There is also an asymmetricality in COR theory that is consistent with cognitive psychology. All things being equal, resource loss is psychologically more injurious to a person than resource gain is beneficial to the individual (cf. Tversky & Kahneman, 1974).

Also important to the JD–R model are a number of corollaries (Hobfoll & Shirom, 2001) that follow from COR theory: (a) people invest some resources to protect existing resources and acquire additional resources; (b) a greater store of resources is protective against resource drain; (c) chains of stressful events (e.g., job loss, followed by loss of income, reduced self-esteem, tension in one's marriage) that strip away resources can be particularly stressful. According to the JD–R model, chronic job stressors are an ongoing drain on resources including personal energetic resources. Chronic resource drain could result in burnout or depression.

Two additional elements of COR theory are also relevant to the JD–R model. First, COR theory underlines the instrumental *and* symbolic value of resources. Second, resource-poor individuals are more vulnerable to stressors. Schaufeli and Taris (2014) identified a number of personal resources that are bulwarks against the impact of job stressors. These include intrinsic work motivation, efficacy beliefs, and optimism.

The Evidence Bearing on the JD–R Model

Demerouti et al. (2001) found that in a sample of German workers ($n > 370$, ½ were women), job demands (e.g., time pressure) were concurrently related to one OLBI burnout dimension, exhaustion; resources (e.g., performance feedback, job control) were related to lower levels of another burnout dimension, disengagement. Both sets of findings were anticipated by the JD–R model. Boyd et al. (2011) evaluated the JD–R model in a longitudinal study of almost 300 Australian academics (48% male). The investigators found that resources (autonomy and procedural justice) but not demands (job pressure, workload) predicted GHQ scores 3 years later, controlling for baseline GHQ.

In another longitudinal test of the JD–R model, Hakanen, Schaufeli, and Ahola (2008) examined more than 2,550 Finnish dentists (74% women) at two points in

---

[8]Halbesleben et al. (2014) refined the definition of a resource, conceptualizing it as anything that is *perceived* to help attain a goal regardless of whether the resource actually facilitates goal attainment. They also suggested that a resource's value depends on the context in which it is available. These ideas have been built into the JD–R model.

time 3 years apart. Hakanen et al. found that, controlling for time 1 burnout, job demands (e.g., inflicting pain) at time 1 were directly related to time 2 burnout (MBI emotional exhaustion and depersonalization), and time 1 resources (e.g., contacts with other practitioners) were inversely related to burnout at time 2. Demands had a negative effect on work engagement and resources. In a study of 201 managers and executives (11% women) who worked for a Dutch telecom company, Schaufeli, Bakker, and Van Rhenen (2009) found that over the course of a year, an increase in job demands and a decrease in resources were related to increased burnout (MBI-GS). A limitation of the finding is that it was not clear whether the changes in demands and resources antedated the changes in burnout, as required in a causal model.

The JD–R Model and Matching

Cohen and Wills (1985) outlined the beginnings of a match hypothesis in their review of research on social support. Drawing from the general literature on stress, they wrote that "instrumental support and social companionship functions are assumed to be effective when the resources they provide are closely linked to the specific need elicited by a stressful event" (p. 314). For example, instrumental (tangible) support would most help at a time of economic hardship. Frese (1999) extended the idea to the workplace. He provided the example that an employee involved in a conflict with a supervisor would likely benefit from emotional support because it communicates to the employee that he or she remains a worthy person. Frese extended the idea further, calling attention to the importance of a triple match. According to the triple match model, the type of support that would most likely reduce the impact of a social stressor (e.g., conflict with a supervisor) on social anxiety would be emotional support. In other words, the type of support that would be optimally effective would match the domain of the stressor *and* the psychological outcome.

The idea of matching took root in an extension of JD–R theory. de Jonge and Dormann (2006) advanced the view that resources are most effective in reducing strain (a) when the resource domain (e.g., company-provided training in Rogerian active listening for call center employees) matches a stressful job demand (e.g., an encounter with an irate customer) and (b) the impact would be most felt in terms of strains that match the domain of the stressor and resource (e.g., in reducing psychological distress in the worker). The investigators called this extension of the JD–R model the "triple match principle" (TMP). In the earlier example, there is a match between an emotionally demanding encounter and the training the employee received and the outcome. The matching domains could be physical, for example, with job demands involving heavy lifting, resources that include a forklift, and protection against back pain. The matching could be cognitive, with job demands involving the smooth running of highly complex supply chains, resources involving sophisticated software applications, and the strain involving lack of engagement. de Jonge and Dormann hypothesized that there is more likely to be a buffering-type interaction between resource and stressors when there is a triple match.

They tested their theory in two separate samples, one comprising more than 280 workers (>80% female) and the other comprising more than 260 workers (>90% female). All participants worked in Dutch nursing homes and were followed over 2 years. In the first sample, the authors detected an interaction between time 1 physical stressors (e.g., heavy lifting) and time 1 physical resources (e.g., instrumental support from coworkers) bearing on time 2 emotional exhaustion (MBI), but found no interaction between emotional stressors and emotional resources. Thus, here there was a double, rather than a triple match. In the second study, however, a significant interaction consistent with the theory was found. Emotional resources (e.g., emotional support from supervisors and colleagues) buffered the impact of emotional stressors (e.g., death of a resident) on emotional exhaustion. Although there are inconsistent results, that is to be expected in such a highly specified theory. That some of the findings are consistent with TMP underlines its utility in motivating research. Chrisopoulos, Dollard, Winefield, and Dormann (2010) examined the JD–R model in the TMP context. In a sample of 179 (90% male) Australian police officers, the investigators identified a number of interactions, only some of which were anticipated by the matching principle, findings that nonetheless emphasize the importance of understanding the contribution of resources to burnout and physical symptoms.

Some of Chrisopoulos et al.'s (2010) findings were consistent with Warr's (1987) vitamin model. Chrisopoulos et al. found that sometimes when demands were low and resources high, officers experienced high levels of strain. For example, when cognitive resources were high and cognitive demands low, officers experienced high levels of professional inefficacy (MBI-GS). Warr pointed out that just as too few vitamins are detrimental to an individual's physical health, so is an excessive amount. Warr's model applies to features of the work environment such as job demands and, in the JD–R parlance, resources. The officers in the foregoing example had high levels of resources but little opportunity to apply the resources. However, some findings were inconsistent with Warr's model. For example, officers with high levels of emotional resources and low levels of emotional demands tended to have few physical symptoms.

Summing Up of the JD–R Model

The JD–R model extends the DC and DCS models. The balance of evidence suggests that demands and resources influence the development of burnout symptoms, although there is inconsistency from study to study. However, other considerations may need to be integrated into the model. The model has not been extensively applied to other types of mental health effects (e.g., depressive symptoms; GHQ scores; clinical depression). Podsakoff, LePine, and LePine (2007) noted that not all work stressors contribute to strains. Podsakoff et al. suggested that some work stressors can be categorized as hindrances, which can have an adverse impact, and others, as challenges, the impact of which can be positive. Schaufeli and Taris (2014) observed that the distinction between job demands and resources is not unambiguous. These authors suggested that "a lack of resources can be construed as a job demand" (p. 56) and that challenge stressors could be reconceptualized as resources. Luchman and González-Morales (2013), in their two-stage meta-analysis, found that compared with the JD–R model, the DCS model provided a better fit (is more useful) in explaining burnout. A limitation of the model-fitting effort was that most of the studies that contributed to the meta-analysis were cross-sectional. The aforementioned challenges to the JD–R model are fixable, and the JD–R model as well as demand-resource matching provides fertile ground for future research.

THE EFFORT–REWARD IMBALANCE MODEL

Johannes Siegrist and Robert Karasek have two things in common. Both earned doctorates in sociology. And both developed models of the impact of psychosocial working conditions that influenced OHP research. Siegrist's (1996) effort–reward imbalance (ERI) model differs from Karasek's DC model. The ERI model recognizes that exchange is the bedrock of social life, and that work reflects socially sanctioned exchange. Work-related efforts refer to exertions issuing from the (a) demands of a job and (b) motivations of the worker. Thus, work efforts have sources that are both extrinsic and intrinsic to the worker. Rewards obtained in exchange for work include money and career opportunities as well as a number of less tangible forms of recompense (e.g., recognition and self-esteem). Siegrist's model connects with ideas that have played an important role in sociology, including those of George Homans, Alvin Gouldner, and George Herbert Mead. Homans (1958) advanced the view that almost all social behavior involves exchange. Gouldner (1960) cogently argued that reciprocity, like the incest taboo, is a norm that is virtually universal in human society. By implication, a violation of such a norm is destabilizing. Mead (1934) suggested that the self is realized in social situations. For Mead, self-respect and self-identity depend on membership in groups (including economic groups).

Building on his forebears in sociology, Siegrist (1996) fostered the idea that disruptions to the "continuity of crucial social roles" such as the work role constitute threats to an individual's self-regulatory functioning, mastery, and self-esteem, and consequently give rise to distress. Examples of job conditions reflective of this kind of disruption include layoffs, job insecurity, jobs in which avenues for advancement are blocked, and work that requires a great deal of effort but provides meager rewards. The ERI model recognizes that work "is spent as part of a contract based on the norm of social reciprocity where rewards are provided in terms of money, esteem, and career opportunities including job security" (Siegrist et al., 2004, p. 1484). These contracts are often asymmetric and unbalanced to the detriment of the worker. Siegrist (1996) questioned why workers in such jobs remain employed in them and thus subject themselves to a chronic imbalance between effort and reward. He went on to observe that workers employed in low-paying jobs and jobs with few tangible benefits often face excessively high costs in relinquishing those jobs because there are few opportunities to obtain more remunerative work. In Siegrist's words, such workers "exhibit a low level of status control" and are at risk for adverse health effects (also see Sinclair, Probst, Hammer, & Schaffer, 2013).

Siegrist (1996; also see Hobfoll, 2001) challenged a view that has been prominent in some circles, namely, that cognitive appraisal is necessary for a particular event to be deemed a threat. Citing neurobiological evidence, he suggested that there are "rapid and direct pathways of affective information processing that bypass neocortical-limbic structure and, thus, are not subjected to conscious awareness" (p. 31). In Siegrist's model, an imbalance between effort and reward at work, especially if chronically recurrent, can have adverse emotional effects without the imbalance being subjected to conscious appraisal.

Siegrist and his colleagues (2004) somewhat revised the model, adding physical demands, depending upon the nature of the job being studied, to the psychological demands the model already considers in the realm of effort. Another addition to the ERI model is the motivational construct of work-related commitment, or intrinsic effort (as distinct from extrinsic efforts that issue from the requirements of the job). People high in work-related commitment (overcommitment) are at greater risk of increasing their effort out of proportion to the job's rewards. Compared with workers who are not overcommitted, overcommitted individuals put themselves at even greater risk for ill health when efforts and rewards are unbalanced (Siegrist et al., 2004). Qualitative research on teachers suggests that the most dedicated educators— teachers who are overcommitted—are at greatest risk for burnout (Farber, 1991).

TABLE 3.4 Longitudinal Studies That Bear on the Relationship of the ERI Model to Psychological Distress

Study Team	Country	Sample	Time Lag	Control Variables	Major Findings	Comments
Godin et al. (2005)	Belgium	<2,000 (½ ♂) SOMSTRESS study	1 y	Sociodemo., threat from global economy, job dissatisfaction, workplace instability	In ♂s combination of no ERI at T1 but ERI at T2 → ↑ T2 depression, anxiety, somatization, & fatigue. In ♀s, combination of ERI at T1 & T2 → ↑ T2 depress., anxiety, somatization, and fatigue	Dimensions of SCL-90 treated dichotomously. Excluded workers with above-cutoff T1 scores. Part of the effect is concurrent.
Head et al. (2004)	U.K.	>7,300 civil servants (²⁄₃ ♂) Whitehall II	5 y	Age, employment grade, health behaviors, negative affectivity, baseline DV	ERI → ↑ alcohol-related problems	Alcohol problems treated dichotomously. Trichotomized ERI.
Kivimäki et al. (2007)	Finland	>4,800 hospital employees (Hospital Personnel Study) + >18,000 municipal employees (10 Town Study) Mostly ♀s	2–4 y	Sociodemo., employment grade	ERI → ↑ GHQ & depression dx in the 10 Town Study ERI→ ↑ depression dx in Hospital Personnel Study	ERI comprised a single item making the findings surprising ordinarily given the weaknesses of a 1-item scale. Dichotomized GHQ used in both studies. Self-reported doctor-dx of depression & GHQ used in both studies. Excluded individuals with disorder or borderline disorder at baseline.
Kuper et al. (2002)	U.K.	>6,800 civil servants (²⁄₃ ♂) Whitehall II	11 y	Sociodemo., coronary risk factors	ERI → ↓ MH	Dichotomized continuous MH DV (SF-36). Trichotomized ERI (but measured differently than in Head et al. [2004]). Did not control baseline DV.
Niedhammer et al. (2015)	France	National sample 4,717 workers (≈ 50% ♂)	4 y	See Table 3.2	Low reward → GAD & MDD	Prospective study. One of few studies to look at GAD. Diagnosed disorder.
Stansfeld et al. (1999)	U.K.	>7,300 civil servants (²⁄₃ ♂) Whitehall II	5 y	T1 GHQ, employment grade, age	ERI → ↑ GHQ, poor social functioning, & worse general mental health	Dichotomized continuous DV. Trichotomized ERI. Excluded baseline cases.

♂, male; ♀, female; Baseline DVs, baseline versions of the dependent variables; ERI, effort–reward imbalance; GAD, generalized anxiety disorder; IVs, principal independent variables; MDD, major depressive disorder; MH, mental health; Sociodemo., sociodemographic variables at baseline.

Although there has been less longitudinal research on the ERI model than on the Karasek models, the extant longitudinal evidence is largely consistent with the ERI model; evidence (see Table 3.4) comes from research in Belgium (Godin, Kittel, Coppieters, & Siegrist, 2005), Finland (Kivimäki et al., 2007), and the U.K. (Head et al., 2004; Kuper, Singh-Manoux, Siegrist, & Marmot, 2002; Stansfeld et al., 1999).

Kuper et al. (2002) underlined a major obstacle to comparing the relative efficacies of the DCS and ERI models within the same study. The investigators cobbled together existing items to create a scale to reflect efforts as per the ERI model. The efforts component of the ERI measure overlapped the DCS demands scale ($r = 0.84$). Kuper et al. (2002) also found modest correlations between decision latitude and ERI effort ($r = 0.59$) and rewards ($r = 0.50$) components. Although it would be difficult to compare the Siegrist and Karasek models (and the JD–R model), it is clear that both models provide useful means for studying the effects of psychosocial working conditions on mental health.

OTHER PSYCHOSOCIAL FACTORS

This section concerns a number of psychosocial working conditions. These conditions include organizational justice, job insecurity, long working hours, shift work, stressful job-related events, and work-related social stressors. One potential protective factor, namely, coping, is briefly noted.

Organizational Justice

It is fitting that we come to organizational justice after a section on the ERI model.[9] An imbalance in which a worker is remunerated disproportionately less than the value of his or her work is a matter of fairness, or justice. Kivimäki et al. (2007) underlined a connection between the ERI model and organizational justice: effort–reward imbalance suggests "injustice of exchange." Kivimäki et al. (2007) found modest correlations between ERI and organizational justice. Organizational injustice, however, differs from ERI in that the former involves ways of "being treated without respect and with bias" regardless of contractual obligations, and does not depend on the contracted balance of the effort–reward exchange (Kivimäki et al., 2007, p. 664).

There are at least two dimensions of organizational justice: procedural and relational. Procedural justice refers to the fairness of decision-making in the organization, and includes welcoming input from employees affected by organizational decisions, efforts to reduce bias, and, more generally, the ethical treatment of people who work for the organization. Procedural justice was one of the two components of the resource factor (autonomy was the other) that affected GHQ scores in the earlier-mentioned study of Australian academics (Boyd et al., 2011). Relational justice includes "polite and considerate treatment" of employees by their supervisors, a factor that overlaps somewhat with supervisor support (Kivimäki et al., 2003).

A portion of the research on organizational justice comes from Finland. Kivimäki et al. (2003) found that among hospital personnel, controlling for baseline confounders,

---

[9] We note that a component of organizational justice, procedural justice, could also be seen as a resource in the JD–R model (Boyd et al., 2011).

procedural justice, but not relational justice, predicted GHQ caseness (scores above a cutoff that demarcates high risk for mental disorder). The impact of procedural justice on the incidence of elevated GHQ scores was partly mediated by sleep disturbance (Elovainio, Kivimäki, Vahtera, Keltikangas-Järvinen, & Virtanen, 2003). Procedural injustice is related to "prolonged negative emotional states" (p. 288), and one of the leading manifestations of such states is sleep disturbance. Relational justice had a slightly different impact on the hospital personnel. Low levels of relational, but not procedural, justice predicted newly incident cases of doctor-diagnosed depression, controlling for high workload combined with low control (Ylipaavalniemi et al., 2005). Using data sets from a study of 10 Finnish towns and the earlier-mentioned hospital worker study, Kivimäki et al. (2007) found that baseline ERI and a combined measure of procedural and relational justice predicted the incidence of GHQ caseness and doctor-diagnosed depression. Using the same combined sample, Elovainio et al. (2013) found that independently assessed procedural and interactional (akin to relational) justice predicted newly incident cases of sickness absence owing to physician-assessed anxiety disorders. There was also modest, but statistically significant, evidence of reverse causality.

The Whitehall II study[10] is a large-scale, ongoing study of nonindustrial British civil servants working in central London. The purpose of the study was to examine the relationship between job stress, SES, and CVD. Investigators have extended the research to include psychological outcomes. Using data from Whitehall II, Ferrie et al. (2006) found that low levels of relational justice (procedural justice was not assessed) were related to the incidence of GHQ caseness over 5 to 8 years postbaseline, controlling for confounders. Ferrie et al. also found that a worsening of relational justice between phase 1 (baseline) and phase 2 (a 3- to 4-year lag) was associated with caseness at phase 3 (5 to 8 years postbaseline). Thus, research findings from Finland and the United Kingdom suggest that workplace justice influences worker mental health. There are also contradictory results. Lang, Bliese, Lang, and Adler (2011), using three samples of U.S. military personnel, found longitudinal evidence of reverse causal processes, with depressive symptoms predicting later perceptions of lower levels of organizational justice, and not the other way around.

Job Insecurity

Job insecurity is a consequence of recessions, global competition, and efforts to make workplaces run more efficiently. In perhaps the best controlled study of the impact of job insecurity, Ferrie et al. (2001) capitalized on events not anticipated when Whitehall II began, an initiative to increase workplace efficiency, an initiative that, in effect, created a natural experiment. An advantage of Whitehall II is that researchers can statistically control baseline levels of the outcome variables, that is, data on the dependent variables collected before the introduction of even the possibility of restructuring. Briefly, a new program was introduced that affected some, but not all, members

---

[10] The original "Whitehall study" showed that SES was inversely related to mortality risk in men. The original study was particularly important because, although highly stratified, the civil service, by its nature, does not include the richest or the poorest members of British society (Ferrie, 2004). The later Whitehall II study was established to explain *why* lower socioeconomic statuses were at greater risk, particularly with regard to cardiovascular mortality. Whitehall II, unlike the original Whitehall study, included women.

of the civil-servant sample. The new program led to increased job insecurity in some members of that sample. In study 1, which assessed the impact of the *anticipation* of job losses, Ferrie et al. (2001) evaluated the effect when functions carried out by existing agencies were being tested against alternative ways of achieving goals (e.g., privatization). The study team found that, compared with male civil-servant controls with assured job security, males anticipating insecurity experienced greater risk of GHQ caseness. A parallel finding did not obtain for females. In a second study, the team examined the impact of one entire department having been sold to the private sector (these participants were excluded from the first study). Ferrie et al. (2001) found no significant effect on GHQ caseness in either male or female civil servants. A study (Ferrie, Shipley, Stansfeld, & Marmot, 2002) that followed these civil servants to a later phase of data collection found that in men and women, job insecurity was related to higher total GHQ and depression (based on a GHQ subscale) scores. Two differences distinguish the publications. First, in contrast to the analyses in the earlier publication (Ferrie et al., 2001), which used a dichotomous measure of mental health, the analyses in the later publication (Ferrie et al., 2002) employed continuous measures (affording greater statistical power). Second, the length of exposure to job insecurity described in the later publication was longer.

In a Canadian study, Marchand et al. (2005), using the National Population Health Survey (NPHS) data, found that job insecurity predicted severe psychological distress 6 years later. Wang (2004), using the same sample, found that over the 6-year follow-up, job insecurity predicted an episode of major depression in workers who were free of the disorder at baseline. In a study conducted in The Netherlands, Bültmann et al. (2002), using data from the Maastrich Cohort Study, found that in men (but not women), job insecurity at baseline predicted newly incident GHQ caseness 1 year later. In the 5-year Danish Work Environment Cohort Study (DWECS), Rugulies et al. (2006) found that job insecurity in men, but not women, predicted future incidence of very high levels of depressive symptoms, adjusting for concurrent alcohol use and leisure time physical activities as well as baseline depressive symptoms. A different Danish study found that the combination of past unemployment and insecurity involving an individual's current job predicted incidence of later use of antidepressant medications over a 3½-year follow-up (Rugulies, Thielen, Nygarrd, & Diderichsen, 2010). In a prospective study involving a nationally representative sample of French workers, Niedhammer et al. (2015) found that insecurity at baseline predicted major depressive disorder (MDD) and generalized anxiety disorder (GAD) 4 years later. In the 2-year Netherlands Mental Health Survey and Incidence Study (NEMESIS), Plaisier et al. (2007) found that job insecurity was related to the incidence of depression and anxiety disorders in Dutch women but not in men.

Job insecurity has been found to be related to alcohol use. Using nationally representative samples of U.S. workers recruited before and during the Great Recession, Frone (2015) found that exposure to the recession was related to a decrease in alcohol use during work hours (presumably to protect the worker's job) but an increase in after-work alcohol consumption. Consistent with a self-medication model, he also found that the impact of the Great Recession lay mainly in increases in heavy drinking among middle-aged and older employees, but not younger workers. In line with the model, older workers, with their workplaces short-staffed and their own work intensifying, their homes depreciating in value, and their retirement accounts shrinking, would be more likely to experience recession-related distress and to turn to alcohol, a legal drug, to alleviate distress.

Research from Canada, Denmark, Finland, France, The Netherlands, the United Kingdom, and the United States indicates that job insecurity is a risk factor for psychological distress, depression, and alcohol consumption, although the results are not perfectly consistent for the sexes. Frone's (2015) alcohol findings held for men and women. The theme of imperfect consistency arises again and again, and should not invalidate the general direction of the findings highlighting the mental health effects of job insecurity.

Long Working Hours

A 22-year-old-man, who was a first-year analyst working 100 hours per week at the San Francisco office of the investment bank Goldman Sachs, jumped to his death in June 2015. Before he committed suicide, he called his parents to tell them, "I have not slept for two days, have a client meeting tomorrow morning, have to complete a presentation, my V.P. is annoyed and I am working alone in my office" (Cohan, 2015).

The Japanese, who have had considerable experience with long working hours, have a word for "death from overwork"—*karoshi*— (Nishiyama & Johnson, 1997). Of course, long work hours can also have other consequences, including lack of time to spend with children, spouse, parents, and friends, and lack of time for recreation or reading for pleasure. With rare exceptions, few studies have prospective data on the psychological consequences of long working hours. Shields (1999), using the NPHS data, found that long working hours in women, controlling for a host of confounding factors, doubled their risk of experiencing a new episode of major depression 2 years later, although she did not obtain a parallel finding in men, in whom depression is somewhat less common. Niedhammer et al. (2015), however, in their prospective study of French workers, found that long hours at baseline failed to predict MDD or GAD 4 years later. In a New Zealand study, long working hours were found to be associated with alcohol problems in men and women, adjusting for a host of covariates including childhood adversities and deviant peers (Gibb, Fergusson, & Horwood, 2012). More research needs to be conducted.

Night Work and Shift Work

Suspicion that certain work shifts have a baleful effect on mental health comes from research indicating that the circadian rhythms of depressed patients differ from those of healthy controls (Scott, Monk, & Brink, 1997). Working at night or on a rotating shift can disrupt a worker's circadian rhythm, which is thought to give rise to neurovegetative symptoms (e.g., disturbance of sleeping patterns, appetite, energy levels) of depression. Night work can disrupt social relationships, which in turn can contribute to psychological distress. In many occupations, individuals work night or rotating shifts. One of those occupations is nursing. It is perhaps the occupation most often targeted for research on the impact of shift work. One of the best controlled studies of the impact of shift work was conducted by Bohle and Tilley (1989), who, over 15 months, followed 60 Australian student nurses—all women—organized into two groups by "routine hospital rostering"; the nurses had no control over the rosters. During the first 6 months, both groups rotated between day and afternoon shifts (two-rotation shifts). However, for the remainder of the study, one group continued with the two-rotation shifts, and the second group added a night shift (three-rotation shift). At 15 months, the three-rotation group showed higher GHQ scores than the two-rotation group, although the two groups were highly similar at baseline and 6 months. Bohle and Tilley also found that support from supervisors was related to lower symptom levels and that the personality factor neuroticism[11] could not explain the 15-month results.

Adeniran et al. (1996) replicated and extended a prior study ($n = 43$) of British student nurses who worked night shifts (Healy, Minors, & Waterhouse, 1993) by following an additional 53 over a similar 3-month period. Unfortunately, neither study included a comparison group comprising student nurses who worked only day shifts. By contrast, both groups of Australian nurses in the study by Bohle and Tilley showed an increase in GHQ scores from baseline to 6 months; it was only after 6 months that the two-rotation group showed a decrement in GHQ scores, but the group that transitioned into three rotations that included a night shift showed a continued increase in symptoms.

Adeniran et al. documented increases in neurovegetative symptoms and cognitive disturbance (problems concentrating and reduced interest in things), irritability, and psychosomatic symptoms after 3 months of night work. Adeniran et al. also found that two person factors, preshift depressive symptoms and sensitivity to criticism, were related to increased postshift symptoms, although without a control group, it is difficult to weigh the preshift factors' effects independently of the effects of working at night. The pattern of depressive and psychosomatic symptoms in a small study ($n = 37$) of Australian student nurses (>60% female) who were followed from baseline to 6 and 12 months later revealed adaptation to shift work over time (West, Ahern, Byrnes, & Kwanten, 2007).

It is difficult to generalize from research findings bearing on shift work in nurses to shift work in other occupations. Thus, the nature of the mental health impact of working at night or on a rotating shift work remains to be clarified further.

Stressful Occupational Events and Work-Related Social Stressors

Niedhammer et al. (1998) in the GAZEL study evaluated the impact of important occupational events on French workers. Occupational events include "major changes in work content or organization." They found that independently of the DCS variables, the number of occupational events (e.g., job change, transfer) occurring between the first and second years was related to increased risk for elevated levels of depressive symptoms, although the researchers had to assess depressive symptoms and events at the same wave of data collection.

In a 5-year, multiwave longitudinal study of a sample of more than 300 German workers, Dormann and Zapf (2002) examined the impact of workplace social stressors, which refer to "social animosities, conflicts with co-workers and supervisors, unfair behavior, and a negative group climate" (p. 35). Using innovative controls for unmeasured third factors, Dormann and Zapf found that social stressors affect depressive symptoms indirectly by provoking feelings of irritation, which in turn give rise to depressive symptoms. Reverse causal effects in which irritation or depressive symptoms precipitate the occurrence of social stressors were ruled out.

---

[11]Neuroticism refers to a fundamental dimension of personality along which individuals differ. It is thought to reflect a stable propensity to experience negative feelings such as anxiety, worry, and moodiness.

Coping

It is widely believed that coping behaviors can be helpful in the workplace. For example, political skill, which refers to an ability to understand coworkers and managers, and to use that understanding to attain one's own and an organization's goals, is thought to be a coping resource (Ferris et al., 2005). In cross-sectional research, political skill was found to buffer the impact of job stressors such as excessive workload and role conflict on strains like anxiety (Perrewé et al., 2005) and burnout (Meurs, Gallagher, & Perrewé, 2010). The literature on coping is vast; coping, as a category of potential protective factors, deserves a larger treatment than the space limitations of this book allow.

Coping refers to an individual's efforts to prevent or reduce a perceived threat, harm, or loss, or to mitigate the associated distress (Carver & Connor-Smith, 2010; Skinner, Edge, Altman, & Sherwood, 2003). Coping efforts, however, must be assessed independently of whether they are effective. Coping efforts have been viewed as involving voluntary, person–environment transactions that can change from one situation to the next (Lazarus & Folkman, 1987), although it is recognized that there are automatic or involuntary (Skinner et al., 2003) and stable or dispositional aspects of coping (Carver & Connor-Smith, 2010). Coping efforts have been classified as either problem- or emotion-focused (Lazarus & Folkman, 1984). Researchers have also employed alternative ways of categorizing such efforts, including approach or avoidant coping (Holahan et al., 2007; Moos & Holahan, 2003).

A line of thought in social science suggests that the effectiveness of individual, work-related coping efforts is limited. Alfred Adler (1994/1898), who is better known for having broken with Sigmund Freud and founding his own school of psychoanalysis, regarded the elimination of occupational disease as an aim of social legislation, and viewed personal efforts as insufficient. C. Wright Mills (1959), the well-known sociologist, advanced the view that occupational problems such as unemployment are embedded in large social and economic structures, making solutions to such problems more than simply a matter of a personal response. To appreciate this line of reasoning, consider a variation on an idea advanced by Jeffery (1989) as applied to a circumstance other than work. Jeffery (1989) wrote that "water sanitation could logically be defined as an individual behavior problem" (p. 1198). Perhaps people can be induced to engage in personal, health-related coping behaviors that involve their individually identifying and decontaminating polluted water in order to make the water drinkable—of course, one mistake in thousands of attempts could lead to a deadly disease such as cholera. By contrast, a more effective way of protecting everyone's health involves an organized, population-based approach to comprehensive sanitation measures. The goal of protecting the health of individuals, although somewhat amenable to personal coping efforts, is often more effectively addressed by organized public health measures.

Pearlin and Schooler (1978) voiced skepticism about the efficacy of coping in the workplace. They hypothesized that an individual's coping efforts are more likely to be effective in close interpersonal contexts in which the individual has considerable control, such as marriage and child-rearing. They reasoned that coping is less likely to be effective in work roles because the often impersonal organization of workplaces is a barrier to successful coping. In a cross-sectional study of more than 2,000 Chicago residents, Pearlin and Schooler found that coping efforts were effective in the context of spousal and parenting roles, and largely ineffective in work roles.

The efficacy of coping in the occupational context has been a problematic area of research. Although there have been a multitude of methodologically weak cross-sectional studies (e.g., Pearlin & Schooler, 1978), González-Morales, Rodríguez, and Peiró (2010) pointed out that "few studies examining coping with work stressors are longitudinal and their results are not consistent" (p. 32). In a 4-year study of more than 500 Chicago residents (two thirds of whom were male), Menaghan and Merves (1984) found that most coping efforts were either ineffective (e.g., selective ignoring or restricting expectations) in reducing work-related problems (e.g., overload, inadequate rewards) or made such problems worse (e.g., direct action coping). In a 6- to 9-month longitudinal study of almost 450 teachers in Spain (two thirds of whom were female), González-Morales et al. (2010) found that coping (direct action and support seeking) had little impact on burnout. In a 1-year longitudinal study of 180 female, first-year New York City teachers, Schonfeld (2001) found only null results for the effects of coping (e.g., direct action, positive comparisons) on strains such as depressive symptoms and self-esteem. Schreuder et al. (2011), in a 1-year longitudinal study of more than 380 female nurses in The Netherlands, found that controlling for ERI, coping (e.g., problem solving, avoidant coping) did not protect against sickness absence, a proxy for a combination of "physical and mental impairments."

In one of the most intriguing studies, Shimazu and Schaufeli (2007) followed 418 male Japanese assembly line workers for 1 year. The investigators reasoned that, based on COR theory (Hobfoll, 1989), problem-focused coping is likely to be helpful in the short run but unhelpful over time because it is effortful, and will drain resources, giving rise to fatigue. Shimazu and Schaufeli argued that combining problem-focused coping with distraction, an emotion-focused type of coping that they suggested would enhance recuperation, would strengthen the effectiveness of problem-focused coping over the long run. They found that the combination predicted reduced levels of a strain.

Coping remains an important area of research. However, more longitudinal research is required to better assess the efficacy of coping strategies in occupational contexts. Research along the lines of Shimazu and Schaufeli (2007) could be helpful, although researchers should also be mindful of the constraints that wider social, organizational, and economic structures place on individual coping efforts.

OTHER RESEARCH CONSIDERATIONS

Considering the research reviewed in this chapter, it is reasonable to conclude that psychosocial working conditions (e.g., decision latitude, psychological workload, job insecurity) have an impact on mental health. Readers, however, should be alert to the fact that research issues remain. Although the chapter does not cover every research issue, six issues are underlined here. The first is the importance of testing reverse causal hypotheses. The second concerns the question of controlling for socioeconomic status (SES). The third concerns the related issue of controlling for stressors occurring outside the domain of work. The fourth concerns the timing of the waves of data collection points in longitudinal studies. The fifth issue concerns decisions regarding which working populations to study. The sixth issue pertains to OHP's reliance on self-report measures. The issues are also pertinent to research on the relation of psychosocial job factors to cardiovascular and musculoskeletal disorders, areas covered in Chapter 4.

Reverse Causality

The first issue concerns a question that has not been sufficiently explored, namely, whether the mental health or personality of workers affects psychosocial workplace characteristics (de Lange, Taris, Kompier, Houtman, & Bongers, 2003; Dormann & Zapf, 2002; Elovainio et al., 2013; Hurrell, Nelson, & Simmons, 1998; Lang et al., 2011; Schonfeld, 2001). We would have a more rounded picture of the dynamics of the workplace if we compiled more evidence bearing on both the impact of workplace characteristics on mental health and personality *and* the reverse (Zapf, Dormann, & Frese, 1996). There are at least three ways in which worker mental health could affect measures of workplace characteristics. First, worker mental health may affect work factors more or less directly. For example, because depressed individuals are often irritable, they may drive away supporters or foment conflict with coworkers and precipitate other problems at work. Conflict and support are ordinarily independent variables rather than dependent variables. Second, a psychologically distressed worker may perceive workplace characteristics more negatively than is warranted, biasing self-report scales. Third, workers suffering from a serious mental illness may drift downward to less prestigious jobs, which offer few resources.

Although the research literature on general stress suggests that stressful life events play a role in the onset of depression, there has also been evidence for personal predispositions to encounter stressful events. Kendler, Karkowski, and Prescott (1999) found that "some individuals have a stable tendency to select themselves into situations with a high probability of producing stressful life events" (p. 838). Lang et al. (2011), who tested standard and reverse causal effects in research on the relation between organizational justice and depressive symptoms, warned that "results from longitudinal analyses require modifying previous assumptions of causality" (p. 613).

de Lange et al. (2004), in the SMASH study,[12] found reverse causal effects from strain to the DCS variables; these effects, however, were weaker than those of the DCS variables on strain. Plaisier et al. (2007), in their 2-year longitudinal study, controlled for reverse causal processes by limiting the follow-up sample to individuals who were free of mental disorder at baseline, in order to examine the relation of workplace factors such as workload to the incidence of mental disorder at follow-up. It would also be of interest to learn whether mental disorder or high levels of psychological distress at baseline influenced workload at follow-up, controlling for baseline workload. Paul and Moser (2009) found that poor mental health is related to increased risk of job loss, although the effect of job loss on mental health was greater. Schonfeld (2001) was able to rule out the reverse causal hypothesis that preexisting distress in teachers gives rise to work-related stressors. The untangling of reverse causal effects helps provide a more nuanced picture of the relations among mental health, job stressors, and resource factors.

Controlling for Socioeconomic Status

The second issue is the question of whether to control for SES when assessing the relation of psychosocial working conditions to mental health, particularly in studies that

---

[12] SMASH stands for Study on Musculoskeletal disorders, Absenteeism, Stress and Health.

cut across large numbers of jobs that virtually assign job incumbents to SES positions. SES is an important determinant of the social contexts (e.g., neighborhood quality, housing quality, exposure to street crime) in which individuals are embedded, social contexts that influence mental health (Tausig & Fenwick, 2011).[13] At the same time, lower-SES jobs ordinarily afford workers less control, less job security, and so forth, underlining the confounding of SES and working conditions. In a 35-year study that began during the childhood of the 500 Finnish participants, Hakanen, Bakker, and Jokisaari (2011) found that the relation of social class of origin to burnout 35 years later was largely mediated by working conditions in the intervening years. In other words, the link between SES of origin and burnout was mediated by psychosocial working conditions entailed in the jobs to which an individual's social class of origin often led by virtue of class-associated hurdles and supports (e.g., resource-poor and -rich schools).

SES often serves as a control variable in a good deal of research on risk factors for ill health (North, Syme, Feeney, Shipley, & Marmot, 1996). Although SES and psychosocial working conditions such as decision authority covary, some Whitehall II researchers provided evidence that the influences of SES and psychosocial working conditions on health can be disentangled (Kuper et al., 2002). An investigator may want to use SES as a control variable in a regression equation in which the investigator aims to assess the impact of a working condition on the mental (or physical) health of workers. However, because SES and working conditions are confounded, a result of including SES as a control variable would be that the regression coefficient for the variable representing a working condition will underestimate the true impact of that working condition (North et al., 1996; Rugulies et al., 2006). An answer to the question of whether to control for SES is not always clear, but three views need to be highlighted: (a) SES (and inequality) has health effects independent of workplace psychosocial risk factors (Marmot & Wilkinson, 2001) and should be controlled; (b) the "true" size of the effect of a psychosocial working condition on a mental health outcome is somewhere between the effect size obtained when SES is included in the regression equation and when it is omitted (North et al. 1996); (c) the true effect size can be found in the regression equation in which SES is omitted (Rugulies et al. 2006).

The third view suggests that the impact of SES on mental health is fully mediated by job conditions to which workers are exposed. An alternative would be to assess stressors occurring at work *and* outside of work. The extensiveness of nonwork stressors (e.g., quality of housing, having been a crime victim) combined with work stressors would more fully (although probably not completely) encompass the impact of SES. This leads us to the third issue.

Nonwork Stressors

Exposure to stressors is not limited to the occupational domain (e.g., unexpected rent increase, major illness in a loved one). Individuals are exposed to stressors in many life roles (e.g., spouse). Analyses of the impact of job stressors on mental health outcomes could benefit from controlling for stressors occurring outside of work (Schonfeld, 2001). Because nonwork stressors are more proximal, they are likely to

---

[13] Chapter 4 takes up the relation of SES to physical health.

embody some of the influence of SES on mental health in a way that is distinct from the influence of psychosocial working conditions.

In addition, controlling for nonwork stressors has two methodological advantages for research on the impact of psychosocial working conditions on mental health. The first is that by controlling for nonwork stressors, an investigator can obtain more precise estimates of the effect of workplace stressors on psychological outcomes (Schonfeld & Bianchi, 2016b).

But what if nonwork stressors are related to mental health outcomes but are uncorrelated with workplace stressors? Will not the effect sizes for workplace stressors remain about the same regardless of whether or not the investigator controls for nonwork stressors? The answer is "Yes." In that case, why control for nonwork stressors? Such a situation puts in relief the second advantage to controlling for nonwork stressors. If nonwork stressors explain additional variance in psychological outcomes beyond what workplace stressors explain—even if work and nonwork stressors are uncorrelated—then the prediction equation will generate less error variance. The result is that standard errors used in testing the significance of regression coefficients will be smaller, providing more power to detect effects of workplace stressors (D. Rindskopf, personal communication, November 2015).

Timing Waves of Data Collection

The fourth issue concerns timing. Although the bulk of the studies included in this chapter are longitudinal, one two-wave longitudinal study was not covered because 24 years elapsed between wave 1 and wave 2. Even if incumbents remained in the same jobs, the working conditions at baseline and 24 years later are likely to be very different. It is also likely that individuals in the sample changed jobs, perhaps multiple times. Although a 24-year lag is an extreme example, workers in studies with shorter time lags are still subject to changes in working conditions and may even change jobs. For example, Ferrie et al. (2002), using Whitehall II data, controlled for civil service grade (a proxy for SES) at baseline; however, some of the individuals in the sample, over time, rose to higher grades. Then what is the influence of grade? Grade at what point in time? What about predicting psychological symptoms from psychosocial working conditions measured during an earlier wave, when psychosocial working conditions during the later wave of data collection have changed?

Kasl (1983) took a critical view of the idea that longitudinal studies supposedly provide a "broad solution to problems of causal inference in stress and disease studies" (p. 89). Most of the longitudinal studies covered in this chapter employed veteran-worker samples. A problem with fielding a study involving veteran workers is the likelihood that the most important effects of stressful working conditions on worker health have occurred before the study begins. There is a second problem that involves scheduling the waves of data collection. Factors that influence the development of chronic diseases may take a long time to act. But the action of psychosocial working conditions is different. de Lange et al. (2004), in the SMASH study, evaluated the suitability of 1-, 2-, and 3-year lags in assessing the effects of earlier-measured DCS variables on later-measured strain (and reverse causal effects). The study team found the 1-year lag to be the most suitable for assessing the influence of the DCS factors on depressive symptoms and emotional exhaustion. In studies involving many different occupational groups, the timing of waves of data collection to reasonably estimate the temporal extent of the causal impact of psychosocial stressors on mental health outcomes cannot be tailored to any more than a handful of those groups, although de Lange et al. used a heterogeneous sample of workers.

Women who recently completed college to become teachers and who were assigned to badly run, chaotic schools almost immediately showed a spike in depressive symptoms (Schonfeld, 2000). The decision about the timing of the waves of data collection in Schonfeld's study derived from preliminary knowledge based on his acquaintance with many teachers. A study with 5 years, or even 2 years or 1 year, between waves of data collection would not have detected the spike in symptoms approximately when it occurred, compromising the study's capacity to generate reasonably accurate estimates of the impact of working conditions on symptoms (cf. de Lange et al., 2004). Schonfeld (2001) decided to collect data on depressive symptoms before the school year began and then again during the fall and spring terms. Otherwise, he would not have been able to document the almost immediate spike in symptoms experienced by teachers in the most chaotic schools. Researchers have to be careful to schedule waves of data collection that maximize the chances of identifying the effects of interest (Frese & Zapf, 1988), which is easier to do for longitudinal studies involving a single occupation about which an investigator can have intimate knowledge than for studies that encompass many different occupations.

Another problem related to timing is that researchers need to know which individuals changed jobs, affecting the chronicity of exposure. The chronicity of the exposure, even in individuals who remain in the same jobs or organizations, needs to be understood in planning research on the impact of exposures to adverse working conditions (Ford et al., 2014). de Lange et al. (2004) limited their sample to workers employed in organizations that were stable, and not subject to reorganization. Sometimes even restricting analyses to individuals who stayed in the same jobs between one wave of data collection and the next is not sufficient. When Schonfeld (2001) regressed depressive symptoms assessed during the spring term on teachers' working conditions during the fall term, he excluded individuals who remained teachers but changed schools, and restricted the analyses to teachers who remained in the same schools. Psychosocial working conditions of the teachers who were transferred to other schools were likely to change.

Researchers have important decisions to make regarding the timing of waves of data collection in longitudinal studies. Preliminary evidence from past research and from the judgments of job incumbents should inform decisions about timing.

Decisions About Study Populations

The fifth issue concerns decisions regarding the working populations to study. Research that encompasses a wide range of occupations is more suited to descriptive than analytic studies (Kristensen, 1995). Kristensen wrote, "In analytical studies where possible causal relationships are elucidated, it is the variation of exposure that matters" (p. 21). To assess the impact of psychosocial working conditions, the so-called exposure variables, investigators can select members of occupational groups for the purpose of contrasting exposures to violence, job insecurity, and so on. These occupational groups can even have the same job titles (e.g., teachers in chaotic and well-run schools) provided the groups have contrasting working conditions, the impact of which is the subject of the research. By limiting the number of occupational groups being studied, investigators can better plan the timing of data collection to detect the impact of targeted working conditions on mental health.

Reliance on Self-Report Measures

The sixth issue concerns the reality that mental health outcomes and psychosocial workplace factors are both often measured by self-report. Kasl (1983) criticized self-report stressor scales of an earlier era because they commonly embedded in the same item a stressor and reference to a consequence of the stressor (e.g., "How disturbed are you by [some condition at work]?"). With such items populating self-report stressor scales, the correlations of the scales with measures of distress are likely to be inflated. Kasl (1987) advanced the idea that items in self-report stressor measures should be neutrally worded. Items should minimize reference to the distress the putative stressors are hypothesized to affect. Spector (1992) provided evidence that self-report scales can be effective in assessing work environments. Each item in such scales should be clear and unambiguous, and ascertain the occurrence of a condition and its frequency without reference to how disturbing the worker completing the scale finds the condition. Schonfeld (1996) and Schonfeld, Rhee, and Xia (1995) showed that stressor scales comprising neutrally worded self-reports can minimize confounding with preexisting depressive symptoms.

In their classic paper on validity, Campbell and Fiske (1959) adduced evidence for the view that the correlation between measures of two constructs is likely to be increased if the constructs are assessed by the same method (e.g., paper-and-pencil self-report). A corollary is that the correlation between workplace stressors and mental health is likely to be increased if measured by common methods. Virtanen et al. (2007) raised this concern, pointing out that some longitudinal studies assessed work stressors and mental health using "subjective assessments." In other words, the relation of work stressors to mental health is partly an artifact of researchers' use of self-reports to assess both types of variables. Virtanen and her colleagues overcame this *potential* source bias by (a) assessing by self-report workplace demands and control and (b) evaluating mental health independently by mining Finland's National Prescription Register for information on study participants' antidepressant prescription records.

In a study involving both self-reports and external ratings of stressors, Semmer, Zapf, and Greif (1996) suggested that "the analyses show that self-reports may be better than is often assumed" (p. 304). Spector (1987, 1992, 2006) challenged the common-methods view, providing empirical evidence that common methods do not necessarily increase the magnitude of the correlation between measures of different constructs, particularly in the area of self-report data (e.g., stressor and strain scales). Karasek (1979) observed that data on his Swedish sample contain both expert ratings and self-reports on job-related discretion, and these were reasonably highly correlated ($r = 0.69$). In Hackman and Lawler's (1971) study of U.S. telephone company employees, the correlation between employees' and researchers' ratings of employee autonomy was 0.91. Dohrenwend et al. (2006) found that soldiers' recall of battlefield events was highly accurate. Leino and Hänninen (1995) showed that workers' "perceptions of psychosocial job factors are not invariant, but are influenced by changes in objective work conditions" (p. 139).

"Objective" measures are not without pitfalls. Frese and Zapf (1988) and Semmer et al. (1996) showed that objective measures of working conditions (e.g., expert observer ratings) suffer from deficiencies. These deficiencies include observations that are time-limited, ratings that bear on unrepresentative sampling of working conditions, observers who inadvertently elicit changes in the workers observed, biases in the observers, and raters who do not have sufficient information to account for conditions affecting an individual worker. Objective measures are sometimes used to characterize the working conditions of several workers who happen to share the same job title (imputation), minimizing genuine within-title variability in exposure to stressors. Schonfeld (1992) and Schonfeld et al. (1995) found serious deficiencies in official, objective measures of school violence because violent incidents were undercounted, making such measures almost unusable in research on teacher stress. Virtanen et al.'s use of official prescription history as a proxy for mental health problems underestimates the problems because many sufferers with depression or anxiety (a) are treated via psychotherapy and not pharmacotherapy or (b) go untreated. All told, a reasonable view is that the quality of the measures used in a study is more important than the types of measures used.

SUMMARY

Much research has examined the impact of psychosocial working conditions on mental health. More studies have examined the impact of unemployment on mental health than any other psychosocial factor. The consensus of that research is that unemployment has a deleterious effect on mental health, and could even lead to suicide. The next most commonly researched area has been the relation of the DC(S) variables to mental health. The research shows that high levels of job demands and/or low job control adversely affect mental health. High demands and low control, singly or in combination, are risk factors for poorer mental health. Evidence suggests that reduced support from coworkers or supervisors is also a risk factor. The JD–R model suggests that demands and resources have an impact on burnout; however, much less research has been conducted on the JD–R than the DC(S) model. Findings tend to be supportive of the ERI model; however, less research has been directed at the ERI than on the DC(S) model.

Other psychosocial factors are likely to influence mental health, although the evidentiary base is not deep. These other psychosocial factors include organizational injustice, long working hours, rotating shift work, and job-related stressful events. Research on the adverse mental health impact of job insecurity has been promising.

OHP researchers face a number of challenges when studying the mental health impact of psychosocial working conditions. One challenge involves estimating the appropriate amount of time between waves of data collection in order to assess the causal impact of working conditions on health. Researchers must identify workers whose jobs have changed between waves because the impact of time-1 working conditions on time-2 outcomes will be different for workers who remained in the same position and workers who changed jobs. It would also be of interest if we could obtain a greater understanding of how the mental health of a worker influences psychosocial working conditions. Because it is also likely that self-report measures will continue to play a role in research on the impact of psychosocial working conditions (cf. Sauter & Murphy, 1995), it is important to ensure that self-report measures are of high quality and minimize confounding. Researchers face the challenge of fathoming the role of SES in understanding the relation of working conditions to mental health. Clearly, SES and working conditions are related. Finally, in research on the impact of job stressors, statistically controlling for stressors occurring in nonwork domains would help investigators obtain more precise estimates of the impact of workplace stressors.

REFERENCES

Aalto, A., Elovainio, M., Kivimäki, M., Uutela, A., & Pirkola, S. (2012). The Beck Depression Inventory and General Health Questionnaire as measures of depression in the general population: A validation study using the Composite International Diagnostic Interview as the gold standard. *Psychiatry Research, 197*, 163–171. doi:10.1016/j.psychres.2011.09.008

Adeniran, R., Healy, D., Sharp, H., Williams, J. M., Minors, D., & Waterhouse, J. (1996). Interpersonal sensitivity predicts depressive symptom response to the circadian rhythm disruption of nightwork. *Psychological Medicine, 26*(6), 1211–1221.

Adler, A. (1994). Health manual for the tailoring trade. In E. Hoffman (Ed.), *The drive for self: Alfred Adler and the founding of individual psychology* (pp. 1–14). Reading, MA: Addison-Wesley. (Original work published 1898)

Adler, D. A., Mclaughlin, T. J., Rogers, W. H., Chang, H., Lapitsky, L., & Lerner, D. (2006). Job performance deficits due to depression. *American Journal of Psychiatry, 163*, 1569–1576. doi:10.1176/appi.ajp.163.9.1569

Bakker, A. B., & Demerouti, E. (2014). Job demands-resources theory. In P. Y. Chen & C. L. Cooper (Eds.), *Work and wellbeing: A complete reference guide* (Vol. 3, pp. 37–64). Chichester, England: Wiley.

Barnett, R. C., & Brennan, R. T. (1997). Change in job conditions, change in psychological distress, and gender: A longitudinal study of dual-earner couples. *Journal of Organizational Behavior, 18*, 253–274. doi:10.1002/(SICI)1099-1379(199705)18:3<253::AID-JOB800>3.0.CO;2-7

Baxter, A., Charlson, F., Somerville, A., & Whiteford, H. (2011). Mental disorders as risk factors: Assessing the evidence for the Global Burden of Disease Study. *BMC Medicine, 9*, 134. doi:10.1186/1741-7015-9-134

Beck, A. T., Ward, C. H., Mendelson, M., Mock, J., & Erbaugh, J. (1961). An inventory for measuring depression. *Archives of General Psychiatry, 4*, 561–571. doi:10.1001/archpsyc.1961.01710120031004

Berkman, L. F., & Syme, S. (1979). Social networks, host resistance, and mortality: A nine-year follow-up study of Alameda County residents. *American Journal of Epidemiology, 109*(2), 186–204.

Berman, A. L. (2009). Depression and suicide. In I. H. Gotlib & C. L. Hammen (Eds.), *Handbook of depression* (2nd ed., pp. 510–530). New York, NY: Guilford Press.

Bianchi, R., Schonfeld, I. S., & Laurent, E. (2014). Is burnout a depressive disorder? A re-examination with special focus on atypical depression. *International Journal of Stress Management, 21*, 307–324. doi:10.1037/a0037906

Bohle, P., & Tilley, A. J. (1989). The impact of night work on psychological well-being. *Ergonomics, 32*, 1089–1099. doi:10.1080/00140138908966876

Bourbonnais, R., Comeau, M., & Vezina, M. (1999). Job strain and evolution of mental health among nurses. *Journal of Occupational Health Psychology, 4*, 95–107. doi:10.1037/1076-8998.4.2.95

Boyd, C. M., Bakker, A. B., Pignata, S., Winefield, A. H., Gillespie, N., & Stough, C. (2011). A longitudinal test of the job demands-resources model among Australian university academics. *Applied Psychology: An International Review, 60*, 112–140. doi:10.1111/j.1464-0597.2010.00429.x

Brand, J. E., Levy, B. R., & Gallo, W. T. (2008). Effects of layoffs and plant closings on subsequent depression among older workers. *Research on Aging, 30*, 701–721. doi:10.1177/0164027508322574

Bromet, E. J., Dew, M. A., Parkinson, M. S., & Schulberg, H. C. (1988). Predictive effects of occupational and marital stress on the mental health of a male work force. *Journal of Organizational Behavior, 9*, 1–13. doi:10.1002/job.4030090102

Bruce, M., Leaf, P. J., Rozal, G. M., & Florio, L. (1994). Psychiatric status and 9-year mortality data in the New Haven Epidemiologic Catchment Area Study. *American Journal of Psychiatry, 151*(5), 716–721.

Bültmann, U., Kant, I., Van den Brandt, P., & Kasl, S. (2002). Psychosocial work characteristics as risk factors for the onset of fatigue and psychological distress: Prospective results from the Maastricht Cohort Study. *Psychological Medicine, 32*(2), 333–345.

Campbell, D. T., & Fiske, D. W. (1959). Convergent and discriminant validation by the multitrait-multimethod matrix. *Psychological Bulletin, 56*, 81–105. doi:10.1037/h0046016

Carver, C. S., & Connor-Smith, J. (2010). Personality and coping. *Annual Review of Psychology, 61*, 679–704. doi:10.1146/annurev.psych.093008.100352

Chrisopoulos, S., Dollard, M. F., Winefield, A. H., & Dormann, C. (2010). Increasing the probability of finding an interaction in work stress research: A two-wave longitudinal test of the triple-match principle. *Journal of Occupational and Organizational Psychology, 83*, 17–37. doi:10.1348/096317909X474173

Clays, E., De Bacquer, D., Leynen, F., Kornitzer, M., Kittel, F., & De Backer, G. (2007). Job stress and depression symptoms in middle-aged workers: Prospective results from the Belstress study. *Scandinavian Journal of Work, Environment & Health, 33*(4), 252–259.

Cohan, W. D. (2015, October 3). Deaths draw attention to Wall Street's grueling pace. *New York Times.*

Cohen, S., & Wills, T. A. (1985). Stress, social support, and the buffering hypothesis. *Psychological Bulletin, 98,* 310–357. doi:10.1037/0033-2909.98.2.310

Coope, C., Donovan, J., Wilson, C., Barnes, M., Metcalfe, C., Hollingworth, W., . . . Gunnell, D. (2015). Characteristics of people dying by suicide after job loss, financial difficulties and other economic stressors during a period of recession (2010–2011): A review of coroners' records. *Journal of Affective Disorders, 183,* 98–105. doi:10.1016/j.jad.2015.04.045

Cooper, M., Russell, M., & Frone, M. R. (1990). Work stress and alcohol effects: A test of stress-induced drinking. *Journal of Health and Social Behavior, 31,* 260–276. doi:10.2307/2136891

Crum, R. M., Muntaner. C., Eaton, W. W., & Anthony, J. C. (1995). Occupational stress and the risk of alcohol abuse and dependence. *Alcoholism, Clinical and Experimental Research, 19,* 647–655. doi:10.1111/j.1530-0277.1995.tb01562.x

de Jonge, J., & Dormann, C. (2006). Stressors, resources, and strain at work: A longitudinal test of the triple-match principle. *Journal of Applied Psychology, 91,* 1359–1374. doi:10.1037/0021-9010.91.5.1359

de Jonge, J., van Vegchel, N., Shimazu, A., Schaufeli, W., & Dormann, C. (2010). A longitudinal test of the demand-control model using specific job demands and specific job control. *International Journal of Behavioral Medicine, 17,* 125–133. doi:10.1007/s12529-010-9081-1

de Lange, A. H., Taris, T. W., Kompier, M. J., Houtman, I. D., & Bongers, P. M. (2003). 'The very best of the millennium': Longitudinal research and the demand-control-(support) model. *Journal of Occupational Health Psychology, 8,* 282–305. doi:10.1037/1076-8998.8.4.282

de Lange, A. H., Taris, T. W., Kompier, M. J., Houtman, I. D., & Bongers, P. M. (2004). The relationships between work characteristics and mental health: Examining normal, reversed and reciprocal relationships in a 4-wave study. *Work & Stress, 18,* 149–166. doi:10.1080/02678370412331270860

Deb, P., Gallo, W. T., Ayyagari, P., Fletcher, J. M., & Sindelar, J. L. (2011). The effect of job loss on overweight and drinking. *Journal of Health Economics, 30,* 317–327. doi:10.1016/j.jhealeco.2010.12.009

Dee, T. (2001). Alcohol abuse and economic conditions: Evidence from repeated cross-sections of individual-level data. *Health Economics, 10*(3), 257–270.

Demerouti, E., Bakker, A. B., Nachreiner, F., & Schaufeli, W. B. (2001). The job demands-resources model of burnout. *Journal of Applied Psychology, 86,* 499–512. doi:10.1037/0021-9010.86.3.499

Derogatis, L. R. (1977). *The SCL-R-90 Manual I: Scoring, Administration and Procedures for the SCL-90.* Baltimore, MD: Clinical Psychometric Research.

Derogatis, L. R. (1983). *SCL-90-R: Administration, scoring and procedures manual-II.* Baltimore, MD: Clinical Psychometric Research.

Dohrenwend, B. P., Shrout, P. E., Egri, G., & Mendelsohn, F. S. (1980). Nonspecific psychological distress and other dimensions of psychopathology. *Archives of General Psychiatry, 37,* 1229–1236. doi:10.1001/archpsyc.1980.01780240027003

Dohrenwend, B. P., Turner, J. B., Turse, N. A., Adams, B. G., Koenen, K. C., & Marshall, R. (2006). The psychological risks of Vietnam for U.S. veterans: A revisit with new data and methods. *Science, 313,* 979–982. doi:10.1126/science.1128944

Dooley, D., Fielding, J., & Levi, L. (1996). Health and unemployment. *Annual Review of Public Health, 17,* 449–465.

Dormann, C., & Zapf, D. (2002). Social stressors at work, irritation, and depressive symptoms: Accounting for unmeasured third variables in a multi-wave study. *Journal of Occupational and Organizational Psychology, 75,* 33–58. doi:10.1348/096317902167630

Durkheim, É. (1951/1912). *Suicide: A study in sociology* (J. A. Spaulding & G. Simpson, Transl.). Glencoe, IL: Free Press.

Elovainio, M., Kivimäki, M., Vahtera, J., Keltikangas-Järvinen, L., & Virtanen, M. (2003). Sleeping problems and health behaviors as mediators between organizational justice and health. *Health Psychology, 22,* 287–293. doi:10.1037/0278-6133.22.3.287

Elovainio, M., Linna, A., Virtanen, M., Oksanen, T., Kivimäki, M., Pentti, J., & Vahtera, J. (2013). Perceived organizational justice as a predictor of long-term sickness absence due to diagnosed mental disorders: Results from the prospective longitudinal Finnish Public Sector Study. *Social Science & Medicine* (1982), *91,* 39–47. doi:10.1016/j.socscimed.2013.05.008

Fandiño-Losada, A., Forsell, Y., & Lundberg, I. (2013). Demands, skill discretion, decision authority and social climate at work as determinants of major depression in a 3-year follow-up study. *International Archives of Occupational and Environmental Health, 86,* 591–605. doi:10.1007/s00420-012-0791-3

Farber, B. A. (1991). *Crisis in education: Stress and burnout in the American teacher*. San Francisco, CA: Jossey-Bass.

Ferrie, J. E. (2004). *Work stress and health: The Whitehall II study*. London, England: Council of Civil Service Unions/Cabinet Office.

Ferrie, J. E., Head, J., Shipley, M. J., Vahtera, J., Marmot, M. G., & Kivimäki, M. (2006). Injustice at work and incidence of psychiatric morbidity: The Whitehall II study. *Occupational and Environmental Medicine, 63*, 443–450. doi:10.1136/oem.2005.022269

Ferrie, J. E., Shipley, M., Marmot, M., Martikainen, P., Stansfeld, S., & Smith, G. (2001). Job insecurity in white-collar workers: Toward an explanation of associations with health. *Journal of Occupational Health Psychology, 6*, 26–42. doi:10.1037/1076-8998.6.1.26

Ferrie, J. E., Shipley, M. J., Stansfeld, S. A., & Marmot, M. G. (2002). Effects of chronic job insecurity and change in job security on self-reported health, minor psychiatric morbidity, physiological measures, and health related behaviours in British civil servants: The Whitehall II study. *Journal of Epidemiology and Community Health, 56*, 450–454. doi:10.1136/jech.56.6.450

Ferris, G. R., Treadway, D. C., Kolodinsky, R. W., Hochwarter, W. A., Kacmar, C. J., Douglas, C., & Frink, D. D. (2005). Development and validation of the political skill inventory. *Journal of Management, 31*, 126–152. doi:10.1177/0149206304271386

Ford, M. T., Cerasoli, C. P., Higgins, J. A., & Decesare, A. L. (2011). Relationships between psychological, physical, and behavioural health and work performance: A review and meta-analysis. *Work & Stress, 25*, 185–204. doi:10.1080/02678373.2011.609035

Ford, M. T., Matthews, R. A., Wooldridge, J. D., Mishra, V., Kakar, U. M., & Strahan, S. R. (2014). How do occupational stressor-strain effects vary with time? A review and meta-analysis of the relevance of time lags in longitudinal studies. *Work & Stress, 28*, 9–30. doi:10.1080/02678373.2013.877096

Frese, M. (1999). Social support as a moderator of the relationship between work stressors and psychological dysfunctioning: A longitudinal study with objective measures. *Journal of Occupational Health Psychology, 4*, 179–192. doi:10.1037/1076-8998.4.3.179

Frese, M., & Zapf, D. (1988). Methodological issues in the study of work stress: Objective vs. subjective measurement of work stress and the question of longitudinal studies. In C. L. Cooper & R. Payne (Eds.), *Causes, coping, and consequences of stress at work* (pp. 375–411). Chichester, England: Wiley.

Freud, S. (1962). *Civilization and its discontents* (J. Strachey, Trans.). New York, NY: W. W. Norton. (Original work published 1930)

Freudenberger, H. J. (1974). Staff burnout. *Journal of Social Issues, 30*(1), 159–165.

Frone, M. R. (2015). The Great Recession and employee alcohol use: A U.S. population study. *Psychology of Addictive Behaviors*. doi:10.1037/adb0000143

Frone, M. R., & Tidwell, M.-C. O. (2015). The meaning and measurement of work fatigue: Development and evaluation of the three-dimensional Work Fatigue Inventory (3D-WFI). *Journal of Occupational Health Psychology, 20*(3), 273–288. doi:10.1037/a0038700

Garcy, A., & Vågerö, D. (2012). The length of unemployment predicts mortality, differently in men and women, and by cause of death: A six year mortality follow-up of the Swedish 1992–1996 recession. *Social Science & Medicine, 74*(1982), 1911–1920. doi:10.1016/j.socscimed.2012.01.034

Gelsema, T. I., Van Der Doef, M., Maes, S., Janssen, M., Akerboom, S., & Verhoeven, C. (2006). A longitudinal study of job stress in the nursing profession: Causes and consequences. *Journal of Nursing Management, 14*, 289–299. doi:10.1111/j.1365-2934.2006.00635.x

Gibb, S. J., Fergusson, D. M., & Horwood, L. J. (2012). Working hours and alcohol problems in early adulthood. *Addiction, 107*, 81–88. doi:10.1111/j.1360-0443.2011.03543.x

Godin, I., Kittel, F., Coppieters, Y., & Siegrist, J. (2005). A prospective study of cumulative job stress in relation to mental health. *BMC Public Health, 5*, 67–76.

Goetzel, R., Ozminkowski, R., Sederer, L., & Mark, T. (2002). The business case for quality mental health services: Why employers should care about the mental health and well-being of their employees. *Journal of Occupational and Environmental Medicine, 44*(4), 320–330.

Goldberg, D. P. (1972). *The detection of psychiatric illness by questionnaire: A technique for the identification and assessment of non-psychotic psychiatric illness*. London, England: Oxford University Press.

Goldberg, D. P., Oldehinkel, T. T., & Ormel, J. J. (1998). Why GHQ threshold varies from one place to another. *Psychological Medicine, 28*, 915–921. doi:10.1017/S0033291798006874

González-Morales, M., Rodríguez, I., & Peiró, J. M. (2010). A longitudinal study of coping and gender in a female-dominated occupation: Predicting teachers' burnout. *Journal of Occupational Health Psychology, 15*(1), 29–44. doi:10.1037/a0018232

Gotlib, I. H., & Hammen, C. L. (2009). *Handbook of depression* (2nd ed.). New York, NY: Guilford Press.

Gouldner, A. W. (1960). The norm of reciprocity: A preliminary statement. *American Sociological Review, 25*(2), 161–178.

Gururaj, G., Isaac, M., Subbakrishna, D., & Ranjani, R. (2004). Risk factors for completed suicides: A case-control study from Bangalore, India. *Injury Control and Safety Promotion, 11*(3), 183–191.

Hackman, J., & Lawler, E. E. (1971). Employee reactions to job characteristics. *Journal of Applied Psychology, 55*(3), 259–286. doi:10.1037/h0031152

Hakanen, J. J., Bakker, A. B., & Jokisaari, M. (2011). A 35-year follow-up study on burnout among Finnish employees. *Journal of Occupational Health Psychology, 16*, 345–360. doi:10.1037/a0022903

Hakanen, J. J., Schaufeli, W. B., & Ahola, K. (2008). The Job Demands-Resources model: A three-year cross-lagged study of burnout, depression, commitment, and work engagement. *Work & Stress, 22*, 224–241. doi:10.1080/02678370802379432

Halbesleben, J. B., Neveu, J., Paustian-Underdahl, S. C., & Westman, M. (2014). Getting to the 'COR': Understanding the role of resources in conservation of resources theory. *Journal of Management, 40*, 1334–1364. doi:10.1177/0149206314527130

Häusser, J. A., Mojzisch, A., Niesel, M., & Schulz-Hardt, S. (2010). Ten years on: A review of recent research on the job demand-control (-support) model and psychological well-being. *Work & Stress, 24*, 1–35. doi:10.1080/02678371003683747

Haw, C., Hawton, K., Gunnell, D., & Platt, S. (2015). Economic recession and suicidal behaviour: Possible mechanisms and ameliorating factors. *International Journal of Social Psychiatry. 61*, 73–81 doi:10.1177/0020764014536545

Head, J., Stansfeld, S., & Siegrist, J. (2004). The psychosocial work environment and alcohol dependence: A prospective study. *Occupational and Environmental Medicine, 61*, 219–224. doi:10.1136/oem.2002.005256

Healy, D., Minors, D. S., & Waterhouse, J. (1993). Shiftwork, helplessness and depression. *Journal of Affective Disorders, 29*, 17–25. doi:10.1016/0165-0327(93)90114-Y

Heikkilä, K., Nyberg, S. T., Fransson, E. I., Alfredsson, L., De Bacquer, D., Bjorner, J. B., ... Kivimäki, M. (2012). Job strain and alcohol intake: A collaborative meta-analysis of individual-participant data from 140,000 men and women. *PLOS ONE, 7*. doi:10.1371/journal.pone.0040101

Hemmingsson, T., & Lundberg, I. (1998). Work control, work demands, and work social support in relation to alcoholism among young men. *Alcoholism, Clinical and Experimental Research, 22*, 921–927. doi:10.1097/00000374-199806000-00024

Hintsa, T., Elovainio, M., Jokela, M., Ahola, K., Virtanen, M., & Pirkola, S. (2016). Is there an independent association between burnout and increased allostatic load? Testing the contribution of psychological distress and depression. *Journal of Health Psychology, 21*, 1576–1586. doi:10.1177/1359105314559619

Hobfoll, S. E. (1989). Conservation of resources: A new attempt at conceptualizing stress. *American Psychologist, 44*, 513-524. doi:10.1037/0003-066X.44.3.513

Hobfoll, S. E. (2001). The influence of culture, community, and the nested-self in the stress process: Advancing Conservation of Resources Theory. *Applied Psychology: An International Review, 50*, 337–421. doi:10.1111/1464-0597.00062

Hobfoll, S. E., & Shirom, A. (2001). Conservation of resources theory: Applications to stress and management in the workplace. In R. T. Golembiewski (Ed.), *Handbook of organizational behavior* (2nd ed., pp. 57–80). New York, NY: Marcel Dekker.

Holahan, C. J., Moos, R. H., Moerkbak, M. L., Cronkite, R. C., Holahan, C. K., & Kenney, B. A. (2007). Spousal similarity in coping and depressive symptoms over 10 years. *Journal of Family Psychology, 21*, 551–559. doi:10.1037/0893-3200.21.4.551

Homans, G. C. (1958). Social behavior as exchange. *American Journal of Sociology, 63*, 597–606. doi:10.1086/222355

House, J., Landis, K., & Umberson, D. (1988). Social relationships and health. *Science, 241*, 540–545. doi:10.1126/science.3399889

Hurrell, J. J., Jr., Nelson, D. L., & Simmons, B. L. (1998). Measuring job stressors and strains: Where we have been, where we are, and where we need to go. *Journal of Occupational Health Psychology, 3*, 368–389. doi:10.1037/1076-8998.3.4.368

Jahoda, M. (1981). Work, employment, and unemployment: Values, theories, and approaches in social research. *American Psychologist, 36*, 184–191. doi:10.1037/0003-066X.36.2.184

Jahoda, M., Lazarsfeld, P. F., & Zeisel, H. (1971). *Marienthal: The sociography of an unemployed community*. Chicago, IL: Aldine. (Original work published 1933)

Jeffery, R. W. (1989). Risk behaviors and health: Contrasting individual and population perspectives. *American Psychologist, 44,* 1194–1202. doi:10.1037/0003-066X.44.9.1194

Johnson, J. V., Hall, E. M., & Theorell, T. (1989). Combined effects of job strain and social isolation on cardiovascular disease morbidity and mortality in a random sample of the Swedish male working population. *Scandinavian Journal of Work, Environment & Health, 15,* 271–279. doi:10.5271/sjweh.1852

Kain, J., & Jex, S. (2010). Karasek's (1979) job demands-control model: A summary of current issues and recommendations for future research. In P. L. Perrewé & D. C. Ganster (Eds.), *New developments in theoretical and conceptual approaches to job stress* (pp. 237–268). Bingley, England: Emerald Group Publishing. doi:10.1108/S1479-3555(2010)0000008009

Karasek, R. A. (1979). Job demands, job decision latitude, and mental strain: Implications for job redesign. *Administrative Science Quarterly, 24*(2), 285–308.

Karasek, R. A. (1985). *Job Content Questionnaire and user's guide.* Los Angeles: Department of Industrial and Systems Engineering, University of Southern California.

Karasek, R. A. (2006). *JCQ version 2.0.* The JCQ Center. Retrieved from www.jcqcenter.org

Karasek, R., Baker, D., Marxer, F., Ahlbom, A., & Theorell, T. (1981). Job decision latitude, job demands, and cardiovascular disease: A prospective study of Swedish men. *American Journal of Public Health, 71*(7), 694–705.

Karasek, R., & Theorell, T. (1990). *Healthy work: Stress, productivity, and the reconstruction of working life.* New York, NY: Basic Books.

Kasl, S. V. (1983) Pursuing the link between stressful life experiences and disease: A time for reappraisal. In C. L. Cooper (Ed.), *Stress research* (pp. 79–102). Chichester, England: Wiley.

Kasl, S. V. (1987). Methodologies in stress and health: Past difficulties, present dilemmas, future directions. In S. V. Kasl & C. L. Cooper (Eds.), *Stress and health: Issues in research methodology* (pp. 307–318). Chichester, England: Wiley.

Kawakami, N., Haratani, T., & Araki, S. (2002). Effects of perceived job stress on depressive symptoms in blue-collar workers of an electrical factory in Japan. *Scandinavian Journal of Work, Environment & Health, 18*(3), 195–200. doi:10.5271/sjweh.1588

Kendler, K., Karkowski, L., & Prescott, C. (1999). Causal relationship between stressful life events and the onset of major depression. *The American Journal of Psychiatry, 156*(6), 837–841.

Kessler, R., Akiskal, H., Ames, M., Birnbaum, H., Greenberg, P., Hirschfeld, R., ... Wang, P. (2006). Prevalence and effects of mood disorders on work performance in a nationally representative sample of U.S. workers. *American Journal of Psychiatry, 163,* 1561–1568. doi:10.1176/appi.ajp.163.9.1561

Kessler, R. C., House, J. S., & Turner, J. B. (1987). Unemployment and health in a community sample. *Journal of Health and Social Behavior, 28*(1), 51–59. doi:10.2307/2137140

Kivimäki, M., Elovainio, M., Vahtera, J., & Ferrie, J. (2003). Organisational justice and health of employees: Prospective cohort study. *Occupational and Environmental Medicine, 60*(1), 27–33.

Kivimäki, M., Vahtera, J., Elovainio, M., Virtanen, M., & Siegrist, J. (2007). Effort-reward imbalance, procedural injustice and relational injustice as psychosocial predictors of health: Complementary or redundant models? *Occupational and Environmental Medicine, 64*(10), 659–665.

Kristensen, T. S. (1995). The demand-control-support model: Methodological challenges for future research. *Stress Medicine, 11,* 17–26. doi:10.1002/smi.2460110104

Kristensen, T. S., Borritz, M., Villadsen, E., & Christensen, K. B. (2005). The Copenhagen Burnout Inventory: A new tool for the assessment of burnout. *Work & Stress, 19,* 192–207. doi:10.1080/02678370500297720

Kuper, H., Singh-Manoux, A., Siegrist, J., & Marmot, M. (2002). When reciprocity fails: Effort-reward imbalance in relation to coronary heart disease and health functioning within the Whitehall II study. *Occupational and Environmental Medicine, 59*(11), 777–784.

Laitinen-Krispijn, S., & Bijl, R. V. (2000). Mental disorders and employee sickness absence: The NEMESIS study. *Social Psychiatry and Psychiatric Epidemiology, 35,* 71–77. doi:10.1007/s001270050010

Lang, J., Bliese, P. D., Lang, J. B., & Adler, A. B. (2011). Work gets unfair for the depressed: Cross-lagged relations between organizational justice perceptions and depressive symptoms. *Journal of Applied Psychology, 96,* 602–618. doi:10.1037/a0022463

Lazarus, R. S., & Folkman. S. (1984). *Stress, appraisal, and coping.* New York, NY: Springer Publishing.

Lazarus, R. S., & Folkman, S. (1987). Transactional theory and research on emotions and coping [Special Issue]. *European Journal of Personality, 1*(3), 141–169. doi:10.1002/per.2410010304

Leino, P., & Hänninen, V. (1995). Psychosocial factors at work in relation to back and limb disorders. *Scandinavian Journal of Work, Environment & Health, 21*(2), 134–142.

Luchman, J. N., & González-Morales, M. (2013). Demands, control, and support: A meta-analytic review of work characteristics interrelationships. *Journal of Occupational Health Psychology, 18*, 37–52. doi:10.1037/a0030541

Lundin, A., Lundberg, I., Allebeck, P., & Hemmingsson, T. (2012). Unemployment and suicide in the Stockholm population: A register-based study on 771,068 men and women. *Public Health, 126*, 371–377. doi:10.1016/j.puhe.2012.01.020

Lundin, A., Lundberg, I., Hallsten, L., Ottosson, J., & Hemmingsson, T. (2010). Unemployment and mortality: A longitudinal prospective study on selection and causation in 49321 Swedish middle-aged men. *Journal of Epidemiology and Community Health, 64*, 22–28. doi:10.1136/jech.2008.079269

Mäki, N., & Martikainen, P. (2012). A register-based study on excess suicide mortality among unemployed men and women during different levels of unemployment in Finland. *Journal of Epidemiology and Community Health, 66*, 302–307. doi:10.1136/jech.2009.105908

Malach-Pines, A. (2005). The Burnout Measure, Short Version. *International Journal of Stress Management, 12*, 78–88. doi:10.1037/1072-5245.12.1.78

Marchand, A., & Blanc, M.-E. (2011). Occupation, work organization conditions, and alcohol misuse in Canada: An 8-year longitudinal study. *Substance Use & Misuse, 46*, 1003–1014. doi:10.3109/108 26084.2010.543249

Marchand, A., Demers, A., & Durand, P. (2005). Do occupation and work conditions really matter? A longitudinal analysis of psychological distress experiences among Canadian workers. *Sociology of Health & Illness, 27*, 602–627. doi:10.1111/j.1467-9566.2005.00458.x

Marmot, M., & Wilkinson, R. (2001). Psychosocial and material pathways in the relation between income and health: A response to Lynch et al. *BMJ (Clinical Research Ed.), 322*(7296), 1233–1236.

Maslach, C., & Jackson, S. E. (1986). *Maslach Burnout Inventory: Second edition*. Palo Alto, CA: Consulting Psychologists Press.

Mausner-Dorsch, H., & Eaton, W. W. (2000). Psychosocial work environment and depression: Epidemiologic assessment of the demand-control model. *American Journal of Public Health, 90*, 1765–1770. doi:10.2105/AJPH.90.11.1765

McEwen, B. S. (2004). Protection and damage from acute and chronic stress: Allostasis and allostatic overload and relevance to the pathophysiology of psychiatric disorders. *Annals of the New York Academy of Sciences, 1032*, 1–7.

McKee-Ryan, F., Song, Z., Wanberg, C. R., & Kinicki, A. J. (2005). Psychological and physical well-being during unemployment: A meta-analytic study. *Journal of Applied Psychology, 90*(1), 53–76. doi:10.1037/0021-9010.90.1.53

McTernan, W. P., Dollard, M. F., & LaMontagne, A. D. (2013). Depression in the workplace: An economic cost analysis of depression-related productivity loss attributable to job strain and bullying. *Work & Stress, 27*, 321–378. doi:10.1080/02678373.2013.846948

Mead, G. H. (1934). *Mind, self, and society*. Chicago, IL: University of Chicago Press.

Meier, S. T. (1984). The construct validity of burnout. *Journal of Occupational Psychology, 57*, 211–219. doi:10.1111/j.2044-8325.1984.tb00163.x

Menaghan, E. G., & Merves, E. S. (1984). Coping with occupational problems: The limits of individual efforts. *Journal of Health and Social Behavior, 25*, 406–423. doi:10.2307/2136379

Meurs, J. A., Gallagher, V. C., & Perrewé, P. L. (2010). The role of political skill in the stressor–outcome relationship: Differential predictions for self- and other-reports of political skill. *Journal of Vocational Behavior, 76*, 520–533. doi:10.1016/j.jvb.2010.01.005

Michélsen, H., & Bildt, C. (2003). Psychosocial conditions on and off the job and psychological ill health: Depressive symptoms, impaired psychological wellbeing, heavy consumption of alcohol. *Occupational and Environmental Medicine, 60*(7), 489–496.

Mills, C. W. (1959). *The sociological imagination*. London, UK: Oxford University Press.

Milner, A., Page, A., & LaMontagne, A. (2013). Long-term unemployment and suicide: A systematic review and meta-analysis. *PLOS ONE, 8*(1), e51333. doi:10.1371/journal.pone.0051333

Mino, Y., Shigemi, J., Tsuda, T., Yasuda, N., & Bebbington, P. (1999). Perceived job stress and mental health in precision machine workers of Japan: A 2 year cohort study. *Occupational and Environmental Medicine, 56*(1), 41–45.

Miret, M., Ayuso-Mateos, J., Sanchez-Moreno, J., & Vieta, E. (2013). Depressive disorders and suicide: Epidemiology, risk factors, and burden. *Neuroscience and Biobehavioral Reviews 37*(10, Pt. 1), 2372–2374. doi:10.1016/j.neubiorev.2013.01.008

Moos, R. H., & Holahan, C. J. (2003). Dispositional and contextual perspectives on coping: Toward an integrative framework. *Journal of Clinical Psychology, 59*, 1387–1403. doi:10.1002/jclp.10229

Mortensen, P., Agerbo, E., Erikson, T., Qin, P., & Westergaard-Nielsen, N. (2000). Psychiatric illness and risk factors for suicide in Denmark. *The Lancet, 355*(9197), 9–12.

Muntaner, C., Tien, A. Y., Eaton, W. W., & Garrison, R. (1991). Occupational characteristics and the occurrence of psychotic disorders. *Social Psychiatry and Psychiatric Epidemiology, 26*, 273–280. doi:10.1007/BF00789219

Nicholson, A., Kuper, H., & Hemingway, H. (2006). Depression as an aetiologic and prognostic factor in coronary heart disease: A meta-analysis of 6362 events among 146 538 participants in 54 observational studies. *European Heart Journal, 27*(23), 2763–2774.

Niedhammer, I., Goldberg, M., Leclerc, A., Bugel, I., & David, S. (1998). Psychosocial factors at work and subsequent depressive symptoms in the Gazel cohort. *Scandinavian Journal of Work, Environment & Health, 24*(3), 197–205.

Niedhammer, I., Malard, L., & Chastang, J. (2015). Occupational factors and subsequent major depressive and generalized anxiety disorders in the prospective French national SIP study. *BMC Public Health, 15*, 200. doi:10.1186/s12889-015-1559-y

Nishiyama, K., & Johnson, J. (1997). Karoshi—death from overwork: Occupational health consequences of Japanese production management. *International Journal of Health Service, 27*(4), 625–641.

North, F., Syme, S., Feeney, A., Shipley, M., & Marmot, M. (1996). Psychosocial work environment and sickness absence among British civil servants: the Whitehall II study. *American Journal of Public Health, 86*(3), 332–340.

Olstad, R., Sexton, H., & Søgaard, A. (2001). The Finnmark Study: A prospective population study of the social support buffer hypothesis, specific stressors and mental distress. *Social Psychiatry and Psychiatric Epidemiology, 36*(12), 582–589.

Parkes, K. R., Mendham, C. A., & von Rabenau, C. (1994). Social support and the demand-discretion model of job stress: Tests of additive and interactive effects in two samples. *Journal of Vocational Behavior, 44*, 91–113. doi:10.1006/jvbe.1994.1006

Paterniti, S., Niedhammer, I., Lang, T., & Consoli, S. M. (2002). Psychosocial factors at work, personality traits and depressive symptoms: Longitudinal results from the GAZEL study. *British Journal of Psychiatry, 181*(2), 111–117.

Paul, K. I., & Moser, K. (2009). Unemployment impairs mental health: Meta-analyses. *Journal of Vocational Behavior, 74*, 264–282. doi:10.1016/j.jvb.2009.01.001

Pearlin, L. I., & Schooler, C. (1978). The structure of coping. *Journal of Health and Social Behavior, 19*, 2–21. doi:10.2307/2136319

Perrewé, P. L., Zellars, K. L., Rossi, A. M., Ferris, G. R., Kacmar, C. J., Liu, Y., … Hochwarter, W. A. (2005). Political skill: An antidote in the role overload–strain relationship. *Journal of Occupational Health Psychology, 10*, 239–250. doi:10.1037/1076-8998.10.3.239

Plaisier, I., de Bruijn, J., de Graaf, R., ten Have, M., Beekman, A., & Penninx, B. (2007). The contribution of working conditions and social support to the onset of depressive and anxiety disorders among male and female employees. *Social Science & Medicine, 64*, 401–410. doi:10.1016/j.socscimed.2006.09.008

Podsakoff, N. P., LePine, J. A., & LePine, M. A. (2007). Differential challenge stressor-hindrance stressor relationships with job attitudes, turnover intentions, turnover, and withdrawal behavior: A meta-analysis. *Journal of Applied Psychology, 92*, 438–454. doi:10.1037/0021-9010.92.2.438

Pratt, L., Ford, D., Crum, R., Armenian, H., Gallo, J., & Eaton, W. (1996). Depression, psychotropic medication, and risk of myocardial infarction: Prospective data from the Baltimore ECA follow-up. *Circulation, 94*(12), 3123–3129.

Qin, P., Agerbo, E., & Mortensen, P. (2003). Suicide risk in relation to socioeconomic, demographic, psychiatric, and familial factors: A national register-based study of all suicides in Denmark, 1981–1997. *American Journal of Psychiatry, 160*, 765–772. doi:10.1176/appi.ajp.160.4.765

Quinn, R. P., & Staines, G. L. (1979). *The 1977 Quality of Employment Survey: Descriptive statistics with comparison data from the 1960–70 and the 1972–73 surveys.* Ann Arbor: University of Michigan.

Radloff, L. S. (1977). The CES-D Scale: A self-report depression scale for research in the general population. *Applied Psychological Measurement, 1*, 385–401. doi:10.1177/014662167700100306

Rihmer, Z. (2001). Can better recognition and treatment of depression reduce suicide rates? A brief review. *European Psychiatry, 16*(7), 406–409.

Robins, L., Wing, J., Wittchen, H., Helzer, J., Babor, T., Burke, J., … Regier, D. (1988). The Composite International Diagnostic Interview: An epidemiologic instrument suitable for use in conjunction with different diagnostic systems and in different cultures. *Archives of General Psychiatry, 45*, 1069–1077. doi:10.1001/archpsyc.1988.01800360017003

Robinson, W. S. (1950). Ecological correlations and the behavior of individuals. *American Sociological Review, 15*, 352–357. doi:10.2307/2087176

Romelsjö, A., Hasin, D., Hilton, M., Boström, G., Diderichsen, F., Haglund, B., … Svanström, L. (1992). The relationship between stressful working conditions and high alcohol consumption and severe alcohol problems in an urban general population. *British Journal of Addiction, 87*(8), 1173–1183.

Rugulies, R., Bültmann, U., Aust, B., & Burr, H. (2006). Psychosocial work environment and incidence of severe depressive symptoms: Prospective findings from a 5-year follow-up of the Danish work environment cohort study. *American Journal of Epidemiology, 163*, 877–887. doi:10.103/aje/kwj119

Rugulies, R., Thielen, K., Nygaard, E., & Diderichsen, F. (2010). Job insecurity and the use of antidepressant medication among Danish employees with and without a history of prolonged unemployment: A 3.5-year follow-up study. *Journal of Epidemiology and Community Health, 64*, 75–81. doi:10.1136/jech.2008.078493

Sauter, S. L., & Murphy, L. R. (1995). Introduction. In S. L. Sauter & L. R. Murphy (Eds.), *Organizational risk factors for job stress* (pp. 321–322). Washington, DC: American Psychological Association.

Schaufeli, W. B., Bakker, A. B., & Van Rhenen, W. (2009). How changes in job demands and resources predict burnout, work engagement and sickness absenteeism. *Journal of Organizational Behavior, 30*, 893–917. doi:10.1002/job.595

Schaufeli, W. B., Leiter, M. P., Maslach, C., & Jackson, S. E. (1996). Maslach burnout inventory—General survey. In C. Maslach, S. E. Jackson, & M. P. Leiter (Eds.), *Maslach burnout inventory* (3rd ed.). Palo Alto, CA: Consulting Psychologists Press.

Schaufeli, W. B., & Taris, T. W. (2014). A critical review of the job demands-resources model: Implications for improving work and health. In G. F. Bauer & O. Hämmig (Eds.), *Bridging occupational, organizational and public health: A transdisciplinary approach* (pp. 43–68). Dordrecht, The Netherlands: Springer. doi:10.1007/978-94-007-5640-3_4

Schonfeld, I. S. (1990). Distress in a sample of teachers. *Journal of Psychology, 123*, 321–338. doi:10.1080/00223980.1990.10543227

Schonfeld, I. S. (1992). Assessing stress in teachers: Depressive symptoms scales and neutral self-reports of the work environment. In J. C. Quick, L. R. Murphy, & J. J. Hurrell, Jr. (Eds.), *Work and well-being: Assessments and instruments for occupational mental health* (pp. 270–285). Washington, DC: American Psychological Association.

Schonfeld, I. S. (1996). Relation of negative affectivity to self-reports of job stressors and psychological outcomes. *Journal of Occupational Health Psychology, 1*, 397–412. doi:10.1037/1076-8998.1.4.397

Schonfeld, I. S. (2000). An updated look at depressive symptoms and job satisfaction in first-year women teachers. *Journal of Occupational and Organizational Psychology, 73*, 363–371. doi:10.1348/096317900167074

Schonfeld, I. S. (2001). Stress in 1st-year women teachers: The context of social support and coping. *Genetic, Social, and General Psychology Monographs, 127*, 133–168.

Schonfeld, I. S. (2006). School violence. In E. K. Kelloway, J. Barling, & J. J. Hurrell, Jr. (Eds.), *Handbook of workplace violence* (pp. 169–229). Thousand Oaks, CA: Sage.

Schonfeld, I. S., & Bianchi, R. (2016a). Burnout and depression: Two entities or one. *Journal of Clinical Psychology, 72*, 22–37. doi:10.1002/jclp.22229

Schonfeld, I. S., & Bianchi, R. (2016b). Burnout in firefighters: A word on methodology. *Occupational Medicine, 66*, 79. doi:10.1093/occmed/kqv184

Schonfeld, I. S., Rhee, J. & Xia, F. (1995). Methodological issues in occupational-stress research: Research in one occupational group and its wider applications. In S. L. Sauter & L. R. Murphy (Eds.), *Organizational risk factors for job stress* (pp. 323–339). Washington, DC: American Psychological Association.

Schreuder, J. H., Plat, N., Magerøy, N., Moen, B. E., van der Klink, J. L., Groothoff, J. W., & Roelen, C. M. (2011). Self-rated coping styles and registered sickness absence among nurses working in hospital care: A prospective 1-year cohort study. *International Journal of Nursing Studies, 48*, 838–846. doi:10.1016/j.ijnurstu.2010.12.008

Scott, A., Monk, T., & Brink, L. (1997). Shiftwork as a risk factor for depression: A pilot study. *International Journal of Occupational and Environmental Health, 3*(Suppl. 2), S2–S9.

Selvin, H. C. (1958). Durkheim's *Suicide* and problems of empirical research. *American Journal of Sociology, 63*, 607–619. doi:10.1086/222356

Semmer, N., Zapf, D., & Greif, S. (1996). 'Shared job strain': A new approach for assessing the validity of job stress measurements. *Journal of Occupational and Organizational Psychology, 69*, 293–310. doi:10.1111/j.2044-8325.1996.tb00616.x

Shields, M. (1999). Long working hours and health. *Health Reports/Statistics Canada, Canadian Centre for Health Information, 11*(2), 33–48.

Shields, M. (2006). Stress and depression in the employed population. *Health Reports, 17*(4), 11–29.

Shimazu, A., & Schaufeli, W. B. (2007). Does distraction facilitate problem-focused coping with job stress? A 1 year longitudinal study. *Journal of Behavioral Medicine, 30*, 423–434. doi:10.1007/s10865-007-9109-4

Shirom, A. (1989). Burnout in work organizations. In C. L. Cooper & I. Robertson (Eds.), *International review of industrial and organizational psychology* (pp. 25–48). Chichester, UK: Wiley.

Shirom, A., & Melamed, S. (2006). A comparison of the construct validity of two burnout measures in two groups of professionals. *International Journal of Stress Management, 13*, 176–200. doi:10.1037/1072-5245.13.2.176

Siegrist, J. (1996). Adverse health effects of high-effort/low-reward conditions. *Journal of Occupational Health Psychology, 1*, 27–41. doi:10.1037/1076-8998.1.1.27

Siegrist, J., Starke, D., Chandola, T., Godin, I., Marmot, M., Niedhammer, I., & Peter, R. (2004). The measurement of effort-reward imbalance at work: European comparisons. *Social Science & Medicine, 58*, 1483–1499. doi:10.1016/S0277-9536(03)00351-4

Sinclair, R. R., Probst, T., Hammer, L. B., & Schaffer, M. M. (2013). Low income families and occupational health: Implications of economic stress for work-family conflict research and practice. In A. G. Antoniou & C. L. Cooper (Eds.), *The psychology of the recession on the workplace* (pp. 308–323). Northampton, MA: Edward Elgar Publishing. doi:10.4337/9780857933843.00030

Skinner, E. A., Edge, K., Altman, J., & Sherwood, H. (2003). Searching for the structure of coping: A review and critique of category systems for classifying ways of coping. *Psychological Bulletin, 129*, 216–269. doi:10.1037/0033-2909.129.2.216

Skipper, J. K., Jr., Jung, F. D., & Coffey, L. (1990). Nurses and shiftwork: Effects on physical health and mental depression. *Journal of Advanced Nursing, 15*(7), 835–842.

Spector, P. E. (1987). Method variance as an artifact in self-reported affect and perceptions at work: Myth or significant problem? *Journal of Applied Psychology, 72*, 438–443. doi:10.1037/0021-9010.72.3.438

Spector, P. E. (1992). A consideration of the validity and meaning of self-report measures of job conditions. In C. L. Cooper & I. T. Robertson (Eds.), *International review of industrial and organizational psychology* (Vol. 7, pp. 123–151). New York, NY: Wiley.

Spector, P. E. (2006). Method variance in organizational research: Truth or urban legend? *Organizational Research Methods, 9*, 221–232. doi:10.1177/1094428105284955

Stansfeld, S., Fuhrer, R., Shipley, M., & Marmot, M. (1999). Work characteristics predict psychiatric disorder: Prospective results from the Whitehall II Study. *Occupational and Environmental Medicine, 56*(5), 302–307.

Stansfeld, S. A., Shipley, M. J., Head, J., & Fuhrer, R. (2012). Repeated job strain and the risk of depression: Longitudinal analyses from the Whitehall II study. *American Journal of Public Health, 102*, 2360–2366. doi:10.2105/AJPH.2011.300589

Steptoe, A., Wardle, J., Lipsey, Z., Mills, R., Oliver, G., Jarvis, M., & Kirschbaum, C. (1998). A longitudinal study of work load and variations in psychological well-being, cortisol, smoking, and alcohol consumption. *Annals of Behavioral Medicine, 20*(2), 84–91.

Tausig, M., & Fenwick, R. (2011). *Work and mental health in social context.* New York, NY: Springer. doi:10.1007/978-1-4614-0625-9

Theorell, T., Hammarström, A., Aronsson, G., Träskman Bendz, L., Grape, T., Hogstedt, C., . . . Hall, C. (2015). A systematic review including meta-analysis of work environment and depressive symptoms. *BMC Public Health, 15*(738). doi:10.1186/s12889-015-1954-4

Tversky, A., & Kahneman, D. (1974). Judgment under uncertainty: Heuristics and biases. *Science, 185*(4157), 1124–1131. doi:10.1126/science.185.4157.1124

Virtanen, M., Honkonen, T., Kivimäki, M., Ahola, K., Vahtera, J., Aromaa, A., & Lönnqvist, J. (2007). Work stress, mental health and antidepressant medication findings from the Health 2000 Study. *Journal of Affective Disorders, 98*, 189–197. doi:10.1186/1471-2458-12-236

Wang, J. L. (2004). Perceived work stress and major depressive episodes in a population of employed Canadians over 18 years old. *Journal of Nervous and Mental Disease, 192*(2), 160–163.

Wang, J., Schmitz, N., Dewa, C., & Stansfeld, S. (2009). Changes in perceived job strain and the risk of major depression: Results from a population-based longitudinal study. *American Journal of Epidemiology, 169*, 1085–1091. doi:10.1093/aje/kwp037

Warr, P. (1987). *Work, unemployment, and mental health.* New York, NY: Oxford University Press.

Warr, P. (1994). A conceptual framework for the study of work and mental health. *Work & Stress, 8*, 84–97. doi:10.1080/02678379408259982

West, S. H., Ahern, M., Byrnes, M., & Kwanten, L. (2007). New graduate nurses adaptation to shift work: Can we help? *Collegian (Royal College of Nursing, Australia), 14*(1), 23–30.

World Health Organization. (2013). *Suicide rates per 100,000 by country, year and sex.* Retrieved from www.who.int/mental_health/prevention/suicide_rates/en

Ylipaavalniemi, J., Kivimäki, M., Elovainio, M., Virtanen, M., Keltikangas-Järvinen, L., & Vahtera, J. (2005). Psychosocial work characteristics and incidence of newly diagnosed depression: A prospective cohort study of three different models. *Social Science & Medicine, 61,* 111–122. doi:10.1016/j.socscimed.2004.11.038

Zapf, D., Dormann, C., & Frese, M. (1996). Longitudinal studies in organizational stress research: A review of the literature with reference to methodological issues. *Journal of Occupational Health Psychology, 1,* 145–169. doi:10.1037/1076-8998.1.2.145

Zung, W. W. K. (1965). A self-rating depression scale. *Archives of General Psychiatry, 12,* 63–70. doi:10.1001/archpsyc.1965.01720310065008

FOUR

Epidemiology, Medical Disease, and OHP

KEY CONCEPTS AND FINDINGS COVERED IN CHAPTER 4

MacMahon and Pugh (1970), in their landmark textbook, wrote, "Epidemiology is the study of the distribution and determinants of disease frequency in man" (p. 1). Their anachronistic use of the word "man," more concretely refers to human populations. Knowledge of disease distribution may yield clues to the mechanisms that bring about disease. Kasl (1978) underlined the applicability of epidemiologic methods to understanding work stress processes. He emphasized the idea that epidemiology and the social sciences share many of the same research methods. Epidemiology's concern with the health of populations is particularly useful in studying work stress.

Some of the research covered in Chapter 3 targeted specific populations (e.g., workers who lost their jobs through no fault of their own and stably employed workers) and involved a type of study associated with epidemiology, the prospective cohort study. The prospective cohort study, the make-up of which was described in Chapter 2, is the bread and butter of epidemiologic research. This chapter examines the impact of psychosocial working conditions on medical-related outcomes, concentrating on cardiovascular disease (CVD). It is important to study CVD because it is the leading cause of death globally (WHO, 2013). In addition, the ramifications of CVD include great economic costs in terms of lost work, disability payments, and medical expenses (Nichols, Bell, Pedula, & O'Keeffe-Rosetti, 2010).

Later in the chapter, the relation of psychosocial working conditions to musculoskeletal problems is explored. Although it is intuitive that working conditions that require heavy lifting or repetitive motion (e.g., typing on a keyboard) are risk factors for musculoskeletal problems, psychosocial factors also play a role in the development of these problems. Finally, the chapter briefly examines three other health-related outcomes—sickness absence, self-rated health, and fatigue.

CARDIOVASCULAR DISEASE

In this chapter, the term "CVD" refers to a set of conditions including atherosclerosis, ischemic heart disease, myocardial infarction, angina pectoris, and hypertension. Atherosclerosis refers to the buildup of plaque on artery walls, thus narrowing the arteries, and consequently reducing or blocking blood flow. Low-density lipoprotein (LDL or the "bad" cholesterol) particles get stuck in the endothelium, the lining of artery walls. The particles can become oxidized, provoking an inflammatory immune response involving white blood cells. The white blood cells, however, are not equipped to process oxidized LDL particles, which break up, creating further damage. Atherosclerosis is an important contributor to the development of ischemia, which refers to inadequate blood flow to tissues. The chapter, however, is exclusively concerned with ischemia as it pertains to the heart.

Myocardial infarction (MI) is the medical term for a heart attack. The blood supplies oxygen to tissues throughout the body. In an MI, heart cells die as a result of being denied sufficient oxygen, often owing to a narrowing or blockage in one or more of the coronary arteries. Often a precursor to an MI, angina refers to chest pains that sometimes occur when coronary ischemia prevents sufficient oxygen and nutrients from getting to cells making up the heart muscle. The heart must pump harder to deliver the oxygen and nutrients throughout the body and to the heart itself. This extra work causes a buildup of lactic acid (the same substance that accumulates in the legs of a runner during a grueling workout). Lactic acid in the heart muscle is the source of the pain. Hypertension, another risk factor for an MI, refers to high blood pressure. With high blood pressure, the heart must also work harder.

A Riddle

There is a riddle that involves CVD. Although the death rates from the disease have declined in recent years, the prevalence rates have remained steady. Research conducted by the American Heart Association and the Centers for Disease Control and Prevention indicates that rates of death attributable to CVD have declined in the United States in recent years (Go et al., 2013). For example, the age-adjusted death rate from CVD in 2009 was 236 per 100,000, a decline of 33% from 1999. However, over the same 10-year period, the prevalence of CVD in the United States has remained relatively stable (Go et al., 2013, Charts 2 to 8). Landsbergis et al. (2011) reported that the United States has experienced reductions in CVD-related mortality over 40 years without a concomitant decline in the incidence of CVD. Improvements in CVD treatment are the likely explanation of this inconsistency between a decline in mortality unaccompanied by a parallel decline in prevalence. Although Go et al. (2013) and Landsbergis et al. (2011) observed a decline in the prevalence of cigarette smoking (a risk factor for CVD), it is possible that the rates of CVD have remained steady because of the influence of other factors such as psychosocial stressors, including work-related stressors.

Psychosocial Working Conditions Could Affect CVD Through Health Behaviors

There are two general pathways by which the psychosocial work environment can affect CVD risk: (a) an indirect pathway in which the work environment influences health behaviors that in turn have an adverse effect on CV health, and (b) a pathway in which the work environment slowly and cumulatively influences biological functioning. In the first general pathway, adverse workplace characteristics drive the worker, perhaps by precipitating psychological distress, to consume alcohol (see Chapter 3), smoke more, or overeat. Job stress may provoke attempts at self-medicating (by overeating, smoking) in response to challenges to homeostasis, or it may diminish the self-control (Ayyagari, & Sindelar, 2010) needed to exercise regularly and regulate other health behaviors. Over time, these behavioral changes erode the physical health of the worker. Smoking contributes to CVD, cancer, and emphysema. Obesity contributes to CVD and diabetes. Reduced leisure time physical exercise contributes to poor CV health and weight gain.

Cigarette Smoking

The research on the relation of psychosocial working conditions to smoking has been mixed (see Table 4.1). Because few people start to smoke after age 22 (Ayyagari, & Sindelar, 2010), the research in this area concerns mainly the relation of working conditions to workers continuing to smoke. The relation of psychosocial working conditions to smoking is unclear, with some studies finding a relation and others not, although, on balance, the evidence suggests that it may be easier to give up smoking if work is less stressful.

Obesity and Weight Gain

Obesity refers to the buildup of excess fat owing to an imbalance between consumption and energy expenditure. It is a risk factor for CVD, stroke, and other serious health problems. Although the causes of obesity are multifactorial (e.g., genetic, cultural), the increase in the prevalence of obesity in the last few decades is too rapid to be explained by genetic and cultural processes (Solovieva, Lallukka, Virtanen, & Viikari-Juntura, 2013), suggesting that these changes in prevalence have other sources, including changes in people's work lives. There are at least two reasons to suspect that psychosocial workplace stressors contribute to obesity. First, job stress, as will be discussed later in the chapter, affects cortisol levels, and excess cortisol secretion is related to the accumulation of abdominal fat and metabolic abnormalities (Björntorp. 2001). Second, overeating or eating unhealthful foods is sometimes a response to stress that makes an individual feel better (Greeno & Wing, 1994; Sproesser, Schupp, & Renner, 2014).

As seen in Table 4.1, research often relies on body mass index (BMI), a quotient equal to weight in kilograms divided by height in meters squared. BMI is a measure of relative weight. BMI removes "the dependency of weight on height," thus indexing relative obesity (Keys, Fidanza, Karvonen, Kimura, & Taylor, 1972). Table 4.1 includes results showing no effects for psychosocial stressors on weight gain (Landsbergis et al., 1998; Reed et al., 1989). Findings showing that psychosocial stressors affect weight gain (the "positive associations") tend to be small, in keeping with the results of a meta-analysis of prospective studies (Solovieva et al., 2013) and the conclusion of a review paper (Wardle, Chida, Gibson, Whitaker, & Steptoe, 2011). Wardle et al. (2011) tended to find positive associations in higher quality studies. Variability in findings has been attributed to factors such as inadequate power, single-item measures, confounding working conditions and SES, and overcontrol of covariates such as mediating variables (Solovieva et al., 2013; Wardle et al., 2011).

Heterogeneity in individuals' responses to job stress may also help account for the absence of more pronounced effects of job stress on weight gain. Gram Quist et al. (2013) hypothesized that some of the variability in research findings results from adverse psychosocial working conditions having a two-way relationship with weight, that is, in some workers, adverse job conditions lead to weight gain, and in others, weight loss, a hypothesis the investigators' findings have borne out. Other investigators have also identified heterogeneous effects of stressors (Block, He, Zaslavsky, Ding, & Ayanian, 2009; Deb, Gallo, Ayyagari, Fletcher, & Sindelar, 2011; Nyberg et al., 2011). Block et al. found that, compared with average-weight coworkers, initially heavier workers were more vulnerable to job stressors precipitating weight gain. Deb et al. found that job loss outside the individual's control was more likely to precipitate weight gain in individuals who already manifested problematic health behaviors. Nyberg et al. found the change over an average of 4 years from a nonstrain to a strain job co-occurred with weight gain in the initially nonobese, and weight loss in the initially obese.

Leisure Time Physical Activity

High-strain jobs (jobs that combine high workload and low control) may create fatigue in workers and require them to devote more time to recovery, tamping down the desire for leisure time physical activity. The research evidence linking adverse psychosocial working conditions to reduced leisure time physical activity is mixed, but

TABLE 4.1 Longitudinal Studies That Bear on the Relation of Psychosocial Workplace Factors on Health Behaviors

Study Team	Country	Sample	Time Lag	Control Variables	Major Findings	Comments
Smoking						
Ayyagari & Sindelar (2010)	U.S.	3,825 current and former smokers (50% ♀); Health & Retirement Survey	At least twice, 2 y apart up to 8 y & 4 waves	Sociodemo., occupation, time, health	High job stress → ↓ smoking cessation.	Nationally representative sample of age 50–64-year-olds at time 1. Controlled time b/c smokers tend to give up smoking over time. Job stress is rough binary measure.
Eriksen (2005)	Norway	2,452 nurses' aides, smokers (96% ♀)	15 mo	Sociodemo., baseline daily cigarette consumption	Long work hrs → ↓ smoking cessation. No effect for DCS variables	Long work hours reflect >36 h/week.
Eriksen (2006)	Norway	1,203 nurses' aides, ex-smokers (97% ♀)	15 mo	Sociodemo.	Poor social climate → relapse Exposure threats & violence → relapse No effect for DCS variables	Social climate reflects a "supportive, trustful, relaxed" work unit No other covariates than sociodemo.
Falba et al. (2005)	U.S.	3,025 (<50% ♀) smokers and former smokers at time 1, age 50–60	2 y	Sociodemo., alcohol use, cancer, spouse smoked	Involuntary job loss → relapse in former smokers Involuntary job loss → ↑ smoking in those who smoked at time 1	Nationally representative sample over cross section of occupations. Past research on smoking mostly limited to single work sites.
Heikkilä et al. (2012b)	6 samples from 5 European countries	>52,000 (50% ♀). one-stage meta-analysis	1–9 y	Sociodemo.	High-strain jobs, support -| smoking. High-strain jobs, support -| smoking cessation.	Treated continuous IVs categorically.
Kouvonen et al. (2009)	Finland	>4,900 smokers (77% ♀); Hospital Study + 10-Town Study	3.6 y	Sociodemo., other health behaviors (e.g., alcohol), anxiety	Low strain jobs → smoking cessation; Control → smoking cessation.	Strain & control divided into quartiles.

(continued)

123

TABLE 4.1 Longitudinal Studies That Bear on the Relation of Psychosocial Workplace Factors on Health Behaviors (*continued*)

Study Team	Country	Sample	Time Lag	Control Variables	Major Findings	Comments
Landsbergis et al. (1998)	U.S.	189 white & blue collar ♂'s	3 y	Sociodemo.	Gain in DL → ↓ smoking No effect for ΨWL or strain	Change–change study; cannot ascertain if the change in DL antedated the change in smoking or vice versa. Treated continuous IVs categorically.
Ota et al. (2010)	Japan	571 ♂ who smoked	2 y	Baseline sciodemo., treatment for CVD, alcohol intake, smoking intensity	High-strain jobs, support ↛ smoking cessation	Treated continuous IVs categorically. Smoking dichotomized.
Reed et al. (1989)	U.S.	>4,700 ♂ of Japanese ancestry	18 y	Age	ΨWL, DA, & strain ↛ smoking	Men largely remained in the same jobs but nature of jobs could have changed over 18 y. IVs were imputed, treated as quartiles.
Sanderson et al. (2005)	Denmark	4,700 ♀ nurses who smoked	6 y	None	Day shift → smoking cessation Perceived control at work → smoking cessation	Control treated categorically.
Slopen et al. (2013)	U.S.	4,938 (≈ 50% ♀)	10 y	Sociodemo.	High work stress at time 1 & 2 → smoking at T1 and T2 Workers attempting to quit between T1 & T2: high work stress → lack of success	Work stress was amalgam of DA, SkD, ΨWL, coworker & supervisor support, & job insecurity. Cannot ascertain temporal priority, particularly with 10 y between data collection waves.
P. Smith et al. (2008)	Canada	>3,400 in variety of sectors (69% ♂) NPHS	2 y	Sociodemo., personal stress, baseline smoking, BMI, distress	Low control → ↑ smoking	Treated continuous IVs categorically. Effect on smoking more apparent in lower SES and less well-educated workers.

Obesity and Weight Gain

Berset et al. (2011)	Switzerland	76 service workers (72% ♂)	2 y	Sociodemo., physical health	Control → ↓ BMI Work-related social stressors → ↑ BMI ΨWL & ERI ↛ BMI	Continuous IVs.
Block et al. (2009)	U.S.	1,300 (53% ♀) representative sample of residents	9 y	Age, gender, and DV assessed the previous wave	Less SkD (♂ only) less DA, more ΨWL, & more financial stress interacted with baseline weight in such a way as to accelerate weight gain in those who were initially heavier	Biased toward the null b/c not clear that workplace stress at baseline characterized the workplaces over the 9 y of the study. Continuous IVs.
Brunner et al. (2007)	U.K.	>10,000 civil servants (⅔ ♂) Whitehall II	Multiple assessments over 19 y	Sociodemo., employment grade, baseline weight, health behaviors	No. of assessment occasions individuals experienced iso-strain → ↑ BMI obesity.	Iso-strain (high ΨWL, low DL. Treated continuous IVs categorically.
Deb et al. (2012)	U.S.	>20,000 (50% ♀); Health & Retirement Survey	9 waves over 18 y	Sociodemo., baseline BMI, job stress, risk aversion	Business closing → ↑ BMI	Results suggest that the impact of job loss on BMI is largely confined to individuals with already unhealthy BMIs.
Gram Quist et al. (2013)	Denmark	3,647 ♀ health care workers	3 y	Sociodemo., physical work, seniority	Role conflicts → ↑ BMI (at least 2 kg/m²) Role clarity → ↑ BMI and ↓ BMI	Small no. of males. Organized analyses to reveal that role clarity can → gain in BMI in some and loss in BMI in others.
Hannerz et al. (2004)	Denmark	1,980 ♂'s DWECS Study	5 y	Sociodemo., employment grade, baseline weight, health behaviors	Job insecurity → ↑ BMI ΨWL & DA ↛ BMI but each IV interacted with initial BMI such that the initially heavier were more affected	Treated continuous IVs categorically.

TABLE 4.1 Longitudinal Studies That Bear on the Relation of Psychosocial Workplace Factors on Health Behaviors (*continued*)

Study Team	Country	Sample	Time Lag	Control Variables	Major Findings	Comments
Iversen et al. (2012)	Denmark	4,700 (58% ♀)	10 y	Sociodemo., physical activity, alcohol, smoking, nonwork stress, childhood adversity	♀s who experienced 3+ major work life events → ↑ weight In ♂s, work LEs ↛ weight	Examples of major work LEs include loss of work & serious conflicts with coworkers. LEs were ascertained retrospectively at follow-up. Temporal ordering of IV & DV could not be ascertained.
Kivimäki et al. (2002)	Finland	800 initially healthy factory workers (⅔ ♂)	10 y	Sociodemo., baseline BMI	ERI → ↑ BMI Control → ↓ BMI No effect for strain	Long follow-up likely attenuated effects (although there were statistical controls for job changes). Treated continuous IVs categorically.
Landsbergis et al. (1998)	U.S.	189 white & blue collar ♂s	3 y	Sociodemo.	Changes in DL, ΨWL, & strain ↛ changes in overweight status or BMI	See the earlier-mentioned entry for Landsbergis et al. (1998).
Nyberg et al. (2012)	Belgium, Finland, U.K.	>42,000 (≈ 50% ♀)	Av. 4 y	Sociodemo., baseline BMI, smoking	Baseline strain ↛ later weight gain at follow-up See comment	One-stage meta-analysis. Change from no-strain to strain co-occurred with change from nonobese to obese. Change–change analysis.
Overgaard et al. (2006)	Denmark	15,000 ♀ nurses	6 y	Familial obesity, smoking, physical activity	ΨWL & control ↛ weight gain	Treated continuous IVs categorically. Marginally sig. trend for ΨWL or control to predict weight gain in nurses who were obese at baseline.

Study	Country	Sample	Follow-up	Controls	Findings	Notes
Reed et al. (1989)	U.S.	>4,700 ♂s of Japanese ancestry	18 y	Age	ΨWL, DA, control, & strain ↛ BMI	See the earlier-mentioned entry for Reed et al. (1989).
Roos et al. (2013)	Finland	7,000 (>80% ♀) municipal workers, >40 y of age	5–7 y	Sociodemo., baseline weight, health behaviors	Physical threats → ↑ weight gain in ♀s; Hazardous exposures (e.g., dirt, solvents, etc.), night shift → ↑ weight in ♂s	IVs in quartiles. Long follow-up could have attenuated effects.

Leisure Time Physical Activity

Study	Country	Sample	Follow-up	Controls	Findings	Notes
Fransson et al. (2012)	6 samples from 5 European countries	>56,000 (50% ♀). one-stage meta-analysis	2–9 y	Baseline PA; Baseline DC quadrants	High-strain or passive jobs → ↓ PA; Low control → ↓ PA; ↓ PA → high- strain or passive jobs	Reverse-causal effect was not as strong as the hypothesized causal effect. Treated continuous IVs and DV categorically.
Popham & Mitchell (2006)	U.K.	9,400 (>50% ♀)	Every 2 y for 8 y	No. of children at home, health	No. of hrs. worked → ↓ PA	The relation of hrs. worked to PA was concurrent.
Reed et al. (1989)	U.S.	>4,700 ♂ of Japanese ancestry	18 y	Age	ΨWL, DA, control, & strain ↛ PA	See the earlier-mentioned entry for Reed et al. (1989).
P. Smith et al. (2008)	Canada	>3,400 (79% ♂) NPHS	Every 2 y for 8 y	Sociodemo., BMI, health, baseline PA, personal stress	Low control → ↓ PA	IV in quartiles.

♂, male; ♀, female; ΨWL, psychological workload or psychological demands; Baseline DVs, baseline versions of the dependent variables; b/c, because; BMI, body mass index; DA, decision authority; DCS, demand–control–support; DL, decision latitude; IVs, principal independent variables; MH, mental health; NPHS, National Population Health Survey; PA, physical activity; sig., significant; SkD, skill discretion; Sociodemo., sociodemographic variables.

on balance is more supportive (Fransson et al., 2012; P. Smith et al., 2008; Popham & Mitchell, 2006) than not (Reed et al., 1989). Based on research on large combined samples (Fransson et al., 2012), it appears that adverse psychosocial working conditions are related to reduced engagement in leisure time physical activity. Fransson et al. (2012) also found a smaller, but significant, reverse-causal association between physical inactivity at baseline and a later shift into high-strain or passive jobs.

Summary[1]

The research findings on smoking are not sufficiently convincing to affirm that psychosocial working conditions contribute to smoking frequency or its cessation. The findings with regard to weight gain and leisure time physical activity are somewhat more persuasive. There is evidence that initially at-risk workers, when exposed to psychosocial job stressors, are more vulnerable to weight gain. Fransson et al.'s (2012) massive study suggests that psychosocial working conditions influence the extent to which individuals engage in leisure time physical activity.

Biological Links From Psychosocial Working Conditions to CVD

The first general pathway from psychosocial working conditions to CVD is potentially through the health behaviors described earlier. The second general pathway involves chains of biological links from psychosocial stressors to CVD. Findings from primate experiments revealed proatherosclerotic effects of social stressors, controlling for dietary cholesterol, blood pressure, and so on (Manuck, Kaplan, Adams, & Clarkson, 1988). In humans, persisting adverse psychosocial work environments have been thought to precipitate bodily changes that, cumulatively, compromise health (Terrill & Garofalo, 2012). The carotid arteries, which originate in the aorta, supply oxygenated blood to the neck and head. The thickness of the intima and the media, the inner two layers of the arteries, is an indicator of the extent of atherosclerosis even in asymptomatic individuals. Job strain, controlling for confounding factors (e.g., SES and early life risk factors), is related, at least cross-sectionally, to carotid intima-media thickness (Hintsanen et al., 2005; Kivimäki et al., 2007), although not all research is in agreement (Rosvall et al., 2002). A reverse-causal effect from intima-media thickness to job strain, however, is not plausible.

Pinning down the exact pathway from psychosocial workplace stressors to CVD is difficult because research in this area requires detailed longitudinal studies on the relation of stressors to small, preclinical physiological changes that accumulate over time. Studies by Cobb (1974) and Chandola et al. (2008) highlight some of those changes. Cobb found evidence that a major psychosocial stressor, involuntary job loss, is related to physiological changes (e.g., serum cholesterol elevations) that can persist over time but are subject to the ameliorative influence of another psychosocial variable, social support. Chandola et al. (2008) found that the link between job strain and CVD is partly mediated by the impact of strain on the components of the metabolic syndrome, a state that encompasses large waist circumference, elevated serum triglycerides, elevated blood pressure, low heart rate variability, and morning rise in cortisol (more on cortisol a little later).

---

[1] Owing to the multifaceted nature of the material covered in this chapter, a summary is placed after each section rather than at the chapter's conclusion.

Workplace Stressors and Human Biology

Workplace stressors are superimposed on a biological system that has evolved over eons. In response to threat, fight-or-flight reactions, with their underlying activation of the hypothalamus–pituitary–adrenal (HPA) axis and the autonomic nervous system, have survival value (Selye, 1976). The hypothalamus signals the autonomic nervous system. HPA-mediated arousal reactions include increased heart rate and respiration, as well as increased blood pressure and the release of glucose from the liver (Cannon, 1929; Walker 20007). The sympathetic nervous system (SNS), a component of the autonomic nervous system, although continually active, will accelerate heart rate and increase blood pressure in response to a major stressor. The activation of another component of the autonomic nervous system, the parasympathetic nervous system, plays an opposite role by tamping down sympathetic activation and maintaining homeostasis, although it is important to note that our conception of homeostasis has changed since the work of Selye (Sterling, 2012).

Although advantageous in rare emergency situations, repeated episodes of HPA-sympathetic arousal are detrimental when provoked by daily workplace conditions. Repeated acute episodes of arousal have been hypothesized to lead to hemodynamic turbulence, the shearing force of which, over time, contributes to the development of endothelial damage (Barnett, Spence, Manuck, & Jennings, 1997). Although there has been contrary evidence (Mann, 2006), the bulk of the evidence suggests that job strain is related to elevated ambulatory blood pressure (Landsbergis, Dobson, Koutsouras, & Schnall, 2013). Ambulatory blood pressure refers to round-the-clock blood pressure, which can be measured by a device that is worn 24 hours a day, even while an individual is asleep.

The occurrence of stressful conditions is processed by the central nervous system (CNS), with nerve impulses exciting the hypothalamus, the pearl-size neural control center located above the brain stem. In response to impulses signaling threat, the hypothalamus secretes corticotropin-releasing hormone (CRH) into the hypophyseal-portal blood vessels. CRH stimulates the pituitary gland, a pea-size organ that extends off the bottom of the hypothalamus at the brain's base, to release adrenocorticotropic hormone (ACTH) into the bloodstream. ACTH, in turn, stimulates the cortex, or outer layer, of the adrenal glands, located atop the kidneys, to release cortisol (hydrocortisone), a steroid hormone that is diffused through the bloodstream. To a lesser extent, ACTH stimulates the adrenal cortex to release aldosterone, a steroid hormone that promotes sodium retention and elevates blood pressure. Excess aldosterone and cortisol have been implicated in the development of hypertension (Kidambi et al., 2007). Homeostatic mechanisms like this include a negative feedback component. Excess cortisol serves to suppress the secretion of CRH and ACTH. In turn, cortisol levels are reduced.

Cortisol and Epinephrine

Cortisol is instrumental in the body's response to stressors. The process of HPA activation is important because it can be stress-protective, with steroids like cortisol stanching "pathophysiological responses to tissue injury and inflammation" (Nijm & Jonasson, 2009). Cortisol also stimulates the liver to create new supplies of glucose. The liver pours these new supplies of glucose into the bloodstream to help the body respond to stressors in at least two important ways. First, because the new supplies of glucose go to the voluntary muscles, which are critical to fight-or-flight, there is no need for glucose to be diverted from the brain to the voluntary muscles. Second, cortisol helps both to direct the newly released glucose to the voluntary muscles and divert glucose away from other organ systems that are not important in fight-or-flight responding (e.g., the digestive system, the immune system, the reproductive system).

In addition to releasing CRH, the hypothalamus also responds to stressors by communicating with the adrenal medulla (the center of each adrenal gland) through the SNS (sympathetic adrenal medullary—SAM—axis). The SAM and HPA axes are activated synergistically and are closely connected. In response to a stressor, the SAM axis is activated more quickly, and its effects recede more quickly than in the case of the HPA axis. SNS signals stimulate the adrenal medulla to secrete epinephrine (adrenaline). Epinephrine increases blood pressure and stimulates the heart to work harder, factors that are likely to be adaptive in fight-or-flight but not necessarily adaptive in the workplace. Chronic workplace stressors have the potential, over time, to lead to the dysregulation of SAM functioning. Schaubroeck and Ganster (1993) found that high levels of chronic exposure to job demands were related to dampened SAM-based CV reactivity, for example, lower levels of blood pressure elevations in response to laboratory challenge, but higher resting blood pressure. In more normally functioning individuals (workers who experience lower levels of chronic demands), one would expect more heightened reactivity to laboratory challenge and lower resting blood pressure.

Allostasis and Allostatic Load

The concept of allostasis refers to the process by which an organism maintains its physiological integrity by changing to meet environmental challenges and demands (McEwen, 1998). Allostatic systems help maintain bodily control by adapting to circumstances, although the thinking regarding allostasis differs from Selye's homeostatic model. The allostatic model is more dynamic than Selye's model. In the allostatic model, a range of set points is allowed as the organism adjusts to new environmental circumstances (Sterling, 2012). For example, in the allostatic model, there is no single blood pressure set point, deviations from which lead to the activation of mechanisms to defend against the change. Sterling observed that "[blood] pressure spends about as much time far below the most frequent level as above it" and that this state of affairs "is not predicted by a model of set-point [plus] arousal-evoked elevation" (p. 7). The process of adapting to adverse conditions has a price that is called "allostatic load" (McEwen, 1998).

The idea of allostatic load includes the concepts of primary mediators, secondary mediators, and a tertiary phase called "allostatic overload" (Ganster & Rosen, 2012). Primary mediators comprise the release of stress hormones such as cortisol and epinephrine as well as pro- and anti-inflammatory proteins known as "cytokines," with the CNS playing a key role in a chain of actions that leads to their release. These substances prepare "the organism to cope with demands that threaten to disrupt homeostatic systems" (p. 1091). Ganster, Fox, and Dwyer (2001) found that elevations in after-work cortisol levels mediated the relation of workload and control to later health care costs, a proxy for a broad range of health conditions. The chronic activation of primary mediators affects secondary mediators, in particular metabolic (e.g., excess glucose, cholesterol), cardiovascular (e.g., higher blood pressure), and immune systems (e.g., excess fibrinogen). If these secondary mediators chronically deviate outside of their normal ranges, they can bring about allostatic overload.

Long-term stimulation constitutes a burden, or an allostatic load on the body, and can lead to persistent problems (Terrill & Garofalo, 2012). A primate study (Kaplan, Manuck, Adams, Weingand, & Clarkson, 1987) examined the impact of long-term arousal via exposure to social stress. Kaplan et al. (1987) found that social stressors, through persistent sympathetic arousal, play a role in the development of atherosclerosis *independently* of heart rate, serum lipid concentrations, and blood pressure. Moreover, the effects of chronic stimulation could persist even after the chronic stimulus situation has receded. Sterling and Eyer (1981) noted that animal research has shown that "when arousal is maintained for long periods, the elevation of blood pressure tends to be sustained even when the arousing stimulus is removed" (p. 19).

Dysregulation of the HPA Axis and Other Harmful Effects

Persistent psychosocial stress can lead to dysregulation of the HPA axis, and can come in the form of a blunted HPA response to new stressors, a condition associated with inflammatory disease (Nijm & Jonasson, 2009). Other research documents the association between atherosclerosis and total cortisol exposure (Dekker et al., 2008), elevated cortisol response to controlled mental stress (Hamer, O'Donnell, Lahiri, & Steptoe, 2010), and a flattening of the expected decline in cortisol levels over the course of a normal day (Matthews, Schwartz, Cohen, & Seeman, 2006). Although locally, the HPA product cortisol has anti-inflammatory effects, its systemic effects can be proinflammatory (Walker, 2007). In summary, the research findings suggest that HPA dysregulation plays a role in the development of atherosclerosis.

Other harmful systemic cortisol-related effects include elevating lipid levels (e.g., cholesterol), promoting abdominal obesity, preventing angiogenesis (the development of new blood vessels out of older ones), and scarring of heart muscle cells (Walker, 2007), all risk factors for CVD. Excess cortisol may also play a role in insulin resistance (Henry Ginsberg, July 4, 2013), a risk factor for type 2 diabetes and CVD.

Summary

The foundation for linking psychosocial stressors, including workplace stressors, to CVD was laid by Cannon and Selye (see Chapter 1). Once signaled via the CNS that a threat is present or, sometimes, anticipated, the HPA and SAM axes play important roles in mobilizing for action. This mobilization has an evolutionary basis, particularly given the survival value of fight-or-flight. However, when there is excessive mobilization, say, as a result of psychosocial stressors chronically experienced in the context of the modern workplace, such mobilization can be harmful. Animal research has linked chronic social stress to coronary disease. Hormonal signals and the SNS drive increases in blood pressure and heart rate, which are thought to be harmful if these increases persist as a result of chronic exposure to stressors.

The concept of allostasis also comes into play. Allostatic systems help maintain bodily control by adapting to circumstances, but a range of set points is allowed as the organism adjusts to new environmental circumstances. However, chronic arousal leads to allostatic overload and, via chains of mediators (e.g., excess cortisol, higher blood pressure), increased risk of the development of CVD.

Depression and CVD

Chapter 3 covered research on the relation of psychosocial working conditions to depression and psychological distress. The relation of psychosocial working conditions to depression and distress is not always acknowledged in research on working conditions and CVD. Although HPA dysregulation has been implicated in the development of CVD,

HPA dysregulation is also associated with depression. High levels of cortisol have been found in depressed individuals, particularly in patients with symptoms of emotional arousal (Sachar, Hellman, Fukushima, & Gallagher, 1970). Gold et al. (1986) found that although cortisol levels were higher in depressed patients than in well controls, cortisol levels in patients who had recovered from depression were no different from levels found in controls. Consistent with the view that disturbance in HPA functioning is associated with depression, Gold et al. found that among the depressed, the pituitary's release of CRH, when experimentally stimulated with ACTH, was weakened.

Musselman et al. (1996) found that depressed patients exhibited exaggerated platelet reactivity, a potential contributor to CVD. Platelets are cell fragments (a platelet does not have a nucleus) that circulate in the blood, and are important in clotting. Psychological stress precipitates HPA and SAM responding, which includes epinephrine release, increased blood flow, and shear stress in arteries, all relevant to platelet activation. Markovits and Matthews (1991) outlined evidence for the view that epinephrine and increased blood flow drive platelet activity to excess, contributing to atherosclerosis. Consistent with this evidence, Nabi et al. (2010), in a 7-year longitudinal study of more than 20,000 workers, found that, controlling for confounders (e.g., smoking, BMI), depression increased the risk of CVD by about two-thirds compared with CVD risk in nondepressed peers.

In a two-stage meta-analysis of 11 incidence studies ($n > 140,000$; the aforementioned study by Nabi et al. was not included), Nicholson, Kuper, and Hemingway (2006) found that depression, adjusting for confounders, almost doubled an individual's risk for developing heart disease. The investigators, however, argued that the effect was likely an overestimate because of factors such as incomplete adjustment for covariates or failure to thoroughly exclude subjects with preclinical disease. Generally speaking, the idea that depression increases the risk of CVD is thought provoking, but more controlled research on the lines of Nabi et al. is needed.

Burnout and CVD

At least two prospective studies (Toker, Melamed, Berliner, Zeltser, & Shapira, 2012; Toppinen-Tanner, Ahola, Koskinen, & Väänänen, 2009) link burnout to CVD. Toppinen-Tanner et al. (2009), who followed almost 7,900 manual and nonmanual workers in the forest products industry in Finland, found that those with high levels of burnout at baseline were more likely to be hospitalized for CVD over the next 10 years in comparison with non–burned-out control workers, adjusting for confounders such as hypertension and diabetes at baseline. Toker et al. (2012), who followed more than 8,800, mostly white collar, Israeli workers for an average of 3.5 years, found that burnout predicted later CVD, controlling for conventional risk factors. When depression and burnout were in the same prediction equation, burnout was the more effective predictor. The 14-item burnout measure used in the study contained three items that tap physical exhaustion (e.g., "I feel physically drained"), which may have also reflected subclinical disease and the early stages of CVD. These findings and the findings of Toppinen-Tanner et al. are nonetheless important, and suggest a fertile area for future research.

Research Linking "Stress at Work" and Demand–Control Variables to CVD

As a preface to this section, it should be noted that, as mentioned in Chapter 3, researchers studying the link between psychosocial working conditions and CVD often converted continuous scales, for example, an independent variable such as decision latitude, into categorical variables, collapsing a great deal of information into a dichotomous or trichotomous factor, leading to underestimates of effect sizes. In this chapter, converting continuous factors into categorical variables (e.g., Kivimäki, Nyberg, et al., 2012) is often limited to the independent variables (e.g., decision latitude) because many of the dependent variables are naturally dichotomous (e.g., the presence or absence of CVD or CVD mortality). These conversions were extremely common.

Karasek and his colleagues extended the demand–control (DC) model beyond its application to mental health, linking the model to the development of CVD. Karasek, Baker, Marxer, Ahlbom, and Theorell (1981) proposed that high psychological workload (e.g., fast pace, high levels of task complexity) and low levels of job control or decision latitude (i.e., little freedom to make work-related decisions) jointly affect the risk of CVD. As noted in Chapter 3, Karasek wrote that high levels of job demands place a worker in "a motivated state of 'stress'" that goes unreleased when bereft of decision latitude. The combination of high workload and little latitude has adverse physiological consequences that pave the way for the development of CVD. Johnson, Hall, and Theorell (1989) advanced the view that workers with jobs in which they experience high workloads but are constrained by low levels of decision latitude are more likely than other workers to experience elevated sympathoadrenal arousal, which, over the long term contributes to the development of CVD. Adrenaline in the aroused individual accelerates heart rate, whereas other hormones precipitate vasoconstriction, which, when combined, lead to elevations in blood pressure.

This introduction to research on work stress and CVD begins with a case-control study involving more than 24,000 individuals living in 52 countries (the Interheart Study). Rosengren et al. (2004) found that in men, but not in women, "permanent stress at work" doubled the risk of a heart attack, controlling for a host of factors (e.g., cholesterol). The investigators also found that severe financial stress was related to increased risk of MI in both men and women.

Studies That Employed Imputation Strategies Linking DC Factors to CVD

Imputation methods assess working conditions independently of how workers in the study sample describe their jobs. Such methods thus eliminate recall and other biases that could affect data derived from interviews and questionnaires. An example of an imputation method would involve the use of averages obtained from workers in an independent sample who have the same job titles as the workers in a study sample. Those averages would be used to describe the jobs of the workers in the study sample. Sometimes, imputation methods involve the use of experts' ratings of the work associated with various job titles, ratings that were completed independently of the research to which the ratings are applied. A limitation of imputation methods is that because the actual jobs of the workers in a study are not directly described, the imputed characteristics at best imperfectly apply to the actual day-to-day activities of workers in the study. Everyone linked to one job title (e.g., middle school teachers) is treated as having the same exposures despite variability in working conditions among individuals holding that job title.

Nine studies (see Table 4.2) used imputation methods to assess psychosocial working conditions, and evaluate the link between those working conditions and CVD. Three had negative findings (Alterman, Shekelle, Vernon, & Burau, 1994; Hemmingsson & Lundberg, 2006; Reed et al., 1989) and six, positive (Andersen et al., 2004; Johnson,

TABLE 4.2 Studies That Used Imputation Methods to Investigate the Relation of Psychosocial Workplace Factors to CVD

Study Team	Country	Sample	Time Lag	Control Variables	Major Findings	Comments
Negative Findings						
Alterman et al. (1994)	U.S.	1,600 blue collar ♂s	10 y & 25 y	Age, BP, serum cholesterol, smoking, alcohol, & FH of CVD	DL, ΨWL, & strain ↛ 10 y incidence of CVD DL, ΨWL, & strain ↛ 25 yr. mortality from CVD	Treated continuous IVs categorically. Western Electric Plant in Cicero, Illinois, made famous in the Hawthorne studies. Workers were stably employed.
Hemmingsson & Lundberg (2006)	Sweden	>39,000 ♂s initially aged 39–41 SHEEP study	Up to 13 y	Initially free of CVD; SC of origin, health behaviors	ΨWL, strain, & low work support ↛ CVD Low control → ↑ smoking, heavy alcohol use, BMI	Treated continuous IVs categorically. Data on SC of origin was controlled. Stressors mediated impact of SC of origin; smoking, alcohol use mediated impact of stressors.
Reed et al. (1989)	U.S.	>4,700 ♂s of Japanese ancestry	18 y	Age; workers initially free of CVD	ΨWL, DA, control, & strain ↛ CVD & CVD mortality	Treated continuous IVs categorically. Worker largely remained in same jobs over follow-up. Absence of effect may reflect regional/cultural differences may have been at work and/or absence of industrial jobs in Hawaii.
Positive Findings						
Andersen et al. (2004)	Denmark	>16,000 (44% ♀)	6–22 y	Sociodemo., CV RFs	Low SkD → ↑ MI Low DL → ↑ MI ΨWL or support ↛ MI	Prospective (incidence) study. Treated continuous IVs categorically. In analyses limited to 5-y follow-up to minimize risk of changes in exposures, only DL → ↑ MI.

Study	Country	Sample	Duration/Design	Controls	Findings	Comments
Johnson et al. (1996)	Sweden	>2,900 ♂s	14 y	Sociodemo., health behaviors	Long-term low control → ↑ CV mortality Low control + low support → ↑ CV mortality	Nested case-control study; similar to retrospective cohort study. IVs divided into quartiles.
Mäntyniemi et al. (2012)	Finland	>69,000 (76% ♀)	4.6 y	Sociodemo., baseline medical conditions	Job strain → ↑ CVD disability	Treated continuous IVs categorically. DV was retirement owing to CVD disability.
Murphy (1991)	U.S.	>9,800 all under age 65. Both genders well represented but exact nos. not clear.	Case-control study	Age	Low control → ↑ CVD disability Active jobs → ↓ CVD disability Hazardous jobs → ↑ CVD disability	IVs treated as quartiles. Used Social Security database to identify severe CVD disability & a 2nd data set comprising a representative sample of Americans.
Steenland et al. (1997)	U.S.	>3,500 ♂s NHANES1	12–16 y	Sociodemo., CV RFs	High control → ↓ CVD Strain ↛ CVD In BC subsample, active jobs → ↓ CVD	Prospective (incidence) study. Treated continuous IVs categorically.
Theorell et al. (1998)	Sweden	>1,000 ♂s 45–64 y old	10 y	Sociodemo., health behaviors, some CV RFs	Low DL → ↑ MI Strain → ↑ MI	Nested case-control study; similar to retrospective cohort study. Treated continuous IVs categorically.

♂, male; ♀, female; ΨWL, psychological workload or psychological demands; BC, blue collar; BP, blood pressure; CVD, cardiovascular disease; DA, decision authority; DL, decision latitude; FH, family history; MI, myocardial infarction; NHANES1, National Health and Nutrition Survey 1; RF, risk factor; SC, social class; SkD, skill discretion; Sociodemo., sociodemographic variables.

Stewart, Hall, Fredlund, & Theorell, 1996; Mäntyniemi et al., 2012; Murphy, 1991; Steenland, Johnson, & Nowlin, 1997; Theorell et al., 1998).

In summary, the results of the studies that used imputed ratings for working conditions were mixed, with most revealing a relation of stressful working conditions to CVD and others not. Hemmingsson and Lundberg's (2006) findings are particularly intriguing because when they statistically adjusted for social class of origin and education, factors that clearly antedated job control, the effect of job control on CVD was reduced to nonsignificance. One interpretation of the finding is that job control partly mediates the link between social class and CVD.[2]

Studies That Involve DC Factors That Were Assessed by Worker Self-Report

This section covers a number of prospective studies in which psychosocial working conditions were assessed by worker self-report, and not imputed (see Table 4.3). The studies should be considered in the context of four broad limitations that bias their results to the null. First, most of the studies, with a few exceptions (André-Petersson, Engström, Hedblad, Janzon, & Rosvall, 2007; Whitehall studies by Bosma et al., 1997 and Kivimäki et al., 2006), assessed the DC variables during a baseline period, and the research participants were followed without regard to whether baseline factors changed over time, potentially underestimating effects on CVD (Ganster & Rosen, 2012; Kivimäki, Singh-Manoux, et al., 2012). Second, in many studies, statistical power was limited; although adjusted odds ratios (see Chapter 2) tended to be greater than 1, they were nonsignificant given the rarity of coronary-related problems (Kivimäki, Singh-Manoux, et al., 2012). In the study by De Bacquer et al. (2005), although the risk-factor adjusted relation of iso-strain to coronary events was significant, the iso-strain group experienced only 14 such events. Third, many of the studies included older adults who were likely to transition into retirement, reducing the continuity of exposures (see, particularly, Kivimäki, Theorell, Westerlund, Vahtera, & Alfredsson, 2008). Fourth, all the studies converted continuous measures of the DC factors into dichotomous or trichotomous variables, reducing power (Landsbergis & Schall, 2013).

At this juncture, we look closely at a Whitehall II study in which investigators evaluated the impact of *cumulative* exposures rather than exposures at one time point. Bosma et al. (1997) found that civil servants who experienced low control at both phases 1 and 2 (about 3 years apart), compared with civil servants who experienced high control at both phases, were at almost twice the risk of developing incident CVD over the subsequent 4 years. Civil servants with intermediate levels of control were at intermediate risk. Other Whitehall II research (Hintsa et al., 2010) indicated that the impact of psychosocial factors on coronary disease in men could not be explained by pre-employment factors such as family history of the disease, social class of origin, and number of siblings (during follow-up too few women experienced CVD for statistical analyses). Although there isn't perfect consistency among the studies in Table 4.3, the balance of the findings, considering their limitations, suggests that psychosocial working conditions exert a modest effect on CVD. Workplace support was not sufficiently studied.

---

[2] A more apt test would involve first regressing CVD occurrence on social class of origin and education, and examining changes in the regression coefficients for those two variables after job control was later controlled. The authors did the reverse, regressing CVD on job control, then adding the social class variables to the equation.

Focus on DC Factors in Women

This section is devoted to research on all-female samples. Some researchers have concluded that the relation of DC factors to CVD risk is "broadly similar for men and women" (Kivimäki et al., 2012, p. 1494). Research from all-female samples, however, suggests that the evidence is not straightforward. A prospective study that followed more than 35,000 U.S. women nurses for 4 years was unable to find a significant link between demands, control, and strain, on the one hand, and CVD, on the other (Lee, Colditz, Berkman, & Kawachi, 2002). That the sample comprised only nurses probably did not bias the results toward the null because nursing is an occupation "characterized by a high level of naturally occurring variation in workload demands and control" (Ganster et al., 2001, p. 956). The study, however, had two limitations that should be underlined. First, the sample included many nurses who at baseline were at or near retirement age, and many of whom were likely retired at follow-up, thus discontinuing exposure to the job conditions being studied. Second, over the 4 years, about half the nurses moved from high-strain jobs to jobs having nonstrain conditions, affecting the cumulative impact of the exposure. Moreover, it was not clear how many nurses who did not have high-strain jobs at baseline moved into high-strain positions at follow-up, a factor that could have muddied the findings.

In a 10-year study of more than 17,000 women health care workers, Slopen et al. (2012) found that controlling for sociodemographic and coronary risk factors, those in high-strain jobs were at elevated risk for MI, but not total CVD. Unexpectedly, women in active jobs (high control and high demands; thought to be cardioprotective) were at elevated risk for CVD. High-strain jobs and active jobs have a factor in common, namely, high levels of demands. Surprisingly, demands, when treated as a single factor, were not related to CVD. Of course, it is possible that, as in the study by Colditz et al. (2002), the nature of the exposures changed over the length of the study. A prospective study of more than 18,000, initially healthy Swedish women who worked full-time (Kuper, Adami, Theorell, & Weiderpass, 2006) found that demands, control, and strain, adjusting for age and CVD risk factors, were not related to the 11-year incidence of CVD, although it is possible that some fraction of the women changed jobs or retired given the length of follow-up. Parallel results were obtained for the more than 14,000 women who worked part-time. Although women more commonly face the double burden of work on a job and work at home (Frankenhaeuser et al., 1989), with rare exceptions (e.g., André-Petersson et al., 2007), domestic workload has not been examined in the studies cited or in most other studies.

Two-Stage Meta-Analysis

In a two-stage meta-analysis involving 11 prospective studies, Kivimäki et al. (2006) found that, controlling for blood glucose, cholesterol, blood pressure, and so forth, components of metabolic syndrome, rendered job strain's once-significant odds ratio nonsignificant. The findings are consistent with the research of Chandola et al. (2008), suggesting that the metabolic syndrome helps mediate the relation between job strain and CVD. Ganster and Rosen (2013) noted that Kivimäki et al.'s (2006) meta-analysis controlled for secondary mediators "that should lead to the CVD outcomes that were assessed. Statistically controlling for [the secondary mediators], then, is essentially partially testing a mediating model" (p. 1107), as per the conceptualization of allostatic load described earlier in this chapter.

The DC and ERI Models Compared

The effort–reward imbalance (ERI) and DC models can be thought of as competing or complementary models of how psychosocial working conditions affect CVD risk. In a nutshell, ERI refers to the extent to which work-related efforts are commensurate with work-related rewards (see Chapter 3 for more detail). Although there has been more research on the DC model in connection with CVD, relatively few studies provide a look at ERI and CVD. In a Finnish study described in Table 4.3, Lynch, Krause, Kaplan, Salonen, and Salonen (1997) found that the combination of high levels of work demands and low financial reward was related to growth in atherosclerotic plaque. In a study of initially healthy Finnish factory employees, Kivimäki et al. (2002) found that, over 25 years, job strain predicted CVD mortality, controlling for other risk factors. A parallel finding was obtained for ERI. In analyses that were limited to workers who remained in the same job for at least 5 years, ensuring a relatively stable exposure history, the link between strain and CVD mortality strengthened. The ERI–CVD link remained about the same. Kivimäki et al. (2002) also found that strain and control but not ERI were related to elevated cholesterol, a secondary mediator, at the 5-year follow-up. In a study of male German blue collar workers, Siegrist, Peter, Junge, Cremer, and Seidel (1990) found that ERI predicted ischemic heart disease over the next 6.5 years controlling for other risk factors. In an 11-year follow-up of British civil servants (Whitehall II), the ERI model predicted CVD in men and women (Kuper, Singh-Manoux, Siegrist, & Marmot, 2002).

In a rare study that directly compared the ERI and DC models by placing them in the same prediction equations, Bosma, Peter, Siegrist, and Marmot (1998) capitalized on Whitehall II data. They found that in men, over the course of a 5-year follow-up, both ERI and job strain increased the risk of CVD adjusting for confounders; in women only ERI predicted CVD, a result that perhaps reflects a degree of overlap in the effort and demand components of the two respective models (see Chapter 3). When strain was replaced in the equation with job control (one of the components of strain; omitting demands), both ERI and low control predicted future CVD in men and women. Social support at work did not predict later CVD.

"Mega-Study" of DC Factors

Many longitudinal studies pertinent to the relation of psychosocial working conditions to health behaviors have had sample sizes that have been too small to detect modest effects—Chapter 2 underlined the view that even small effect sizes can be important when health and mortality are at stake. One-stage meta-analyses (see Chapter 2) can be "mega-studies." Kivimäki and Kawachi (2013) advanced the view that mega-studies, with statistical power obtained from pooling individual-level data from multiple studies, can help to answer research questions bearing on risk factors that have small effect sizes but are nevertheless medically important. Individual studies, with their welter of site- or study-specific results, could hide small effects. Pooling helps to balance out local study effects, and provides the statistical power needed to assess the impact of the risk factors in question.

In a massive ($n > 197,000$), one-stage meta-analysis (a "mega-study") that combined individual-participant data from 13 independent studies, Kivimäki, Nyberg, et al. (2012) followed for, on average, 7.5 years workers who at baseline were CVD free. Controlling for conventional risk factors (e.g., body mass, cholesterol), the study team found that job strain independently increased the risk of CVD by about

TABLE 4.3 Studies That Link Self-Reported DCS Factors to CVD in Mixed-Sex and All-Male Samples

Study Team	Country	Sample	Time Lag	Control Variables	Major Findings	Comments
André-Petersson et al. (2007)	Finland	7,770 (61% ♀) Malmö Diet & Cancer Study	7.8 y	Sociodemo., CV RFs, nonwork, support	Low work support → ↑ MI in ♀s, not ♂s Strain & iso-strain ↛ MI Passive job + low support → ↑ MI in ♀s, not ♂s Domestic ΨWL ↛ MI	Prospective study. Treated continuous IVs categorically. Workers employed same site ≥4 y. Rare study that evaluated domestic ΨWL affected ♀s more than ♂s.
Bosma et al. (1997)	U.K.	>7,300 civil servants (²⁄₃ ♂) Whitehall II	7 y	Sociodemo., CV RFs	Low control twice 3 y apart → ↑ CVD Intermediate control over 3 y → intermediate risk High control → lowest risk ΨWL & support ↛ CVD	Prospective study. Treated continuous IVs categorically. Low control at phases 1 & 2 → ↑ CVD at phase 3, over subsequent 4 y.
De Bacquer et al. (2005)	Belgium	>14,000 ♂s Belstress study	3.2 y	Sociodemo., CV RFs, occupational level	ΨWL, DL, & strain ↛ coronary events Iso-strain → ↓ coronary events Work support → ↑ coronary events	Prospective study. Treated continuous IVs categorically.
Karasek et al. (1981)	Sweden	>1,400 ♂s	6 y	Age, education, smoking, BMI	ΨWL → ↑ CVD indicator Low DL → ↑ CVD indicator	Prospective study. Treated continuous IVs categorically. Although CVD indicator was based on self-report, the indicator was validated against objective data. Results supported in a 2nd study, a case-control CVD mortality study.
Kivimäki et al. (2008)	Sweden	3,160 ♂s; 2,800 excluding ♂s 56–65 y old WOLF Study	9.7 y	Sociodemo., CV RFs	Strain → ↑ CVD	Prospective study. Treated continuous IVs categorically. Finding was for 19–55 subsample but was reduced 70% to nonsig. when 56–65-yr.-olds were included.

(continued)

TABLE 4.3 Studies That Link Self-Reported DCS Factors to CVD in Mixed-Sex and All-Male Samples (*continued*)

Study Team	Country	Sample	Time Lag	Control Variables	Major Findings	Comments
Kuper & Marmot (2003)	U.K.	>10,000 civil servants (2/3 ♂) Whitehall II	Up to 11 y over 5 phases of data collection	Sociodemo., CV RFs	Baseline ΨWL → ↑ CVD Baseline low DL → ↑ CVD Baseline support ↛ CVD	Prospective study. Treated continuous IVs categorically. Analyses serially adjusted for change in employment grade.
Lynch et al. (1997)	Finland	≈2,300 ♂s Kupio Study	6.1 y for MI 8.1 y for mortality	Soc:odemo, CV ♀Fs, depr., hopelessness, illnesses	High ΨWL + low resources + low income ↛ all-cause mortality, CV mortality, MI Also relevant to ERI model	Prospective study. Treated continuous IVs categorically. Sig. effects became nonsig. adjusting for many covariates. Authors suggested it was a case of "overadjustment."
Netterstrøm et al. (2006)	Denmark	>650 ♂s	14 y	Sociodemo., CV RFs	ΨWL → ↑ IHD DL ↛ IHD Job strain → ↑ IHD	Prospective study. Treated continuous IVs categorically. IHD assessed by hospital records. When work factors were imputed, no effects on IHD except for workers in passive jobs being at high risk for IHD.
Schnall et al. (1998)	U.S.	>138 stably employed ♂s	2–4 y	Sociodemo., employment grade	Stable high-strain jobs → ↑ ABP Shifted from high to low or low to high strain → intermediate changes in BP Stable nonstrain → lowest BP	Treated continuous IVs categorically. The evidence is at best suggestive b/c linking time-1–time-2 changes in the IV & DV cannot establish temporal ordering required in establishing a cause–effect relation.
Trudel et al. (2016)	Canada	>1,390 white collar workers (59% ♀)	5 y; assessed at years 1, 3, & 5	Sociodemo., CV RFs	Active jobs over 5 y → ↑ risk of hypertension in ♂s but not ♀s Onset ERI → ↑ABP in ♀s but not in ♂s	Prospective study. Finding in ♂s may be related to downsizing & other changes that led to work intensification.

Note: Findings bearing on all-female samples are described in detail in the text.

♂, male; ♀, female; ΨWL, psychological workload or psychological demands; ABP, ambulatory blood pressure; BC, blue collar; b/c, because; BP, blood pressure; CVD, cardiovascular disease; DA, decision authority; DCS, demand–control–support; depr., depression; DL, decision latitude; DV, dependent variable; FH, family history; IHD, ischemic heart disease; IV, independent variable; MI, myocardial infarction; nonsig., nonsignificant; RF, risk factor; SC, social class; Sig., significant; SkD, skill discretion; Sociodemo., sociodemographic variables.

20% to 30%. The effect of job strain was similar in both men and women and in older and younger workers; the impact of job strain was stronger than the impact of either of its components, job demands and control. In further analyses designed to rule out reverse-causal explanations (subclinical CVD affecting self-reports of job conditions at baseline), the authors excluded workers who experienced CVD during the first years of follow-up, strengthening the link between job strain and CVD. Tests of interactions indicated that the risk associated with job strain did not vary by sex, SES, age, or region in which the original study was conducted. It should be noted that because continuous measures of working conditions were converted to categorical measures, the effect sizes were likely underestimates. The conclusions of a more recent, two-stage meta-analysis ($n > 168,000$) (Xu et al., 2015) are largely consistent with the findings of Kivimäki, Nyberg, et al. (2012) regarding the modestly elevated CVD risk associated with job strain. Xu et al. (2015) also found an even more modestly (but still statistically significant) elevated risk for CVD among individuals with passive jobs (low control combined with few demands).

Summary of Studies Bearing on the DC and ERI Factors

Taking into consideration findings from the imputation studies, the longitudinal and prospective research, longitudinal studies that examined the ERI models, and the mega-study, the evidence, although far from perfect, suggests that job strain or its components can reasonably be thought to modestly increase the risk for CVD. Although the reduction in heart disease risk that comes from preventing job strain is modest compared, say, with the effect of preventing exposure to cigarette smoke, the issue of whether it is important to prevent job strain is separable from the research findings. The authors of the one-stage meta-analysis advanced a worthy idea: exposing workers to job strain and other adverse working conditions is unethical regardless of the impact of strain on heart disease (Kivimäki et al., 2015).

The Relation of Job Loss to CVD Mortality

Chapter 3 showed that job loss can have a harmful effect on mental health. What about physical health and longevity? In research on the relation of unemployment to mortality, investigators have been concerned with the possibility that selection effects explain the relation of job loss to premature death. A plausible selection-based explanation is that people who develop health problems become less able to work and lose or give up their jobs. The antecedent health problems, not job loss, underlie mortality. In view of selection-causation concerns, the studies summarized in Table 4.4 are limited to research on involuntary job loss. The research suggests that involuntary job loss is a risk factor for premature death. Although the pathways from unemployment to poor health are unclear, unemployment creates a host of burdens that threaten health, and subsequently increase mortality risk: financial hardships, depression, demoralizing effects that lead to self-neglect, and so on.

A two-stage meta-analysis ($n > 20$ million) involving samples from many countries indicates that involuntary job loss increases the risk of all-cause mortality by about 60%, controlling for confounders (Roelfs, Shor, Davidson, & Schwartz, 2011). The impact of involuntary job loss on mortality was unlikely to result from preexisting health problems. Roelfs et al. found men and workers in their early or middle but not late careers to be most vulnerable to the impact of job loss. What about the causal

TABLE 4.4 Studies That Link Involuntary Job Loss and Job Insecurity to CVD

Involuntary Job Loss

Study Team	Country	Sample	Time Lag	Control Variables	Major Findings	Comments
Drivas et al. (2013)	Greece	>4,400 ♂ employees of a bus company	13 mo	Age	Job loss → ↑ all-cause mortality, mostly through IHD	Drivas et al. could not control for RFs other than age; confounders → excess mortality b/c the sample was relatively young (mean age = 43) & probably did not self-select into organization that would lay off a large fraction of employees.
Gallo et al. (2006)	U.S.	4,301 age 51–61 (50% ♀)	10 y	Sociodemo., CV RFs, physical illnesses, depression	Job loss → ↑MI, stroke ♀s and ♂s combined in analysis	Study of late career involuntary job loss. Late career job loss… "exceptionally stressful."
Garcy & Vågerö (2012)	Sweden	≈3.4 million (≈ 50% ♀)	5 y	Sociodemo., CV RFs	In ♂s length of unemployment during a recessionary period in which there were mass layoffs → ↑ all-cause, CVD, & cerebrovascular mortality In ♀s length of unemployment → ↑ all-cause mortality only	Prospective study. Unemployment exp. treated as an interval-level variable. To rule out selection explanation, excluded individuals who were unemployed before recession.
Lundin et al. (2010)	Sweden	>37,000 ♂s	8 y	Sociodemo., including childhood SES, health behaviors, psychiatric hospitalization	Unemployment >89 days during a 3-year recession → ↑ all-cause & CVD mortality	Prospective study. Effect sizes greater during the 1st 4 y than the next 4.
Morris et al. (1994)	U.K.	6,000 ♂s	10 y	Sociodemo., baseline health, health behaviors	Job loss → ↑ all-cause, CV, & cancer mortality	Unemployed limited to ♂s who lost jobs for reasons other than illness (e.g., business closings) compared to stably employed ♂s. Cancer deaths least plausible effect.

Study	Country	Sample	Duration	Controls	Findings	Comments
Sullivan & von Wachter (2009)	U.S. (Penn.)	>21,000 ♂s	26 y	Stably employed over 5 y	Job loss b/c of mass layoffs → ↑ all-cause mortality; effect pronounced in first y. Although risk declines over time, the job losers remained at elevated risk	Conservative estimate b/c referee insisted authors not include deaths occurring same year as job loss.
Vahtera et al. (2004)	Finland	20,000 (≈¾ ♀) municipal workers; 10 Towns Study	7.5 y	Sociodemo., type of employment	Job loss → ↑ CV mortality	Although study concerned impact of downsizing on its survivors (see later entry on Vahtera et al., 2004), CV deaths were higher among those who lost jobs.
Job Insecurity						
Dupre et al. (2012)	U.S.	>13,000 (>50% ♀)	8 y	Sociodemo., CV RFs, health behaviors	Each additional job loss → ↑ MI	The risk is cumulative.
Ferrie et al. (2001)	U.K.	>10,300 (⅔ ♂) Whitehall II	7 y	Sociodemo., baseline health	Study 1 Anticipation → ↓ self-rated health in ♂s; Anticipation → ↑ physical symptoms in ♂s, ♀s. Study 2 Chronic insecurity → ↑ BP & BMI	Natural experiment. In Study 1, some civil service units anticipated privatization. In Study 2, later privatization was clearly going to occur. BP & BMI are mediators of CVD.
Vahtera et al. (2004)	Finland	20,000 (≈ ¾ ♀) municipal workers; 4 towns from 10 Towns Study	7.5 y	Sociodemo., absence rate before recession	Units experiencing highest levels of downsizing → ↑ CV deaths. Units experiencing intermediate levels of downsizing → intermediate death rates. Lowest levels → lowest rates	All participants kept their jobs through a recession. Natural experiment in that different government units experienced downsizing to different extents; self-selection unlikely.

♂, male; ♀, female; b/c, because; BP, blood pressure; CVD, cardiovascular disease; IHD, ischemic heart disease; MI, myocardial infarction; RF, risk factor; Sociodemo., sociodemographic variables.

pathways? For example, does job loss influence CV health by contributing to the dysregulation of the HPA axis and autonomic nervous system? The research reviewed underlines just how unhealthy job loss can be without necessarily disentangling the causal pathways. The findings, nonetheless, suggest that government policies that work toward the goal of full employment and provide safety nets for those who lose their jobs protect the public's health.

Job Insecurity and CVD

What about workers who do not lose their jobs but are subject to job insecurity or the threat of job loss? Perhaps the workers who remain on the job have much more overtime (because they now have fewer coworkers) and insufficient sleep, putting them at risk for heart disease (Liu & Tanaka, 2002). In addition to examining the effect of job loss on mental health, Chapter 3 also examined the impact of job insecurity. Table 4.4 includes three studies that demonstrate job insecurity's adverse effect on physical health.

A study by Vahtera et al. (2004) is worth spotlighting. The research team examined the extent to which layoffs in four municipalities—a result of a recession—varied among organizational units. The study, for reasons enumerated in Table 4.5, convincingly demonstrated that downsizing-related changes occurring for those workers *who*

TABLE 4.5	The Strengths of the Study by Vahtera et al. (2004)
Strength	
1	The study was a natural experiment, and the individuals in the various workplaces could not have self-selected on the basis of future exposure to different intensities of the recession, downsizing, and future CV health.
2	The impact of downsizing on mortality reflected a dose–response trend. Dose–response relationships suggest causality in that intensity of exposure is directly related to size of effect.
3	The impact of downsizing was greatest during the first half of follow-up. In many instances, exposure to typical workplace hazards (e.g., chemicals) is stable, and the adverse health impact is stable. By contrast, the downsizing was a one-off event with less impact in the second half of the follow-up period.
4	The impact of downsizing was specific to CV mortality and not related to other causes of death (see Noel, 2002). As far as we know, psychosocial work factors are implicated in CVD, but not in other diseases such as cancer (although Morris et al. [1994] found unemployment was predictive of both CV- *and* cancer-related mortality). In a one-stage meta-analysis that in effect created a massive prospective study involving more than 116,000 men and women, Heikkilä et al. (2013) found that another psychosocial stressor, namely job strain, did not predict lung, breast, prostate, or colorectal cancer.
5	Workers who lost jobs in the downsizing, or who voluntarily withdrew from their jobs, were deliberately excluded from the analyses. The findings applied only to those who worked, contradicting the hypothesis that selection explained the excess of unhealthy workers in workplaces most exposed to downsizing.
6	As expected, CV mortality was higher among those who lost their jobs than among workers who retained theirs.
7	SES and the material conditions of life that SES underwrites were controlled because the study was limited to workers who retained their jobs.
8	There was very little job shifting over the course of the study, suggesting that the effect of downsizing was a signal event for workers who remained.

CV, cardiovascular; CVD, cardiovascular disease; SES, socioeconomic status.

remained on the job contributed to the risk of premature death. Vahtera et al. (2004) noted that the workers who remained on the job in downsized units experienced at least three changes: (a) increased insecurity, (b) increased job demands, and (c) reduced control. The latter two changes were the result of legislation that did not permit the municipalities to reduce services commensurately with reductions in personnel. It is not clear which change or changes precipitated by the downsizing were responsible for the increased risk of premature death, but only that downsizing had this effect.

In a two-stage meta-analysis that combined data ($n > 170,000$ men and women) from 17 independent prospective cohort studies, Virtanen et al. (2013) found that initially healthy workers who experienced job insecurity at baseline were, over a 10-year follow-up, at modestly elevated risk of CVD (30% higher than comparison subjects). When the estimates were adjusted for covariates such as SES, excess risk was reduced to 20%. Individuals with low-SES jobs experienced more job insecurity than others. It is also likely that CVD risk was underestimated because (a) job insecurity was assessed only at baseline (more harmful chronic exposures were not assessed) and (b) the meta-analysis did not statistically control for different intensities of exposure to insecurity as economic conditions changed or participants changed jobs.

Although the mechanisms by which job insecurity and unemployment affect physical health are unclear, the balance of evidence supports the hypothesis that job insecurity and involuntary job loss adversely affect CV health and mortality risk.

Long Working Hours and CVD

In Chapter 3, the Japanese word *karoshi* was mentioned. The word translates to "death from overwork" (Nishiyama & Johnson, 1997). Although not getting the attention that the DC factors have received, long work days have been thought to have adverse health effects. A case-control study (Sokejima & Kagamimori, 1998) conducted in Japan, a country in which long hours of work are common, found that working 11 or more hours a day is a risk factor for MI in men, adjusting for covariates (e.g., history of hypertension). Another case-control study (Liu & Tanaka, 2002) involving Japanese men found that overwork and reduced sleep increased the risk of MI, adjusting for confounders. Longitudinal data from the Canadian National Population Health Survey (Shields, 1999) suggest that moving from standard (35 to 40) to long hours (>41 hours per week) 2 years later influenced factors that can have adverse health implications: weight gain in men, increased smoking in men and women, and increased alcohol consumption in women.

Murphy (1991) found that bus driving involves psychosocial hazards that predict CVD-related disability. Urban drivers, like the drivers in the study described next, must contend with the time pressure of a schedule, yet ensure rider safety. A longitudinal study (Johansson et al., 2012) of Stockholm trainees (88% male) who went on to become bus drivers found that, controlling for blood pressure before obtaining the job, the average number of hours of driving per week was related to elevations in diastolic blood pressure during the drivers' fifth year at work. This study was of particular significance because it began with trainees who were healthy (applicants with health problems were selected out of the candidate pool).

Finally, a two-stage meta-analysis ($n > 600,000$) involving 25 mostly unpublished prospective studies (Kivimäki et al., 2015) indicated long working hours, controlling for confounding factors, modestly but reliably increases the risk of CVD over an average of 8.5 years. A companion finding indicated that long hours had an even greater impact on the risk of stroke. The available evidence suggests that extensive exposure to long work days has adverse implications for health.

Bullying

Chapter 5 covers the psychological impact of workplace aggression, including bullying. Here we briefly look at its relation to CVD. Workplace bullying refers to perpetrators who (a) have a power advantage over their victim and (b) act aggressively toward the victim over a prolonged period of time. In the study of predominantly female Finnish hospital workers, Kivimäki, Virtanen, et al. (2003) found that prolonged workplace bullying was related to the development of CVD in workers in whom CVD was absent at baseline. Reverse causality, namely, that CVD at baseline predicted bullying at follow-up, was ruled out.

Work Schedules and CVD

The shifts that comprise work schedules can vary. In the developed world, the traditional shift is the 8- or 9-a.m. to 5 p.m. work schedule. Alternate shifts include work schedules that begin at 4 p.m. and last until midnight (the night shift), and thus overlap with most individuals' dinnertime. Another alternate shift begins at about midnight and continues till about 8 a.m. (the so-called graveyard shift). There are shifts that rotate such that some weeks they start at one hour, say 8 a.m., and during other weeks, very different hours (4 p.m. or midnight). There are many ways shift work can affect cardiovascular health. Alternate work schedules can disrupt circadian rhythms, giving rise to sleep problems (Karlsson, Alfredsson, Knutsson, Andersson, & Torén, 2005) and metabolic syndrome (Frost, Kolstad, & Bonde, 2009). Alternate schedules can produce the social stress that comes from isolation from friends and family who work standard schedules. Social relationships generally benefit an individual's health (House, Landis, & Umberson, 1988). Orth-Gomer (1983) observed that "most biological functions, e.g., heart rate, blood pressure, and catecholamine excretion rates as well as many behavioral patterns such as sleep and wakefulness exhibit a 24-hour rhythmicity, and that these functions partly depend on work schedules as well as clocks, social engagements, the natural environment (daylight), etc." (p. 407).

There is some evidence that alternate shiftwork adversely affects CVD risk (Fujino et al., 2006; Kawachi et al., 1995; Karlsson et al., 2005; Knutsson, Akerstedt, Jonsson, & Orth-Gomer, 1986; Taylor & Pocock, 1972; van Amelsvoort, Schouten, Maan, Swenne, & Kok, 2001). The preponderance of evidence, however, points in another direction. In a review of 14 prospective studies (7 included mortality findings), relating shiftwork to ischemic heart disease, Frost et al. (2009) found that estimates of relative risk hovered around 1 (no effect). Methodological problems (e.g., inadequate control for confounding factors) in the studies were also an obstacle to drawing firm cause–effect conclusions. A 22-year, Finnish prospective study (Hublin et al., 2010) involving more than 20,000 same-sex twins was unable to establish a link between shift work and CVD, adjusting for sociodemographic, psychosocial, behavioral, and biomedical covariates. In addition, in analyses that capitalized on twin-pairs discordant for CVD, no effect for shift work was found.

Socioeconomic Status and Health

In Chapter 3, it was noted that socioeconomic status (SES) is related to mental health. It has long been known that SES is related to physical health, including CVD risk (Antonovsky, 1968). In the original Whitehall Study ($n > 17,000$ men), or Whitehall I, Rose and Marmot (1981) found that, compared with male civil servants in the highest class, those in the lowest civil service grades were, over the 7.5-year follow-up, more likely to die from CVD, controlling for known risk factors (e.g., smoking, BMI), even if disease-free at baseline. The investigators observed that "a man's employment status was a stronger predictor of his risk of dying from coronary heart disease than any of the more familiar risk factors" (p. 17). Link and Phelan (1995) observed that lower SES translates into less money, fewer resources, fewer social connections, and so on, factors that play a key role in personal and family health.

The findings bearing on the relation of the DC and ERI factors and economic insecurity to CVD at least partly explain why SES is inversely related to CV morbidity and mortality. Marmot and Theorell (1988) showed that job strain is more common in lower status jobs. Jobs on the lower economic rungs tend to offer workers less skill discretion, less autonomy, and uneven support. Andersen et al. (2004) found that skill discretion partially mediated the impact of social position on MI. Adjusting for unmeasured family background characteristics (by using sibling controls) and health behaviors, physical and psychosocial work factors help explain the relation between SES and CVD (Brand, Warren, Carayon, & Hoonakker, 2007).

Summary of Research on the Relation of Psychosocial Workplace Factors to CVD

Psychosocial working conditions can affect the risk of CVD by two routes. One route involves the effects of working conditions on health behaviors that ultimately influence the development of CVD. Evidence that the DC variables influence health risk behaviors such as smoking, weight gain, and reduced leisure time physical activity is mixed. Evidence on weight gain suggests that job stressors affect to a greater extent individuals who are initially heavier. There is evidence that psychosocial stressors, including long hours of work, increase the risk of leisure time physical inactivity.

The second route involves psychosocial working conditions cumulatively exerting biological effects more directly. This more direct pathway involves working conditions that affect CVD risk by first affecting the HPA axis and the autonomic nervous system, although mapping out how the cumulative impact of working conditions affects human biology is challenging.

Evidence that the DC variables affect CV health comes from a number of sources such as case-control and prospective studies, including research that employed imputed measures of working conditions. Not all research, however, has been supportive, especially research on women. However, a mega-study involving almost 200,000 participants suggests that the DC variables affect CV health in both men and women. Prospective studies involving the ERI and DC models have also been supportive of the conclusion that the DC variables and imbalance affect CV health.

Other candidate psychosocial factors that potentially influence CVD include unemployment, job insecurity, long working hours, and bullying. The evidence that job loss and job insecurity adversely affect CV health has been solid. There is some evidence that long hours of work can also compromise health. Research on bullying has been sparse. Taken together, the evidence from research on unemployment and the DC model help to explain, at least partly, the relation between SES and health. Lower status jobs more commonly offer less control over work activities. The balance of evidence suggests that workplace psychosocial stressors influence CVD risk, particularly in men (Backé, Seidler, Latza, Rossnagel, & Schumann, 2012).

MUSCULOSKELETAL PROBLEMS

According to the European Agency for Safety and Health at Work (2013), musculo-skeletal disorders (MSDs) "can affect the body's muscles, joints, tendons, ligaments, bones and nerves." Work-related MSDs often develop slowly as a result of "the work itself or by the employees' working environment." Of course, accidents leading to fractures, and so forth, can also be a source of MSDs; occupational safety and accidents are covered in Chapter 8. The European Agency for Safety and Health at Work reported that MSDs occur principally in the back, neck, shoulders, and upper limbs. In addition to harming individual workers, MSDs also harm a country's economy. Warren, Dillon, Morse, Hall, and Warren (2000) found that about 9% of the representative sample of 3,200 Connecticut residents suffered from work-related musculoskeletal pain. In 2011, almost 2.5 million U.S. workers were receiving disability pensions on account of MSDs, costing the government an average of $13,000 per person per year (Social Security Administration, 2012). Moreover, Warren et al. noted that a great many cases of work-related MSDs go undetected. Musculoskeletal disability made up 26% of all disability pensions, almost twice the proportion of the next most frequent category, mood disorders. In 2011 alone, more than 330,000 workers filed for disability benefits, representing a third of all workers who filed for such benefits that year.

Psychosocial Working Conditions and Musculoskeletal Problems

Much of the literature on musculoskeletal problems is devoted to the relation of such problems to physical work (e.g., lifting cement bags, typing on a keyboard). Postural factors, repetitive movement effects, and heavy lifting contribute to the development of MSDs. The relation of physical work to MSDs is *not* the subject of this section, although it is widely recognized that the physical requirements of jobs largely contribute to the development of MSDs (Andersen, Haahr, & Frost, 2007; Lipscomb, Kucera, Epling, & Dement, 2008). This section examines the impact of psychosocial workplace stressors on musculoskeletal problems.

Bigos et al. (1991) observed that a musculoskeletal problem such as a back injury is "an event that may be influenced by a complex set of factors that cannot be understood solely in terms of biomechanic or ergonomic considerations" (p. 5). How can mental stress be related to musculoskeletal pain? Some answers come from Westgaard (1999), Lundberg (2002), and Theorell (2008).

Westgaard observed that the trapezius (a large muscle that extends from the occipital bone at the lower part of the back of the head down the back to lower thoracic vertebrae and to the shoulder) has been shown to be sensitive to cognitive stress in experimental situations. He went on to suggest that heavy psychological demands precipitate tension in the trapezius, and reduce momentary micro-breaks that briefly rest the muscle, leading to fatigue and pain. This effect is plausible because components of the brain's limbic system, which control the autonomic nervous system (the hypothalamus of the HPA axis is a component of the limbic system), also influence the spinal motor system. Lundberg hypothesized that psychosocial stressors such as lack of control create tension and impede the worker's ability to relax after work and during rest breaks, preventing the worker from experiencing lower physiological activation levels. These periods of relaxation are crucial to physical well-being, as they amount to periods of "anabolism," or the regeneration of tissues (Theorell, 2008). Skeletal muscles can weaken from overwork; however, psychosocial stress (e.g., worries provoked by a tyrannical supervisor, high psychological workload) may hinder restorative sleep and anabolism, increasing muscle vulnerability (Theorell, Hasselhorn, Vingård, & Andersson, 2000). Although this section emphasizes the impact of psychosocial working conditions on musculoskeletal problems, workplace psychosocial factors are interconnected with organizational design, physical and mental tasks, tools and technologies, the physical environment, and the worker's personal characteristics (Carayon, 2009; Carayon, Smith, & Harris, 1999; M.J. Smith & Carayon-Sainfort, 1989).

Evidence That Psychosocial Working Conditions Affect Musculoskeletal Problems

Before reviewing some of the evidence, it is worth noting that research on the relation of psychosocial workplace factors to MSDs and CVD share a characteristic that leads to underestimates of effect sizes. Psychosocial factors are often dichotomized (occasionally trichotomized), leading to such underestimates (Lang, Ochsmann, Kraus, & Lang, 2012). The findings summarized in Table 4.6 suggest that psychosocial working conditions influence the development of musculoskeletal problems including problems that drive workers into disability retirement.

Lundberg (2002) underlined the fact that women are more vulnerable to musculoskeletal problems, which is consistent with their having, on average, less control in their jobs and a greater unpaid workload at home. He noted that, compared with their male colleagues, women in white collar positions are twice as likely to experience neck and shoulder problems. These problems are largely *not* the result of differences in physical strength because physical strength is not relevant to white collar work. Lundberg attributed the higher rates of musculoskeletal problems in women to their greater exposure to psychosocial stressors, with the stressors' additive impact on activation levels. Lundberg wrote that "mental stress may contribute to increased muscle tension, although with considerable individual variability" (p. 387).

Two Meta-Analyses and a Systematic Review

Two sets of two-stage meta-analyses (Hauke, Flintrop, Brun, & Rugulies, 2011; Lang et al., 2012) summarized a great deal of longitudinal research on the relation of psychosocial stressors to MSDs. In two-stage meta-analyses, Lang et al. (2012) provided estimates of the "stability-controlled lagged effects" of baseline psychosocial stressors on later musculoskeletal outcome measures (either by statistical control for baseline problems or by limiting a sample to individuals who were problem free at baseline). A number of key findings emerged. Low workplace support and highly monotonous work were related to increased risk of later low back problems. Job strain and monotonous work increased the risk of neck and shoulder pain. Monotonous work was related to increased risk of upper extremity problems (e.g., arms, wrists,). Given that the studies did not control for physical workload (J. Lang, personal communication, April 2014), the omission is at least partly remedied because the

TABLE 4.6 Studies That Link Psychosocial Workplace Factors to Musculoskeletal Problems and MSD-Related Disability Retirements

Study Team	Country	Sample	Time Lag	Control Variables	Major Findings	Comments
Musculoskeletal Problems						
Andersen et al. (2007)	Denmark	>1,500 (60% ♀)	2 y	Sociodemo., physical baseline RFs (e.g., repetitive motion, long hrs. standing)	Low control → ↑ severe low back pain; Low coworker support → ↑ lower body pain; Low job satisfaction → ↑ neck/shoulder & lower limb pain, lower body pain	Individuals who changed jobs between waves continued in the study.
Ariëns et al. (2001)	Netherlands	>970 (75% ♂) SMASH Study	3 y	Age, gender, initial neck pain, ΦWL	ΨWL → neck pain; Low coworker support → ↑ neck pain; Low DA → ↑ neck pain	Initial neck pain was controlled.
Bergqvist (1995)	Sweden	350 mostly visual display users (≈¾ ♀)	6 y	Hand/wrist problems absent at wave 1	Increases in monotonous work at visual display terminals → ↑ hand/wrist problems	Prospective study. Change-change analyses. Monotony & immobility confounded.
Bergström et al. (2007)	Sweden	>1,500 mostly ♂s in 4 industries	18 mo and 3 y	Sociodemc., baseline neck/back pain, health behaviors, lifting	Control → ↓ sick leave for neck/back pain	Control assessed in terms of positive challenges. Mostly blue collar sample.
Bigos et al. (1991)	U.S.	3,000 aircraft workers (75% ♂)	4 y	Sociodemo., past back injury	Enjoy job → ↓ back pain; MMPI hypochondriasis scale → ↑ back injury	Controlled for past back injury.
Cassou et al. (2002)	France	>18,000 (≈40% ♀)	5 y	Sociodemo., ΦWL, work repetitiveness	ΨWL → ↑ neck & shoulder pain; Low ΨWL → disappearance of pain in workers who had pain initially	Prospective study. Workers without neck & shoulder pain at wave 1. Separate analyses for workers with pain at wave 1.
Johansson et al. (2012)	Sweden	88 bus trainees (88% ♂)	5 y	Musc. problems at baseline	No. hrs. driving → ↑ musc. problems	Followed from trainees to drivers. Trainees were healthy at baseline.
Kivimäki et al. (2001)	Finland	604 municipal workers (¾ ♀)	5 y	Prospective part of study. Sociodemo., ΦWL	Job insecurity → ↑ absences owing to pain; In ♀s but not ♂s, job insecurity → ↑ severe musc. pain	The 604 participants refer to those without musc. pain at wave 1. Insecurity refers to workers still on job after downsizing.
Leino & Magni (1993)	Finland	n > 600 workers (65% ♂) in metal plant	3 times in 15 y	Age, SC, ΦWL, previous sympt. levels	Depressive sympts. → ↑ MSDs; MSDs ↛ depressive sympts.; ΨΦ sympts. → ↑ MSDs; MSDs → ↑ ΨΦ sympts.	Assessed reverse-causal models. ΨΦ refers to headaches, nausea, etc. MSDs involved neck/shoulder, lower back, etc.

Study	Country	Sample	Duration	Controls	Findings	Comments
Leino & Hänninen (1995)	Finland	n >400 workers (65% ♂) in metal plant	See Leino & Magni (1993)	Age, SC, gender, ΦWL	Monotony, control, & poor work social relations → ↑ MSDs	Findings are independent of ΦWL. No reverse-causal models as in Leino & Magni (1993).
Rugulies & Krause (2005)	San Francisco, U.S.	>1,200 (86% ♂) transit operators	7.5 y	Sociodemo., yrs. operating, hrs. per week, musc. problems & ΦWL at baseline	Low coworker/supervisor support, strain, & iso-strain → ↑ nontraumatic neck	Injury was physician diagnosed.
Rugulies & Krause (2008)	San Francisco, U.S.	>1,200 (86% ♂) transit operators	7.5 y	See Rugulies & Krause (2005).	ERI → ↑ lower back pain, neck injury	See Rugulies & Krause (2005).
Shannon et al. (2001)	Canada	>700 hospital employees (87% ♀)	3 y, 3 waves	Sociodemo., initial neck & back pain	ΨWL, job influence, & job interference with family → ↑ neck & back pain	Initial ΦWL (e.g., lifting) was not controlled.
Stansfeld et al. (1998)	U.K.	≈ 9,300 civil servants (⅔ ♂). Whitehall II	5 y	Sociodemo., physical & psychiatric characteristics	In ♀s ΨWL, ERI → ↑ limitations ERI in ♂s & ♀s → ↑ limitations Low emotional support in ♂s → ↑ limitations	Limitations include problems in lifting, stairs, bending, etc. Low emotional support is a nonwork factor.
Trinkoff et al. (2006)	U.S.	500 nurses (95% ♀)	15 mo, 3 waves	Age, ΦWL	Working during time off → ↑ neck/shoulder problems	ΨWL was borderline significant. No effect for job change.
Van den Heuvel et al. (2005)	Netherlands	787 (75% ♂?) SMASH Study	3 y	Age, gender, ΦRFs, emotional exhaustion, NA	ΨWL → ↑ wrist/elbow/hand sympts. ΨWL & strain → ↑ neck/shoulder sympts. Low coworker support → ↑ all the aforementioned sympts.	Differs from Ariens et al. (2001) b/c this study is prospective. Removed affected workers at baseline. Cumulative incidence of problems
Disability Retirement Owing to MSDs						
Lahelma et al. (2012)	Finland	<9,000 (80% ♀)	7 y	Sociodemo., ΦWL	Low job control → ↑ MSD-related retirement	Heavy ΦWL was strong predictor of disability retirement.
Mäntyniemi et al. (2012)	Finland	>69,000 (¾ ♀) 10 Town Study	4.6 y	Sociodemo., baseline physical & mental health	Strain → ↑ MSD-related retirement	Strain had greater impact on MSD than CVD retirement.
Ropponen et al. (2013)	Sweden	>24,000 same-sex twins; 50% ♀	12 y	Sociodemo., genetic make-up	High ΨWL, passive job, iso-strain → ↑ MSD-related retirement	Rare study that controls genetic make-up. Imputed IVs.

♂, male; ♀, female; ΦWL, physical workload; ΨΦ sympts., psychophysiological symptoms; ΨWL, psychological workload; ΨΦ sympts., ΨΦ sympts.; BC, blue collar; b/c, because; BP, blood pressure; DA, decision authority; depr., depression; DL, decision latitude; DV, dependent variable; FH, family history; IV, independent variable; musc., musculoskeletal; NA, negative affectivity; RF, risk factor; SC, social class; SkD, skill discretion; Sociodemo., sociodemographic variables; sympt., symptom; sympts., symptoms.

investigators statistically adjusted for baseline musculoskeletal problems or limited the sample to individuals who were initially free of such problems.

In most of the studies in the meta-analyses conducted by Hauke et al. (2011), physical load was statistically controlled. Low workplace support was related to future pain in several body regions—neck/shoulder, upper extremities, and the lower back—as well as to composite measures of all regions. Low job control, low decision latitude, high job strain, and low job satisfaction were each related to pain in two of the three regions as well as to the composite measures.

Finally, Kraatz, Lang, Kraus, Münster, and Ochsmann (2013) published a systemic review involving 18 high-quality prospective/longitudinal studies that examined neck and shoulder disorders. Kraatz et al. found that workplace psychosocial factors, including high workload, low control, low coworker support, and high job strain, incrementally predicted neck and shoulder injury above what would be predicted by physical job factors.

Summary

The proposed pathways from psychosocial workplace stressors to MSDs include the excitation of the limbic system, the inability to take advantage of momentary work breaks, interference with rest outside of work, and the precipitation of tension and worries that interfere with restorative sleep. Research findings suggest that psychosocial factors, apart from the physical demands of the workplace, play a role in the development of musculoskeletal problems. A limitation in much of the research on the impact of psychosocial factors on MSDs is that reverse-causal processes have rarely been examined (Lang et al., 2012).

OTHER HEALTH-RELATED OUTCOMES

In the interest of rounding out the chapter, and given space limitations, this section briefly covers three other health-related outcomes: sickness absence from work, self-reported health, and fatigue. In their study of Finnish hospital workers, described in Chapter 3, Kivimäki, Elovainio, Vahtera, and Ferrie (2003) found that low levels of skill discretion, high psychological workload, and low levels of organizational justice (the extent to which a worker is treated fairly and with respect) predicted sickness absence over 2 years.

Self-rated health reflects "a combination of different aspects of health and has proved to be a robust and reliable measure of a person's overall health status and a strong predictor of mortality" (Ahnquist, Wamala, & Lindstrom, 2012, p. 931; also see Idler & Benyamini, 1997). Low levels of procedural justice, low skill discretion, and high workload predicted poor self-reported health (Kivimäki, Elovainio, et al., 2003). Longitudinal research conducted in Canada (P. Smith et al., 2008) suggests that low job control has a direct adverse effect on self-rated health as well as an indirect effect through reduced physical activity.

Fatigue is not often the subject of prospective research. One exception is the Maastrich Cohort Study (Bültmann et al., 2002). In that study men having work characterized by high levels of psychological and emotional demands, low levels of decision latitude, low levels of supervisor and coworker support, and high levels of physical demands predicted newly incident cases of severe fatigue 1 year later. In women, high levels of psychological demands, low levels of latitude, low levels of coworker support, and high levels of conflict with supervisors predicted newly incident cases of severe fatigue.

Although more research is needed, based on the aforementioned findings, the DC factors likely influence health beyond their impact on depression, heart disease, and musculoskeletal problems.

REFERENCES

Ahnquist, J., Wamala, S. P., & Lindstrom, M. (2012). Social determinants of health—A question of social or economic capital? Interaction effects of socioeconomic factors on health outcomes. *Social Science & Medicine, 74*, 930–939. doi:10.1016/j.socscimed.2011.11.026

Alterman, T., Shekelle, R., Vernon, S., & Burau, K. (1994). Decision latitude, psychologic demand, job strain, and coronary heart disease in the Western Electric Study. *American Journal of Epidemiology, 139*(6), 620–627.

Andersen, I., Burr, H., Kristensen, T., Gamborg, M., Osler, M., Prescott, E., & Diderichsen, F. (2004). Do factors in the psychosocial work environment mediate the effect of socioeconomic position on the risk of myocardial infarction? Study from the Copenhagen Centre for Prospective Population Studies. *Occupational and Environmental Medicine, 61*(11), 886–892.

Andersen, J., Haahr, J., & Frost, P. (2007). Risk factors for more severe regional musculoskeletal symptoms: A two-year prospective study of a general working population. *Arthritis and Rheumatism, 56*(4), 1355–1364.

André-Petersson, L., Engström, G., Hedblad, B., Janzon, L., & Rosvall, M. (2007). Social support at work and the risk of myocardial infarction and stroke in women and men. *Social Science & Medicine, 64*(4), 830–841.

Antonovsky, A. (1968). Social class and the major cardiovascular diseases. *Journal of Chronic Diseases, 21*(2), 65–106.

Ariëns, G., Bongers, P., Hoogendoorn, W., Houtman, I., van der Wal, G., & van Mechelen, W. (2001). High quantitative job demands and low coworker support as risk factors for neck pain: Results of a prospective cohort study. *Spine, 26*(17), 1896–1901.

Ariëns, G., Bongers, P., Hoogendoorn, W., van der Wal, G., & van Mechelen, W. (2002). High physical and psychosocial load at work and sickness absence due to neck pain. *Scandinavian Journal of Work, Environment & Health, 28*, 222–231. doi:10.5271/sjweh.669

Ayyagari, P., & Sindelar, J. L. (2010). The impact of job stress on smoking and quitting: Evidence from the HRS. *B.E. Journal of Economic Analysis and Policy: Contributions to Economic Analysis and Policy, 10*. doi:10.2202/1935-1682.2259

Backé, E., Seidler, A., Latza, U., Rossnagel, K., & Schumann, B. (2012). The role of psychosocial stress at work for the development of cardiovascular diseases: A systematic review. *International Archives of Occupational and Environmental Health, 85*, 67–79. doi:10.1007/s00420-011-0643-6

Ball, K., & Crawford, D. (2005). Socioeconomic status and weight change in adults: A review. *Social Science & Medicine, 60*, 1987–2010. doi:10.1016/j.socscimed.2004.08.056

Barnett, P., Spence, J., Manuck, S., & Jennings, J. (1997). Psychological stress and the progression of carotid artery disease. *Journal of Hypertension, 15*(1), 49–55.

Bergqvist, U. (1995). Visual display terminal work: A perspective on long-term changes and discomforts. *International Journal of Industrial Ergonomics, 16*(3), 201–209.

Bergström, G., Bodin, L., Bertilsson, H., & Jensen, I. B. (2007). Risk factors for new episodes of sick leave due to neck or back pain in a working population: A prospective study with an 18-month and a three-year follow-up. *Occupational and Environmental Medicine, 64*(4), 279–287.

Berset, M., Semmer, N., Elfering, A., Jacobshagen, N., & Meier, L. (2011). Does stress at work make you gain weight? A two-year longitudinal study. *Scandinavian Journal of Work, Environment & Health, 37*, 45–53. doi:10.5271/sjweh.3089

Bigos, S., Battié, M., Spengler, D., Fisher, L., Fordyce, W., Hansson, T., . . . Wortley, M. (1991). A prospective study of work perceptions and psychosocial factors affecting the report of back injury. *Spine, 16*(1), 1–6.

Björntorp, P. (2001). Do stress reactions cause abdominal obesity and comorbidities? *Obesity Reviews, 2*(2), 73–86.

Block, J., He, Y., Zaslavsky, A., Ding, L., & Ayanian, J. (2009). Psychosocial stress and change in weight among US adults. *American Journal of Epidemiology, 170*, 181–192. doi:10.1093/aje/kwp104

Bosma, H., Marmot, M., Hemingway, H., Nicholson, A., Brunner, E., & Stansfeld, S. (1997). Low job control and risk of coronary heart disease in Whitehall II (prospective cohort) study. *BMJ (Clinical Research Ed.), 314*(7080), 558–565.

Bosma, H., Peter, R., Siegrist, J., & Marmot, M. (1998). Two alternative job stress models and the risk of coronary heart disease. *American Journal of Public Health, 88*, 68–74. doi:10.2105/AJPH.88.1.68

Brand, J. E., Warren, J. R., Carayon, P., & Hoonakker, P. (2007). Do job characteristics mediate the relationship between SES and health? Evidence from sibling models. *Social Science Research, 36*, 222–253. doi:10.1016/j.ssresearch.2005.11.004

Brunner, E., Chandola, T., & Marmot, M. (2007). Prospective effect of job strain on general and central obesity in the Whitehall II Study. *American Journal of Epidemiology, 165*, 828–837. doi:10.1093/aje/kwk058

Bültmann, U., Kant, I., Van den Brandt, P., & Kasl, S. (2002). Psychosocial work characteristics as risk factors for the onset of fatigue and psychological distress: Prospective results from the Maastricht Cohort Study. *Psychological Medicine, 32*(2), 333–345.

Cannon, W. B. (1929). Organization for physiological homeostasis. *Physiological Review, 9*, 399–431.

Carayon, P. (2009). The balance theory and the work system model . . . twenty years later. *International Journal of Human-Computer Interaction, 25*, 313–327. doi:10.1080/10447310902864928

Carayon, P., Smith, M. J., & Haims, M. C. (1999). Work organization, job stress, and work-related musculoskeletal disorders. *Human Factors, 41*, 644–663. doi:10.1518/001872099779656743

Cassou, B., Derriennic, F., Monfort, C., Norton, J., & Touranchet, A. (2002). Chronic neck and shoulder pain, age, and working conditions: Longitudinal results from a large random sample in France. *Occupational and Environmental Medicine, 59*(8), 537–544.

Chandola, T., Britton, A., Brunner, E., Hemingway, H., Malik, M., Kumari, M., . . . Marmot, M. (2008). Work stress and coronary heart disease: What are the mechanisms? *European Heart Journal, 29*, 640–648. doi:10.1093/eurheartj/ehm58

Chida, Y., & Hamer, M. (2008). Chronic psychosocial factors and acute physiological responses to laboratory-induced stress in healthy populations: A quantitative review of 30 years of investigations. *Psychological Bulletin, 134*, 829–885. doi:10.1037/a0013342

Cobb, S. (1974). Physiologic changes in men whose jobs were abolished. *Journal of Psychosomatic Research, 18*(4), 245–258.

De Bacquer, D., Pelfrene, E., Clays, E., Mak, R., Moreau, M., de Smet, P., . . . De Backer, G. (2005). Perceived job stress and incidence of coronary events: 3-year follow-up of the Belgian Job Stress Project cohort. *American Journal of Epidemiology, 161*, 434–441. doi:10.1093/aje/kwi040

Deb, P., Gallo, W. T., Ayyagari, P., Fletcher, J. M., & Sindelar, J. L. (2011). The effect of job loss on overweight and drinking. *Journal of Health Economics, 30*, 317–327. doi:10.1016/j.jhealeco.2010.12.009

Dekker, M., Koper, J., van Aken, M., Pols, H., Hofman, A., de Jong, F., . . . Tiemeier, H. (2008). Salivary cortisol is related to atherosclerosis of carotid arteries. *Journal of Clinical Endocrinology and Metabolism, 93*, 3741–3747. doi:10.1210/jc.2008-0496

Drivas, S., Rachiotis, G., Stamatopoulos, G., Hadjichristodoulou, C., & Chatzis, C. (2013). Company closure and mortality in a Greek bus company. *Occupational Medicine, 63*, 231–233. doi:10.1093/occmed/kqs235

Dupre, M., George, L., Liu, G., & Peterson, E. (2012). The cumulative effect of unemployment on risks for acute myocardial infarction. *Archives of Internal Medicine, 172*(22), 1731–1737.

Eriksen, W. (2005). Work factors and smoking cessation in nurses' aides: A prospective cohort study. *BMC Public Health, 5*, 142.

Eriksen, W. (2006). Work factors as predictors of smoking relapse in nurses' aides. *International Archives of Occupational and Environmental Health, 79*(3), 244–250.

European Agency for Safety and Health at Work. (2013). *Musculoskeletal disorders.* Retrieved from https://osha.europa.eu/en/topics/msds

Falba, T., Teng, H., Sindelar, J. L., & Gallo, W. T. (2005). The effect of involuntary job loss on smoking intensity and relapse. *Addiction, 100*(9), 1330–1339.

Ferrie, J., Shipley, M., Marmot, M., Martikainen, P., Stansfeld, S., & Smith, G. (2001). Job insecurity in white-collar workers: Toward an explanation of associations with health. *Journal of Occupational Health Psychology, 6*, 26–42. doi:10.1037//1076-8998.6.1.26

Frankenhaeuser, M., Lundberg, U., Fredrikson, M., Melin, B., Tuomisto, M., Myrsten, A., . . . Wallin, L. (1989). Stress on and off the job as related to sex and occupational status in white-collar workers. *Journal of Organizational Behavior, 10*, 321–346. doi:10.1002/job.4030100404

Fransson, E., Heikkilä, K., Nyberg, S., Zins, M., Westerlund, H., Westerholm, P., . . . Kivimäki, M. (2012). Job strain as a risk factor for leisure-time physical inactivity: An individual-participant meta-analysis of up to 170,000 men and women: the IPD-Work Consortium. *American Journal of Epidemiology, 176*, 1078–1089. doi:10.1093/aje/kws336

Frost, P., Kolstad, H. A., & Bonde, J. P. (2009). Shift work and the risk of ischemic heart disease: A systematic review of the epidemiologic evidence. *Scandinavian Journal of Work, Environment & Health, 35*, 163–179.

Fujino, Y., Iso, H., Tamakoshi, A., Inaba, Y., Koizumi, A., Kubo, T., & Yoshimura, T. (2006). A prospective cohort study of shift work and risk of ischemic heart disease in Japanese male workers. *American Journal of Epidemiology, 164*, 128–135. doi:10.1093/aje/kwj185

Gallo, W. T., Teng, H. M., Falba, T. A., Kasl, S. V., Krumholz, H. M., & Bradley, E. H. (2006). The impact of late career job loss on myocardial infarction and stroke: A 10 year follow up using the Health and Retirement Survey. *Occupational and Environmental Medicine, 63*, 683–687. doi:10.1136/oem.2006.026823

Ganster, D. C., Fox, M. L., & Dwyer, D. J. (2001). Explaining employees' health care costs: A prospective examination of stressful job demands, personal control, and physiological reactivity. *Journal of Applied Psychology, 86*, 954–964. doi:10.1037/0021-9010.86.5.954

Ganster, D. C., & Rosen, C. C. (2013). Work stress and employee health: A multidisciplinary review. *Journal of Management, 39*, 1085–1122. doi: 10.1177/0149206313475815

Garcy, A., & Vågerö, D. (2012). The length of unemployment predicts mortality, differently in men and women, and by cause of death: A six year mortality follow-up of the Swedish 1992–1996 recession. *Social Science & Medicine, 74*, 1911–1920. doi:10.1016/j.socscimed.2012.01.034

Go, A., Mozaffarian, D., Roger, V., Benjamin, E., Berry, J., Borden, W., . . . Turner, M. (2013). Heart disease and stroke statistics—2013 update: A report from the American Heart Association. *Circulation, 127*, e6–e245. doi:10.1161/CIR.0b013e31828124ad

Gold, P., Loriaux, D., Roy, A., Kling, M., Calabrese, J., Kellner, C., . . . Gallucci, W. (1986). Responses to corticotropin-releasing hormone in the hypercortisolism of depression and Cushing's disease: Pathophysiologic and diagnostic implications. *New England Journal of Medicine, 314*(21), 1329–1335.

Gram Quist, H., Christensen, U., Christensen, K. B., Aust, B., Borg, V., & Bjorner, J. B. (2013). Psychosocial work environment factors and weight change: A prospective study among Danish health care workers. *BMC Public Health, 1*, 343. doi:10.1186/1471-2458-13-43

Greeno, C. G., & Wing, R. R. (1994). Stress-induced eating. *Psychological Bulletin, 115*, 444–464. doi:10.1037/0033-2909.115.3.444

Hamer, M., O'Donnell, K., Lahiri, A., & Steptoe, A. (2010). Salivary cortisol responses to mental stress are associated with coronary artery calcification in healthy men and women. *European Heart Journal, 31*, 424–429. doi:10.1093/eurheartj/ehp386

Hannerz, H., Albertsen, K., Nielsen, M., Tuchsen, F., & Burr, H. (2004). Occupational factors and 5-year weight change among men in a Danish national cohort. *Health Psychology, 23*, 283–288. doi:10.1037/0278-6133.23.3.283

Hauke, A., Flintrop, J., Brun, E., & Rugulies, R. (2011). The impact of work-related psychosocial stressors on the onset of musculoskeletal disorders in specific body regions: A review and meta-analysis of 54 longitudinal studies. *Work & Stress, 25*, 243–256. doi:10.1080/02678373.2011.614069

Heikkilä, K., Nyberg, S. T., Fransson, E. I., Alfredsson, L., De Bacquer, D., Bjorner, J. B., . . . Kivimäki, M. (2012). Job strain and tobacco smoking: An individual-participant data meta-analysis of 166,130 adults in 15 European studies. *PLOS ONE, 7*(7), e35463. doi:10.1371/journal.pone.0035463

Heikkilä, K., Nyberg, S., Theorell, T., Fransson, E., Alfredsson, L., Bjorner, J., . . . Kivimäki, M. (2013). Work stress and risk of cancer: Meta-analysis of 5700 incident cancer events in 116,000 European men and women. *BMJ (Clinical Research Ed.), 346*, f165. doi:10.1136/bmj.f165

Hemmingsson, T., & Lundberg, I. (2006). Is the association between low job control and coronary heart disease confounded by risk factors measured in childhood and adolescence among Swedish males 40–53 years of age? *International Journal of Epidemiology, 35*, 616–622. doi:10.1093/ije/dyi308

Hintsa, T., Shipley, M., Gimeno, D., Elovainio, M., Chandola, T., Jokela, M., . . . Kivimäki, M. (2010). Do pre-employment influences explain the association between psychosocial factors at work and coronary heart disease? The Whitehall II study. *Occupational and Environmental Medicine, 67*, 330–334. doi:10.1136/oem.2009.048470

Hintsanen, M., Kivimäki, M., Elovainio, M., Pulkki-Råback, L., Keskivaara, P., Juonala, M., . . . Keltikangas-Järvinen, L. (2005). Job strain and early atherosclerosis: The Cardiovascular Risk in Young Finns study. *Psychosomatic Medicine*, 67, 740–747. doi:10.1097/01.psy.0000181271.04169.93

House, J. S., Landis, K. R., & Umberson, D. (1988). Social relationships and health. *Science*, 241, 540–545. doi:10.1126/science.3399889

Hublin, C., Partinen, M., Koskenvuo, K., Silventoinen, K., Koskenvuo, M., & Kaprio, J. (2010). Shiftwork and cardiovascular disease: A population-based 22-year follow-up study. *European Journal of Epidemiology*, 25, 315–323. doi:10.1007/s10654-010-9439-3

Idler, E., & Benyamini, Y. (1997). Self-rated health and mortality: A review of twenty-seven community studies. *Journal of Health and Social Behavior*, 38(1), 21–37.

Iversen, L., Strandberg-Larsen, K., Prescott, E., Schnohr, P., & Rod, N. (2012). Psychosocial risk factors, weight changes and risk of obesity: The Copenhagen City Heart Study. *European Journal of Epidemiology*, 27, 119–130. doi:10.1007/s10654-012-9659-9

Johansson, G., Evans, G., Cederström, C., Rydstedt, L., Fuller-Rowell, T., & Ong, A. (2012). The effects of urban bus driving on blood pressure and musculoskeletal problems: A quasi-experimental study. *Psychosomatic Medicine*, 74, 89–92. doi:10.1097/PSY.0b013e31823ba88f

Johnson, J. V., Hall, E. M., & Theorell, T. (1989). Combined effects of job strain and social isolation on cardiovascular disease morbidity and mortality in a random sample of the Swedish male working population. *Scandinavian Journal of Work, Environment & Health*, 15, 271–279. doi:10.5271/sjweh.1852

Johnson, J. V., Stewart, W., Hall, E. M., Fredlund, P. & Theorell, T. (1996). Long-term psychosocial work environment and cardiovascular mortality among Swedish men. *American Journal of Public Health*, 86(3), 324–331.

Kagan, A., Harris, B., Winkelstein, W., Johnson, K., Kato, H., Syme, S., . . . Tillotson, J. (1974). Epidemiologic studies of coronary heart disease and stroke in Japanese men living in Japan, Hawaii and California: Demographic, physical, dietary and biochemical characteristics. *Journal of Chronic Diseases*, 27(7–8), 345–364.

Kaplan, J., Manuck, S., Adams, M., Weingand, K., & Clarkson, T. (1987). Inhibition of coronary atherosclerosis by propranolol in behaviorally predisposed monkeys fed an atherogenic diet. *Circulation*, 76(6), 1364–1372.

Karasek, R., Baker, D., Marxer, F., Ahlbom, A., & Theorell, T. (1981). Job decision latitude, job demands, and cardiovascular disease: A prospective study of Swedish men. *American Journal of Public Health*, 71(7), 694–705.

Karlsson, B., Alfredsson, L., Knutsson, A., Andersson, E., & Torén, K. (2005). Total mortality and cause-specific mortality of Swedish shift- and dayworkers in the pulp and paper industry in 1952–2001. *Scandinavian Journal of Work, Environment & Health*, 31(1), 30–35.

Kasl, S. V. (1978). Epidemiological contributions to the study of work stress. In C. L. Cooper & R. L. Payne (Eds.), *Stress at work* (pp. 3–38). Chichester, UK: Wiley.

Kawachi, I., Colditz, G., Stampfer, M., Willett, W., Manson, J., Speizer, F., & Hennekens, C. (1995). Prospective study of shift work and risk of coronary heart disease in women. *Circulation*, 92(11), 3178–3182.

Keys, A., Fidanza, F., Karvonen, M., Kimura, N., & Taylor, H. (1972). Indices of relative weight and obesity. *Journal of Chronic Diseases*, 25(6), 329–343.

Kidambi, S., Kotchen, J., Grim, C., Raff, H., Mao, J., Singh, R., & Kotchen, T. (2007). Association of adrenal steroids with hypertension and the metabolic syndrome in Blacks. *Hypertension*, 49(3), 704–711.

Kivimäki, M., Elovainio, M., Vahtera, J., & Ferrie, J. (2003). Organisational justice and health of employees: Prospective cohort study. *Occupational and Environmental Medicine*, 60(1), 27–33.

Kivimäki, M., Head, J., Ferrie, J. E., Brunner, E., Marmot, M. G., Vahtera, J., & Shipley, M. J. (2006). Why is evidence on job strain and coronary heart disease mixed? An illustration of measurement challenges in the Whitehall II study. *Psychosomatic Medicine*, 68(3), 398–401.

Kivimäki, M., Hintsanen, M., Keltikangas-Järvinen, L., Elovainio, M., Pulkki-Råback, L., Vahtera, J., . . . Raitakari, O. (2007). Early risk factors, job strain, and atherosclerosis among men in their 30s: The Cardiovascular Risk in Young Finns Study. *American Journal of Public Health*, 97, 450–452. doi:10.2105/AJPH.2005.078873

Kivimäki, M., Jokela, M., Nyberg, S. T., Singh-Manoux, A., Fransson, E. I., Alfredsson, L., . . . Virtanen, M. (2015). Long working hours and risk of coronary heart disease and stroke: A systematic review and meta-analysis of published and unpublished data for 603,838 individuals. *The Lancet*, 386(10005), 1739–1746. doi:10.1016/S0140-6736(15)60295-1

Kivimäki, M., & Kawachi, I. (2013). Need for more individual-level meta-analyses in social epidemiology: Example of job strain and coronary heart disease. *American Journal of Epidemiology, 177*, 1–2. doi:10.1093/aje/kws407

Kivimäki, M., Leino-Arjas, P., Luukkonen, R., Riihimäki, H., Vahtera, J., & Kirjonen, J. (2002). Work stress and risk of cardiovascular mortality: Prospective cohort study of industrial employees. *British Medical Journal, 325*(7369), 857–860.

Kivimäki, M., Nyberg, S., Batty, G., Fransson, E., Heikkilä, K., Alfredsson, L., . . . Theorell, T. (2012). Job strain as a risk factor for coronary heart disease: A collaborative meta-analysis of individual participant data. *The Lancet, 380*, 1491–1497. doi:10.1016/S0140-6736(12)60994-5

Kivimäki, M., Singh-Manoux, A., Batty, D., Vertanen, M., Ferrie, J. E., & Vahtera, J. (2012). Psychosocial factors at work: The epidemiological perspective. In P. Hjemdahl, A. Rosengren, & A. Steptoe (Eds.), *Stress and cardiovascular disease* (pp. 195–209). London, UK: Springer.

Kivimäki, M., Singh-Manoux, A., Virtanen, M., Ferrie, J. E., Batty, G. D., & Rugulies, R. (2015). IPD-Work consortium: Pre-defined meta-analyses of individual-participant data strengthen evidence base for a link between psychosocial factors and health. *Scandinavian Journal of Work, Environment & Health, 41*, 312–321. doi:10.5271/sjweh.3485

Kivimäki, M., Theorell, T., Westerlund, H., Vahtera, J., & Alfredsson, L. (2008). Job strain and ischaemic disease: Does the inclusion of older employees in the cohort dilute the association? The WOLF Stockholm Study. *Journal of Epidemiology and Community Health, 62*, 372–374. doi:10.1136/jech.2007.063578

Kivimäki, M., Vahtera, J., Ferrie, J., Hemingway, H., & Pentti, J. (2001). Organisational downsizing and musculoskeletal problems in employees: A prospective study. *Occupational and Environmental Medicine, 58*(12), 811–817.

Kivimäki, M., Virtanen, M., Elovainio, M., Kouvonen, A., Väänänen, A., & Vahtera, J. (2006). Work stress in the etiology of coronary heart disease: A meta-analysis. *Scandinavian Journal of Work, Environment & Health, 32*(6), 431–442.

Kivimäki, M., Virtanen, M., Vartia, M., Elovainio, M., Vahtera, J., & Keltikangas-Järvinen, L. (2003). Workplace bullying and the risk of cardiovascular disease and depression. *Occupational and Environmental Medicine, 60*(10), 779–783.

Knutsson, A., Akerstedt, T., Jonsson, B., & Orth-Gomer, K. (1986). Increased risk of ischaemic heart disease in shift workers. *The Lancet, 2*(8498), 89–92.

Kouvonen, A., Vahtera, J., Väänänen, A., De Vogli, R., Heponiemi, T., Elovainio, M., . . . Kivimäki, M. (2009). Relationship between job strain and smoking cessation: The Finnish Public Sector Study. *Tobacco Control, 18*, 108–114. doi:10.1136/tc.2008.025411

Kraatz, S., Lang, J., Kraus, T., Münster, E., & Ochsmann, E. (2013). The incremental effect of psychosocial workplace factors on the development of neck and shoulder disorders: A systematic review of longitudinal studies. *International Archives of Occupational and Environmental Health, 86*, 375–395. doi:10.1007/s00420-013-0848-y

Kuper, H., Adami, H., Theorell, T., & Weiderpass, E. (2006). Psychosocial determinants of coronary heart disease in middle-aged women: A prospective study in Sweden. *American Journal of Epidemiology, 164*, 349–357. doi:10.1093/aje/kwj212

Kuper, H., & Marmot, M. (2003). Job strain, job demands, decision latitude, and risk of coronary heart disease within the Whitehall II study. *Journal of Epidemiology and Community Health, 57*, 147–153. doi:10.1136/jech.57.2.147

Kuper, H., Singh-Manoux, A., Siegrist, J., & Marmot, M. (2002). When reciprocity fails: Effort-reward imbalance in relation to coronary heart disease and health functioning within the Whitehall II study. *Occupational and Environmental Medicine, 59*(11), 777–784.

Lahelma, E., Laaksonen, M., Lallukka, T., Martikainen, P., Pietiläinen, O., Saastamoinen, P., . . . Rahkonen, O. (2012). Working conditions as risk factors for disability retirement: A longitudinal register linkage study. *BMC Public Health, 12*, 309. doi:10.1186/1471-2458-12-309

Landsbergis, P., Dobson, M., Koutsouras, G., & Schnall, P. (2013). Job strain and ambulatory blood pressure: A meta-analysis and systematic review. *American Journal of Public Health, 103*, e61–e71. doi:10.2105/AJPH.2012.301153

Landsbergis, P., & Schnall, P. (2013). Job strain and coronary heart disease. *The Lancet, 381*, 448. doi:10.1016/S0140-6736(13)60242-1

Landsbergis, P., Schnall, P., Deitz, D., Warren, K., Pickering, T., & Schwartz, J. (1998). Job strain and health behaviors: Results of a prospective study. *American Journal of Health Promotion, 12*(4), 237–245.

Landsbergis, P., Sinclair, R. R., Dobson, M., Hammer, L. B., Jauregui, M., LaMontagne, A. D., . . . Warren, N. (2011). Occupational health psychology. In D. H. Anna (Ed.), *The occupational environment: Its evaluation, control, and management* (3rd ed., pp. 1087–1130). Fairfax, VA: American Industrial Hygiene Association.

Lang, J., Ochsmann, E., Kraus, T., & Lang, J. W. B. (2012). Psychosocial work stressors as antecedents of musculoskeletal problems: A systematic review and meta-analysis of stability-adjusted longitudinal studies. *Social Science & Medicine, 75,* 1163–1174. doi:10.1016/j.socscimed.2012.04.015

Lee, S., Colditz, G., Berkman, L., & Kawachi, I. (2002). A prospective study of job strain and coronary heart disease in US women. *International Journal of Epidemiology, 31*(6), 1147–1153.

Leino, P., & Hänninen, V. (1995). Psychosocial factors at work in relation to back and limb disorders. *Scandinavian Journal of Work, Environment & Health, 21*(2), 134–142.

Leino, P., & Magni, G. (1993). Depressive and distress symptoms as predictors of low back pain, neck-shoulder pain, and other musculoskeletal morbidity: A 10-year follow-up of metal industry employees. *Pain, 53,* 89–94. doi:10.1016/0304-3959(93)90060-3

Link, B., & Phelan, J. (1995). Social conditions as fundamental causes of disease. *Journal of Health and Social Behavior, Spec No.,* 80–94.

Lipscomb, H., Kucera, K., Epling, C., & Dement, J. (2008). Upper extremity musculoskeletal symptoms and disorders among a cohort of women employed in poultry processing. *American Journal of Industrial Medicine, 51*(1), 24–36.

Liu, Y., & Tanaka, H. (2002). Overtime work, insufficient sleep, and risk of non-fatal acute myocardial infarction in Japanese men. *Occupational and Environmental Medicine, 59*(7), 447–451.

Lundberg, U. (2002). Psychophysiology of work: Stress, gender, endocrine response, and work-related upper extremity disorders. *American Journal of Industrial Medicine, 41*(5), 383–392.

Lundin, A., Lundberg, I., Hallsten, L., Ottosson, J., & Hemmingsson, T. (2010). Unemployment and mortality: A longitudinal prospective study on selection and causation in 49321 Swedish middle-aged men. *Journal of Epidemiology and Community Health, 64,* 22–28. doi:10.1136/jech.2008.079269

Lynch, J., Krause, N., Kaplan, G. A., Salonen, R., & Salonen, J. T. (1997). Workplace demands, economic reward, and progression of carotid atherosclerosis. *Circulation, 96*(1), 302–307.

Lynch, J., Krause, N., Kaplan, G. A., Tuomilehto, J., & Salonen, J. T. (1997). Workplace conditions, socioeconomic status, and the risk of mortality and acute myocardial infarction: The Kuopio Ischemic Heart Disease Risk Factor Study. *American Journal of Public Health, 87,* 617–622. doi:10.2105/AJPH.87.4.617

MacMahon, B., & Pugh, T. F. (1970). *Epidemiology: Principles and methods.* Boston, MA: Little, Brown.

Mann, S. J. (2006). Job stress and blood pressure: A critical appraisal of reported studies. *Current Hypertension Reviews, 2*(2), 127–138.

Mäntyniemi, A., Oksanen, T., Salo, P., Virtanen, M., Sjösten, N., Pentti, J., . . . Vahtera, J. (2012). Job strain and the risk of disability pension due to musculoskeletal disorders, depression or coronary heart disease: A prospective cohort study of 69,842 employees. *Occupational and Environmental Medicine, 69,* 574–581. doi:10.1136/oemed-2011-100411

Manuck, S., Kaplan, J., Adams, M., & Clarkson, T. (1988). Studies of psychosocial influences on coronary artery atherogenesis in cynomolgus monkeys. *Health Psychology, 7,* 113–124. doi:10.1037/0278-6133.7.2.113

Markovitz, J., & Matthews, K. (1991). Platelets and coronary heart disease: Potential psychophysiologic mechanisms. *Psychosomatic Medicine, 53*(6), 643–668.

Marmot, M., & Theorell, T. (1988). Social class and cardiovascular disease: The contribution of work. *International Journal of Health Services, 18*(4), 659–674.

Matthews, K., Schwartz, J., Cohen, S., & Seeman, T. (2006). Diurnal cortisol decline is related to coronary calcification: CARDIA study. *Psychosomatic Medicine, 68*(5), 657–661.

McEwen, B. (1998). Stress, adaptation, and disease. Allostasis and allostatic load. *Annals of the New York Academy of Sciences, 840,* 33–44.

Morris, J., Cook, D., & Shaper, A. (1994). Loss of employment and mortality. *BMJ (Clinical Research Ed.), 308*(6937), 1135–1139.

Murphy, L. R. (1991). Job dimensions associated with severe disability due to cardiovascular disease. *Journal of Clinical Epidemiology, 44*(2), 155–166.

Musselman, D., Tomer, A., Manatunga, A., Knight, B., Porter, M., Kasey, S., . . . Nemeroff, C. (1996). Exaggerated platelet reactivity in major depression. *American Journal of Psychiatry, 153*(10), 1313–1317.

Nabi, H., Kivimäki, M., Suominen, S., Koskenvuo, M., Singh-Manoux, A., & Vahtera, J. (2010). Does depression predict coronary heart disease and cerebrovascular disease equally well? The Health and Social Support Prospective Cohort Study. *International Journal of Epidemiology, 39,* 1016–1024. doi:10.1093/ije/dyq050

Netterstrøm, B., Kristensen, T., & Sjøl, A. (2006). Psychological job demands increase the risk of ischaemic heart disease: A 14-year cohort study of employed Danish men. *European Journal of Cardiovascular Prevention and Rehabilitation, 13*(3), 414–420.

Nichols, G., Bell, T., Pedula, K., & O'Keeffe-Rosetti, M. (2010). Medical care costs among patients with established cardiovascular disease. *American Journal of Managed Care, 16*(3), e86–e93.

Nicholson, A., Kuper, H., & Hemingway, H. (2006). Depression as an aetiologic and prognostic factor in coronary heart disease: A meta-analysis of 6362 events among 146 538 participants in 54 observational studies. *European Heart Journal, 27*, 2763–2774. doi:10.1093/eurheartj/ehl338

Nijm, J., & Jonasson, L. (2009). Inflammation and cortisol response in coronary artery disease. *Annals of Medicine, 41*, 224–233. doi:10.1080/07853890802508934

Nishiyama, K., & Johnson, J. (1997). Karoshi--death from overwork: Occupational health consequences of Japanese production management. *International Journal of Health Services: Planning, Administration, Evaluation, 27*(4), 625–641.

Nyberg, S. T., Heikkilä, K., Fransson, E. I., Alfredsson, L., De Bacquer, D., Bjorner, J. B., . . . Kivimäki, M. (2012). Job strain in relation to body mass index: Pooled analysis of 160 000 adults from 13 cohort studies. *Journal of Internal Medicine, 272*, 65–73. doi:10.1111/j.1365-2796.2011.02482.x

Orth-Gomér, K. (1983). Intervention on coronary risk factors by adapting a shift work schedule to biologic rhythmicity. *Psychosomatic Medicine, 45*(5), 407–415.

Ota, A., Masue, T., Yasuda, N., Tsutsumi, A., Mino, Y., Ohara, H., & Ono, Y. (2010). Psychosocial job characteristics and smoking cessation: A prospective cohort study using the demand-control-support and effort-reward imbalance job stress models. *Nicotine & Tobacco Research, 12*, 287–293. doi:10.1093/ntr/ntp212

Overgaard, D. B. (2004). Psychological workload is associated with weight gain between 1993 and 1999: Analyses based on the Danish Nurse Cohort Study. *International Journal of Obesity and Related Metabolic Disorder, 28*, 1072–1081. doi:10.1093/occmed/kqg135

Oxford English Dictionary. (n.d.). *Allostasis.* Retrieved from www.oed.com/view/Entry/326643?redirectedFrom=allostasis#eid

Popham, F., & Mitchell, R. (2006). Leisure time exercise and personal circumstances in the working age population: Longitudinal analysis of the British household panel survey. *Journal of Epidemiology and Community Health, 60*, 270–274. doi:10.1136/jech.2005.041194

Reed, D., LaCroix, A., Karasek, R., Miller, D., & MacLean, C. (1989). Occupational strain and the incidence of coronary heart disease. *American Journal of Epidemiology, 129*(3), 495–502.

Roelfs, D., Shor, E., Davidson, K., & Schwartz, J. (2011). Losing life and livelihood: A systematic review and meta-analysis of unemployment and all-cause mortality. *Social Science & Medicine, 72*, 840–854. doi:10.1016/j.socscimed.2011.01.005

Roos, E., Lallukka, T., Rahkonen, O., Lahelma, E., & Laaksonen, M. (2013). Working conditions and major weight gain: A prospective cohort study. *Archives of Environmental & Occupational Health, 68*, 166–172. doi:10.1080/19338244.2012.686931

Ropponen, A., Samuelsson, Å., Alexanderson, K., & Svedberg, P. (2013). Register-based data of psychosocial working conditions and occupational groups as predictors of disability pension due to musculoskeletal diagnoses: A prospective cohort study of 24,543 Swedish twins. *BMC Musculoskeletal Disorders, 14*, 268. doi:10.1186/1471-2474-14-268

Rose, G., & Marmot, M. (1981). Social class and coronary heart disease. *British Heart Journal, 45*(1), 13–19.

Rosengren, A., Hawken, S., Ounpuu, S., Sliwa, K., Zubaid, M., Almahmeed, W., . . . Yusuf, S. (2004). Association of psychosocial risk factors with risk of acute myocardial infarction in 11119 cases and 13648 controls from 52 countries (the INTERHEART study): Case-control study. *The Lancet, 364*(9438), 953–962.

Rosvall, M., Ostergren, P., Hedblad, B., Isacsson, S., Janzon, L., & Berglund, G. (2002). Work-related psychosocial factors and carotid atherosclerosis. *International Journal of Epidemiology, 31*(6), 1169–1178.

Rugulies, R., & Krause, N. (2005). Job strain, iso-strain, and the incidence of low back and neck injuries: A 7.5-year prospective study of San Francisco transit operators. *Social Science & Medicine, 61*, 27–39. doi:10.1016/j.socscimed.2004.11.042

Rugulies, R., & Krause, N. (2008). Effort-reward imbalance and incidence of low back and neck injuries in San Francisco transit operators. *Occupational and Environmental Medicine, 65*, 525–533. doi:10.1136/oem.2007.035188

Sachar, E., Hellman, L., Fukushima, D., & Gallagher, T. (1970). Cortisol production in depressive illness: A clinical and biochemical clarification. *Archives of General Psychiatry, 23*(4), 289–298.

Sanderson, D., Ekholm, O., Hundrup, Y., & Rasmussen, N. (2005). Influence of lifestyle, health, and work environment on smoking cessation among Danish nurses followed over 6 years. *Preventive Medicine, 41*(3–4), 757–760.

Schaubroeck, J., & Ganster, D. C. (1993). Chronic demands and responsivity to challenge. *Journal of Applied Psychology, 78*, 73–85. doi:10.1037/0021-9010.78.1.73

Schnall, P., Schwartz, J., Landsbergis, P., Warren, K., & Pickering, T. (1998). A longitudinal study of job strain and ambulatory blood pressure: Results from a three-year follow-up. *Psychosomatic Medicine, 60*(6), 697–706.

Selye, H. (1976). *The stress of life* (Rev. ed.). New York, NY: McGraw-Hill.

Shannon, H. S., Woodward, C. A., Cunningham, C. E., McIntosh, J., Lendrum, B., Brown, J., & Rosenbloom, D. (2001). Changes in general health and musculoskeletal outcomes in the workforce of a hospital undergoing rapid change: A longitudinal study. *Journal of Occupational Health Psychology, 6*, 3–14. doi:10.1037//1076-8998.6.1.3

Shields, M. (1999). Long working hours and health. *Health Reports, 11*(2), 33–48.

Siegrist, J., Peter, R., Junge, A., Cremer, P., & Seidel, D. (1990). Low status control, high effort at work and ischemic heart disease: Prospective evidence from blue-collar men. *Social Science & Medicine, 31*, 1127–1134. doi:10.1016/0277-9536(90)90234-J

Slopen, N., Glynn, R. J., Buring, J. E., Lewis, T. T., Williams, D. R., & Albert, M. A. (2012). Job strain, job insecurity, and incident cardiovascular disease in the Women's Health Study: Results from a 10-year prospective study. *PLOS ONE, 7*, e40512. doi:10.1371/journal.pone.0040512

Slopen, N., Kontos, E. Z., Ryff, C. D., Ayanian, J. Z., Albert, M. A., & Williams, D. R. (2013). Psychosocial stress and cigarette smoking persistence, cessation, and relapse over 9–10 years: A prospective study of middle-aged adults in the United States. *Cancer Causes & Control, 24*, 1849–1863. doi:10.1007/s10552-013-0262-5

Smith, M. J., & Carayon-Sainfort, P. (1989). A balance theory of job design for stress reduction. *International Journal of Industrial Ergonomics, 4*(1), 67–79.

Smith, P., Frank, J., Mustard, C., & Bondy, S. (2008). Examining the relationships between job control and health status: A path analysis approach. *Journal of Epidemiology and Community Health, 62*, 54–61. doi:10.1136/jech.2006.057539

Social Security Administration. (2012). *Annual statistical report on the Social Security Disability Insurance Program, 2011.* Washington, DC: Author. Retrieved from www.ssa.gov/policy/docs/statcomps/di_asr/2011/di_asr11.pdf

Sokejima, S., & Kagamimori, S. (1998). Working hours as a risk factor for acute myocardial infarction in Japan: Case-control study. *BMJ (Clinical Research Ed.), 317*(7161), 775–780.

Solovieva, S., Lallukka, T., Virtanen, M., & Viikari-Juntura, E. (2013). Psychosocial factors at work, long work hours, and obesity: A systematic review. *Scandinavian Journal of Work, Environment & Health, 39*, 241–258. doi:10.5271/sjweh.3364

Sproesser, G., Schupp, H. T., & Renner, B. (2014). The bright side of stress-induced eating: Eating more when stressed but less when pleased. *Psychological Science, 25*, 58–65. doi:10.1177/0956797613494849

Stansfeld, S., Bosma, H., Hemingway, H., & Marmot, M. (1998). Psychosocial work characteristics and social support as predictors of SF-36 health functioning: The Whitehall II study. *Psychosomatic Medicine, 60*(3), 247–255.

Steenland, K., Johnson, J., & Nowlin, S. (1997). A follow-up study of job strain and heart disease among males in the NHANES1 population. *American Journal of Industrial Medicine, 31*(2), 256–260.

Sterling, P. (2012). Allostasis: A model of predictive regulation. *Physiology & Behavior, 106*, 5–15. doi:10.1016/j.physbeh.2011.06.004

Sterling, P., & Eyer, J. (1981). Biological basis of stress-related mortality. *Social Science & Medicine. Part E, Medical Psychology, 15*(1), 3–42.

Sullivan, D., & von Wachter, T. (2009). Job displacement and mortality: An analysis using administrative data. *Quarterly Journal of Economics, 124*(3), 1265–1306.

Taylor, P., & Pocock, S. (1972). Mortality of shift and day workers 1956–68. *British Journal of Industrial Medicine, 29*(2), 201–207.

Terrill, A. L., & Garofalo, J. P. (2012). Cardiovascular disease and the workplace. In R. J. Gatchel & I. Z. Schultz (Eds.), *Handbook of occupational health and wellness* (pp. 87–103). New York, NY: Springer. doi:10.1007/978-1-4614-4839-6_5

Theorell, T. (2008). Anabolism and catabolism: Antagonistic partners in stress and strain. *Scandinavian Journal of Work, Environment & Health, 34*(6, Suppl.), 136–143.

Theorell, T., Hasselhorn, H., Vingård, E., & Andersson, B. (2000). Interleukin 6 and cortisol in acute musculoskeletal disorders: Results from a case-referent study in Sweden. *Stress Medicine, 16*, 27–35. doi:10.1002/(SICI)1099-1700(200001)16:1

Theorell, T., Tsutsumi, A., Hallquist, J., Reuterwall, C., Hogstedt, C., Fredlund, P., . . . Johnson, J. (1998). Decision latitude, job strain, and myocardial infarction: A study of working men in Stockholm. *American Journal of Public Health, 88*, 382–388. doi:10.2105/AJPH.88.3.382

Toker, S., Melamed, S., Berliner, S., Zeltser, D., & Shapira, I. (2012). Burnout and risk of coronary heart disease: A prospective study of 8838 employees. *Psychosomatic Medicine, 74*, 840–847. doi:10.1097/PSY.0b013e31826c3174

Toppinen-Tanner, S., Ahola, K., Koskinen, A., & Väänänen, A. (2009). Burnout predicts hospitalization for mental and cardiovascular disorders: 10-year prospective results from industrial sector. *Stress and Health, 25*, 287–296. doi:10.1002/smi.1282

Trinkoff, A., Le, R., Geiger-Brown, J., Lipscomb, J., & Lang, G. (2006). Longitudinal relationship of work hours, mandatory overtime, and on-call to musculoskeletal problems in nurses. *American Journal of Industrial Medicine, 49*(11), 964–971.

Trudel, X., Brisson, C., Milot, A., Masse, B., & Vézina, M. (2016). Adverse psychosocial work factors, blood pressure and hypertension incidence: Repeated exposure in a 5-year prospective cohort study. *Journal of Epidemiology & Community Health.* doi:10.1136/jech-2014-204914

Vahtera, J., Kivimäki, M., Pentti, J., Linna, A., Virtanen, M., Virtanen, P., & Ferrie, J. (2004). Organisational downsizing, sickness absence, and mortality: 10-town prospective cohort study. *BMJ (Clinical Research Ed.), 328*(7439), 555.

van Amelsvoort, L., Schouten, E., Maan, A., Swenne, C., & Kok, F. (2001). Changes in frequency of premature complexes and heart rate variability related to shift work. *Occupational and Environmental Medicine, 58*(10), 678–681.

van den Heuvel, S. G., van der Beek, A. J., Blatter, B. M., Hoogendoorn, W. E., & Bongers, P. M. (2005). Psychosocial work characteristics in relation to neck and upper limb symptoms. *Pain, 114*(1–2), 47–53.

Virtanen, M., Nyberg, S., Batty, G., Jokela, M., Heikkilä, K., Fransson, E., . . . Kivimäki, M. (2013). Perceived job insecurity as a risk factor for incident coronary heart disease: Systematic review and meta-analysis. *BMJ (Clinical Research Ed.) 347*, f4746. doi:10.1136/bmj.f4746

Walker, B. (2007). Glucocorticoids and cardiovascular disease. *European Journal of Endocrinology, 157*(5), 545–559.

Wardle, J., Chida, Y., Gibson, E. L., Whitaker, K. L., & Steptoe, A. (2011). Stress and adiposity: A meta-analysis of longitudinal studies. *Obesity, 19*, 771–778. doi:10.1038/oby.2010.241

Warren, N., Dillon, C., Morse, T., Hall, C., & Warren, A. (2000). Biomechanical, psychosocial, and organizational risk factors for WRMSD: Population-based estimates from the Connecticut Upper-extremity Surveillance Project (CUSP). *Journal of Occupational Health Psychology, 5*, 164–181. doi:10.1037/1076-8998.5.1.164

Weiss, N. (2002). Can the "specificity" of an association be rehabilitated as a basis for supporting a causal hypothesis? *Epidemiology, 13*(1), 6–8.

Westgaard, R. (1999). Effects of physical and mental stressors on muscle pain. *Scandinavian Journal of Work, Environment & Health, 25*(Suppl. 4), 19–24.

World Health Organization. (2013, March). *Cardiovascular diseases (CVDs)* (Fact sheet no. 317). Retrieved from www.who.int/mediacentre/factsheets/fs317/en/index.html

Xu, S., Huang, Y., Xiao, J., Zhu, W., Wang, L., Tang, H., . . . Liu, T. (2015). The association between job strain and coronary heart disease: A meta-analysis of prospective cohort studies. *Annals of Medicine, 47*, 512–518. doi:10.3109/07853890.2015.1075658

Workplace Violence and Psychological Aggression

KEY CONCEPTS AND FINDINGS COVERED IN CHAPTER 5

Workplace violence and its threat are both physically and psychologically disabling. In 1978, Bloch reported on 253 Los Angeles teachers who were referred for psychiatric evaluation. The teachers were exposed to a continuum of assaultive behavior ranging from threats of rape and murder to unprovoked physical assault. Students who acted out were sometimes sent to an administrator's office but often returned to class within minutes. Administrators compounded problems by discouraging teachers from reporting incidents and casting blame on teachers, although searches of student lockers revealed guns, knives, dynamite, and the like. Teachers suffered "lacerations, bruises, head injuries, and deafness." Bloch, however, found that the threats of brutal attack were often more disabling than an actual attack. The teachers experienced very high levels of anxiety and depressive and PTSD-like symptoms.

Greenberg and Barling (1999) conceptualized workplace violence on a continuum that ranged from "the least harmful behaviors," such as shouting at a coworker, to the most injurious, murder. Although a concern of this chapter is physical violence and its threat, the chapter also examines psychological aggression at the workplace. Psychological aggression does not include physical injury or its threat. One form of psychological aggression is known as "mobbing" (Leymann, 1990, 1996). Mobbing,[1] or bullying, involves one or more perpetrators with a power advantage over their victim systematically directing hostile behaviors toward their target over a sustained period of time. Just below the threshold of psychological aggression or, sometimes, barely overlapping with it, is the concept of incivility, a term that reflects disrespectful behavior. For example, incivility may take the form of a demeaning comment in which harmful intentions are not clear or can be attributed to the ignorance of the doer (Cortina, Magley, Williams, & Langhout, 2001).

Although conceptual differences among various forms of workplace mistreatment exist, there is often overlap in the content of the measures researchers use to assess various forms of mistreatment (Aquino & Thau, 2009; Hershcovis, 2011). Aggression can also be conceptualized as either reactive (e.g., driven by anger arising from a perceived insult) or proactive (e.g., planned in terms of attaining a goal by harming a coworker who is a rival for the same goal). The distinction between reactive and proactive aggression, however, is far from clear-cut because "aggression can have multiple motives" (Spector, 2011).

This chapter contains five sections devoted to violence and psychological aggression in the workplace.[2] The first section examines large cross-sectional studies that provide estimates of the extent of the problem of workplace aggression and identify jobs in which incumbents are at increased risk. The second section covers factors that increase violence exposure, and a subsection is devoted to theory and research on risk factors for engaging in aggressive behavior. The third section provides a close-up look at three occupational groups that have been subject to the threat of

---

[1] The term "mobbing" was borrowed from the work of ethologist Konrad Lorenz (1967) who used it to describe the counteroffensive of social animals that are ordinarily prey to a predator. As a group, the social animals turn on the predator to kill, wound, or "drive it so far away that it will hunt somewhere else" (p. 23). The term in ethology does not accurately translate to the context of human behavior because among humans, the individuals who engage in mobbing are typically more powerful than their victims.

[2] For reasons of space, the chapter does not cover other important types of workplace transgressions such as deliberate property damage and theft or aggression against the organization for which an individual works.

violence: nurses, teachers, and bus drivers. Although there are other occupational groups that are also at elevated risk, practical limitations led us to narrow our focus to three. The fourth section examines the consequences of violence, and the fifth, the consequences of psychological aggression. The second to fifth sections focus on longitudinal evidence, although some case-control and cross-sectional studies are included owing to the relative scarcity of longitudinal research.

It would be helpful from a methodological standpoint if every longitudinal study of violence were to begin at a point in time before an episode of workplace violence were to occur. Such longitudinal studies, however, have been rare. Another limitation of the longitudinal research on workplace violence is the frequent absence of assessments of the nature (e.g., pushing, hitting, kicking, use of a blunt object) and dangerousness of violent events (Høgh & Viitasara, 2005). The lack of precise definitions of the violent events is also a problem for case-control studies (whom to include in the case group; Høgh & Viitasara, 2005). The fifth section of the chapter includes some higher quality longitudinal studies on the impact of bullying. In such studies, bullying at baseline is a predictor of mental health outcomes at follow-up, controlling for baseline mental health (Nielsen & Einarsen, 2012).

EXTENT OF WORKPLACE VIOLENCE AND PSYCHOLOGICAL AGGRESSION

This section examines research on the prevalence of each of three types of aggression: homicide (the rarest), more common types of aggression (e.g., assault), and psychological aggression.

Prevalence of Homicide in the Workplace

Homicide is relatively rare in the workplace. In the United States between 2006 and 2010, 551 workers, on average, have been murdered annually (Bureau of Labor Statistics, 2013b). In 2010, 78% of the homicides were the result of shootings. More than 80% of the homicides occurred in private sector workplaces, although workplace shootings accounted for a tiny fraction of nonfatal workplace injuries. In 2010, 80% of the homicide victims were men. In 2011, there were 458 homicides (and 242 suicides) in U.S. workplaces (Bureau of Labor Statistics, 2012). Extrapolating from the BLS's (2013a) estimate that 139,869,000 people were employed in the United States in 2011, the homicide rate is 3.27 per million workers per year.

Prevalence of Workplace Violence, Excluding Homicide

This section examines the extensiveness of workplace violence and relies on findings from surveys of representative samples of workers. A national survey ($n \approx 600$, 43% female; Budd, Arvey, & Lawless, 1996) found that 2.5% of U.S. workers were attacked over the course of a single year, while 7.4% of workers were threatened with physical harm. Service employees and individuals who worked *other* than eight-to-five were at higher risk of violence exposure. Workers who handled cash, dealt with the public, and were between the ages of 19 and 24 were at increased risk of threat. Gender and ethnicity were not risk factors for either violence or its threat.

Schat, Frone, and Kelloway (2006), using data from a large representative sample of U.S. workers ($n = 2,508$), found that 6% of respondents had experienced some kind of physical violence at work in the previous year. Extrapolating to the U.S. population, the investigators estimated that 7 million U.S. workers are exposed to violence each year and that 1.3% are exposed to violence on a weekly basis. Violent events included (a) pushing, grabbing, and slapping; (b) kicking, biting, and punching; (c) being hit with an object or having an object thrown at but missing the respondent; and (d) being attacked with a knife, gun, or other weapons. According to the British Crime Survey, during 2010 and 2011 about 1.5% of the British work force, or 331,000 workers, experienced at least one incident of violence at work, a 4% increase over the previous data-collection cycle (Cookson & Buckley, 2012). Results of a study of a large ($n > 13,700$) representative sample of workers in Finland (Salminen, 1997) indicated that acts of violence at the workplace—these ranged from threats of harm to being hit hard enough to inflict a bruise or being stabbed—occurred at a rate of about 41 acts per 1,000 workers per year. Although men and women were equally likely to be victims, men were more likely to be the perpetrators. About half of the acts counted were threats.

Schat et al. (2006) identified occupation-related differences in exposure, with managers, business, and financial people least exposed and professionals (includes teachers), service workers, and workers involved in installation, maintenance, and production most exposed. The investigators also found differences by industry sector, with low rates of exposure in manufacturing and finance and high rates in the service industry (which in these data include nurses and teachers) and public administration (which includes police officers and firefighters) sectors.[3] Salminen (1997) found that in Finland, prison guards, police officers, and mental health nurses were at greatest risk.

Health care workers are particularly at high risk. More than 20% of nurses from eight European countries ($n > 34,000$; mostly female) were subject to physical violence initiated by patients or patients' relatives at a monthly or more frequent rate (Camerino, Estryn-Behar, Conway, van Der Heijden, & Hasselhorn, 2008). In Canada, there were approximately 4.4 officially recognized violent incidents per 100 health care workers (mainly nurses) per year (Yassi, Gilbert, & Cvitkovich, 2005). The study, of course, did not include incidents that went unreported. By contrast, Camerino et al. (2008) specifically asked nurses about the occurrence of violent incidents (but not the seriousness of the incidents).

Using official reports over a 4-month period in California, Peek-Asa, Howard, Vargas, and Kraus (1997) found that the occupations in which workers were most at risk for assault included police ($>6,000$ per 100,000 per year) and corrections officers ($>1,700$ per 100,000). Hospital workers (≈465 per 100,000) and individuals who worked in schools (≈270 per 100,000) were also at high risk. School bus drivers (≈518 per 100,000) were at twice the risk of teachers, although the student perpetrators were likely to overlap. Mass transit bus drivers were also at risk (≈445 per 100,000). Although not every occupational category was covered, Hashemi and Webster (1998), using violence-related U.S. Workers Compensation claims from 51 jurisdictions, found that the highest number of assault-related claims came from the education, banking, and health care sectors. The perpetrators

---

[3] I thank Michael Frone for helping to place specific occupations within the larger groups.

were mainly patients, clients, customers, and students. In a study of workers' compensation in Minnesota, LaMar, Gerberich, Lohman, and Zaidman (1998) found the highest rates of compensated assault-related injury were in public administration (a combination of police, corrections, fire, and general government employees), the social services, the health services, interurban transit, educational services, and, surprisingly, cultural institutions like museums. Women were more vulnerable to assault.

A study of a general population sample ($n = 4,961$) of Danes found that 8% had recently been subjected to either workplace violence or its threat (Høgh, Borg, & Mikkelsen, 2003). Of the almost 4,000 workers who were still employed 5 years later, the same percentage had been subjected to violence or its threat. Another study based on the same Danish sample found that workers in teaching and health care were at the highest risk (Wieclaw et al., 2006), which is consistent with analyses by Høgh et al., who found that jobs in which incumbents had a great deal of client contact were at high risk. In the United Kingdom, the highest rates of assault were found in the protective service occupations ($\approx$7%), health and social welfare workers ($\approx$2%), teachers (1.4%), and transport workers (1.4%; Fitzpatrick & Grant, 2012). Arnetz and Arnetz (2000), in a study involving 1,500 workers in 47 health-related workplaces in greater Stockholm, found that 63% of the entire sample experienced at least one episode of violence in the previous 12 months and 22% experienced episodes of violence several times. Some workplaces were emergency departments and geriatric care facilities; most, however, were psychiatric care facilities.

In general, nurses, teachers, bus drivers, and retail workers are at high risk. Workers in protective services, such as police and firefighters, are at very high risk.

Prevalence of Psychological Aggression in the Workplace

Psychological aggression is more common than physical aggression. Leymann (1996) found that 3.5% of Swedish workers ($n \approx 2,400$) were victims of mobbing, with about 40% victimized by multiple mobbers. Schat et al. (2006) estimated that the 1-year prevalence of psychological aggression (in this study, a broad category that ranged from being insulted in front of others to threats of violence) exceeded 40% of the U.S. workforce. Lahelma, Lallukka, Laaksonen, Saastamoinen, and Rahkonen (2012) found that, in their large ($n > 8,900$), mostly female sample of Helsinki municipal employees, the point prevalence[4] of bullying at baseline was 5%. In a Japanese sample ($n \approx 600$), women were found to be regularly bullied at almost twice the rate as men (9% vs. 5%; Giorgi, Ando, Arenas, Shoss, & Leon-Perez, 2013).

Research designed to estimate the incidence of new cases of psychological aggression is rare. In a longitudinal study of a large sample of Norwegian workers ($n = 1,775$), Nielsen, Hetland, Matthiesen, and Einarsen (2012) found that over 2 years, 5% of the sample that had not been bullied at baseline became new targets of bullying. In other words, the 2-year incidence of bullying was 5%.

---

[4] Point prevalence here refers to the percentage of workers experiencing bullying contemporaneously with data collection.

Epidemiologic findings bearing on Swedish workers indicate that victims of bullying were more likely to work in hospitals and schools than in other organizations (Leymann, 1996). Women and younger workers were slightly more likely to be victims. Cortina et al. (2001) found that incidents involving incivility are common: More than 70% of a representative sample ($n > 1,100$) of workers in a U.S. federal court experienced incivility over the previous 5 years, with individuals holding important positions often being the sources of these acts. Women were more commonly victimized than were men.

Workplace Violence and Psychological Aggression Commonly Occur

The research thus shows that violence in the workplace is common, with up to 10% of workers exposed during any 1 year, although there are a few exceptions. Violence is more prevalent in some sectors of the economy (e.g., police, nursing, teaching) than in others (e.g., finance). Furthermore, women are more likely to be victimized than are men. Psychological aggression in the workplace is more common than outright violence, with estimates of psychological aggression being as high as 40% per year in certain occupations.

RISK FACTORS FOR VIOLENCE IN THE WORKPLACE AND WORKER-ON-WORKER PSYCHOLOGICAL AGGRESSION

A number of large studies (Høgh et al., 2003; Schat et al., 2006; Ta et al., 2009) shed some light on the risk factors for aggression in the workplace. Schat et al. (2006) found that in the United States, neither race nor educational attainment were risk factors for workplace violence exposure. By contrast, age had a curvilinear relation to violence exposure with both the youngest (18 to 25) and oldest (41 to 50 and 51 to 65) age groups least exposed, and the ages in between most exposed. Day-shift workers were less exposed than were workers on evening and night shifts. Høgh et al. (2003) found that earlier exposure to violence and its threat was related to a 12-fold higher risk of violence- and threat-exposure 5 years later. A likely reason for the higher risk associated with past exposures "may be that employees tend to stay in the same types of job in [service work]" (Høgh et al., 2003, p. 191). Ecological factors are also evident in workplace violence risk. A North Carolina study indicated that workers in jobs located in census tracts characterized by poverty and instability are at higher risk of violence exposure than are workers in jobs located elsewhere (Ta et al., 2009).

The set of findings underline a number of risk factors for violence exposure. These factors include being aged 26 to 40, evening- and night-shift work, working for an organization located in unstable areas, and past exposures. Past exposure is partly reflective of having remained at the same job (or same type of job) with continuing levels of violence exposure.

Risk Factors for Psychological Aggression by Workers Against Other Workers

The focus of this section is research devoted to understanding worker-on-worker aggression (Hershcovis et al., 2007) rather than aggression committed by outsiders (e.g., customers, students). A meta-analysis found that role conflict, role ambiguity, role overload, and work constraints[5] are concurrently related to victim-reported harassment/aggression (Bowling & Beehr, 2006) although the study did not break out the findings by type of perpetrator (e.g., coworker, supervisor, customer). Luksyte, Spitzmueller, and Maynard (2011) found that holding a job for which one is overqualified[6] is associated with counterproductive workplace behavior.[7] The association is consistent with person–environment (P–E) fit theory (see Chapter 1), which holds that a mismatch between an individual's skills and the skills his or her job requires leads to strain. Superimposed on the P–E fit notion is the idea that an individual bringing relatively advanced skills to a job that requires few of those skills represents an unequal social exchange (see Chapter 3), an exchange that increases the likelihood of a frustration-laden, angry response.

Theories that attempt to explain worker-initiated aggression, however, can be built around the idea that negative emotions (e.g., anger, frustration) mediate the relation of undesirable work-related situations to the expression of workplace aggression (Spector, Fox, & Domagalski, 2006). Examples of provoking situational factors include a worker being treated unfairly, subjected to an insult, or denied resources needed to complete a task. In contrast to the emotion of anger, which is a state that dissipates over time, trait anger is a personality dimension that represents a stable propensity to become angry and is a risk factor itself. The aforementioned stressors may also be more likely to affect a worker who is high in trait anger than a comparable worker who is low in that trait.

Another personality trait, negative affectivity (NA), is characterized by a long-term tendency to experience dysphoric emotions. NA, low self-esteem, and low levels of agreeableness in a worker are thought to put that worker at risk for becoming a target for workplace aggression (Aquino & Thau, 2009; Milam, Spitzmueller, & Penney, 2009; Spector, 2011). Individuals high in NA may evoke psychological aggression because they tend to be irritable and that irritability provokes a negative response. On the other hand, they are also sensitive to a perceived discourtesy or can observe a slight when there was none. Low levels of agreeableness may invite uncivil interactions with others (Milam et al., 2009). Why low self-esteem is a risk factor may reflect (a) the impact of accumulated victimization over time or (b) an inability to defend oneself, making the individual a tempting target for another worker's aggressiveness (Aquino & Thau, 2009).

The vast majority of research on factors that help to explain workplace aggression has been cross-sectional (Spector, 2011). The cross-sectional nature of this research is an obstacle to establishing the temporal priority of the provoking situational factor and an aggressive act. Cross-sectional designs are problematic even for establishing the temporal priority of stable traits (e.g., NA in the victim), which presumably

---

[5] Role ambiguity refers to an information deficiency in the work environment, making the duties required to perform one's job unclear (Beehr, 1995). Role conflict refers to conflicting demands being placed on the worker. Role overload refers to excessive demands on the worker; it is akin to psychological workload, which was discussed in Chapter 3. Work constraints refer to workplace factors (e.g., lack of supplies) that are obstacles to completing one's job.

[6] This is a state of affairs that is more likely to arise during an economic downturn than other times.

[7] There will be more on CWB later. In the study by Luksyte et al. (2011), aggression directed against coworkers and aggression directed against the organization were lumped together because they tend to be highly correlated.

antedate the aggressive act. Although, theoretically, a stable trait antedates recent acts of aggression, it is possible that a recent act of aggression influenced how a worker regards himself or herself, affecting the worker's responses on a trait scale administered contemporaneously with measures of aggression. With these caveats in mind, some cross-sectional research is described next.

Much research on workplace aggression relies on reporting by the victim rather than the perpetrator (Bowling & Beehr, 2006), although there are exceptions (e.g., Douglas & Martinko, 2001; Greenberg & Barling, 1999). In a study of 151 U.S. education and transportation workers, Douglas and Martinko (2001) found that trait anger, favorable attitudes toward revenge, and long-term difficulties (e.g., history of alcohol abuse) were related to psychological aggression at the workplace (e.g., "Saying unkind things to purposely harm other coworkers while at work"). Hershcovis et al. (2007) noted that the combination of situational and personality factors, perhaps in interaction, is more likely to climax in the anger that can fuel aggressive acts. Greenberg and Barling (1999), using a cross-sectional sample of male, nonfaculty employees ($n = 136$) at a Canadian university, found that a history of aggression and alcohol use put an employee at risk for *committing* acts of psychological aggression (e.g., malicious gossip, rude gestures) against a coworker, particularly when workers perceived procedural justice in the organization to be weak. A history of aggression and alcohol use predicted aggression against subordinates under conditions of job insecurity. Procedural injustice and workplace surveillance (e.g., timed lunch) were related to aggression against supervisors. Thus, factors related to aggression against coworkers, subordinates, and supervisors differed somewhat (also see Hershcovis et al., 2007; Inness, LeBlanc, & Barling, 2008).

Alcohol is also implicated in sexual harassment. Sexual harassment of female workers is more likely to occur in work units in which (a) a high proportion of males are heavy drinkers (assessed independently of the females' reports on harassment) and (b) permissive drinking norms prevail (Bacharach, Bamberger, & McKinney, 2007).

A line of research that sheds additional light on risk factors for employee aggression is research on counterproductive workplace behavior (CWB). CWB refers to "intentional acts by employees that harm organizations or their stakeholders" (Spector et al., 2006, p. 30). CWB covers a spectrum of behavior that ranges from violence directed at a coworker to bullying to destroying the employer's property to stealing supplies, and thus overlaps with some of the behaviors already discussed. Moreover, it is sometimes difficult to distinguish acts of aggression against property from acts of aggression against an individual (Spector, 2011). A limitation of CWB research has been that "the vast majority of CWB studies" has relied on cross-sectional designs, limiting conclusions that can be drawn regarding temporal priority and duration of effects (Meier & Spector, 2013). An exception is Meier and Spector's longitudinal study. They followed a sample of mostly Swiss workers ($n > 660$) every 2 months for 10 months. The investigators found that having experienced workplace constraints (e.g., getting incorrect instructions, lack of equipment or supplies) increased the risk of later psychological aggression (e.g., cursing at someone, saying something hurtful to someone). Meier and Spector (2013) also found that engaging in psychological aggression increased the later risk of both experiencing organizational constraints and being on the receiving end of workplace incivility. The research, thus, underlines "a vicious cycle with negative consequences for all parties" (p. 535).

Workplace factors that are thought to contribute to coworker aggression include role conflict, role ambiguity, unfair treatment, a work unit climate that is permissive with regard to alcohol use, and workplace constraints that impede the attainment of work goals. Person factors in perpetrators include a history of aggression, favorable attitudes toward revenge, trait anger, and excessive alcohol use. NA and self-esteem are person factors in victims.

FOCUS ON THREE OCCUPATIONAL GROUPS

Although violence and psychological aggression can be a problem at any job, three occupations, namely, nursing, teaching, and bus driving, are examined. Research suggests that these three occupations are particularly vulnerable. These groups experience higher-than-average risk of violence exposure (Wieclaw et al., 2006). Unlike police work and the military, exposure to violence is not part of nurses', teachers', or bus drivers' job descriptions; research, however, indicates that members of these occupational groups are more highly exposed to violence than are members of most other occupational groups. In the case of bus drivers, there has not been as much research as there has been on nurses and teachers.

Nurses

In research on workplace violence, obtaining accurate data on assaults in nursing, as in any occupation, is critical to understanding factors that put workers at risk. Lion, Snyder, and Merrill (1981) found that as many as four-fifths of all assaults on staff at a large state mental hospital in Maryland were not formally reported. To obtain accurate data on violence and psychological aggression in nurses, it is therefore important to go beyond official reports. In an epidemiologic survey involving a random sample of almost 5,000 Minnesota nurses, Gerberich et al. (2005) found that more than 13% of nurses were assaulted over the course of 12 months. A study (Zhou, Yang, & Spector, 2015) conducted in the southeastern United States found that 7% of new entrants to the nursing profession were assaulted (mainly by patients) over the course of their first 6 months on the job and 16% over the course of the next 6 months. Verbal aggression was more common, experienced by between 28% and 40% of the nurses, depending on the time period. Gerberich et al. (2005), in a case-control study built into their epidemiologic survey, found that emergency room (ER) and psychiatric nurses were at significantly higher risk than the study's reference group, surgical nurses. Nurses who worked in a psychiatric department or a long-term care facility were at elevated risk for psychological aggression (e.g., unwelcome sexual remarks and other verbal abuse; Nachreiner et al., 2007). The rates of assault are particularly high in psychiatric wards (Chen, Sun, Lan, & Chiu, 2009; Harrell, 2011). Using a decade of data from a study (Flannery, Stone, Rego, & Walker, 2001) of assaultive behavior directed at mental health workers in Massachusetts state facilities, the assault rate can be calculated to be about 8% per year in both inpatient and community settings.

Data from Europe (Camerino et al., 2008), Japan (Fujita et al., 2012), and Taiwan (Chen et al., 2009) indicate that violence initiated by patients or their relatives is an occupational hazard. Bearing in mind that these data likely involve underreporting, in the United States, the rate of workplace assault between 2005 and 2009 was

8.1 per 1,000 nurses, which compares unfavorably with the national rate of 5.1 for all workplace assaults (Harrell, 2011); data from OSHA[8] logs parallel these findings (Bureau of Labor Statistics, 2013b).

Crilly, Chaboyer, and Creedy (2004) found that ER nurses in Australia are at risk for both physical and verbal aggression, with 70% over the course of 5 months exposed to episodes of either physical or verbal aggression or both. Verbal aggression may be considered a prophetic event because in the ER context, each patient is a stranger to the nurse, and verbal aggression has to be considered a potential prelude to physical violence. The most common type of verbal aggression was swearing and the most common type of physical violence was pushing. Risk factors for exposure to physical violence included working on the evening shift, excessive alcohol or drug use in perpetrators, perpetrator mental illness, and long waiting times. Particularly noteworthy in this study was that nurses reliably estimated the timing of when an episode of aggression occurred.

Estimates from a meta-analysis (Spector, Zhou, & Che, 2014) that combined data from both representative and convenience samples ($n > 50,000$) from many different countries indicated that, over the course of a year, more than 30% of nurses were victims of physical assault, and almost two-thirds, of nonphysical aggression. Patients and, sometimes, their families were mostly responsible for physical aggression. A variety of individuals (patients, families, doctors, other staff members) were responsible for nonphysical aggression. Spector et al. (2014) found the highest rates of victimization in emergency departments, geriatric treatment facilities, and psychiatric units.

Hospital Climate

Although there has been research on violence exposure among nurses, there has not been much longitudinal research with controls for baseline status. An exception is the study by Yang, Spector, Chang, Gallant-Roman, and Powell (2012). In their two-wave study involving 176 Florida nurses, Yang et al. found that management's lack of violence prevention pressure (e.g., perceived pressure on nurses to complete work quickly even if it means ignoring violence prevention procedures) predicted violence exposure 6 months later in nurses who had not been exposed at time 1. In a study of U.S. nurses ($n = 126$) at the outset of their careers, Spector, Yang, and Zhou (2015) found that violence prevention climate, measured during the nurses' first few months on the job, was related to reduced levels of exposure to violence and verbal abuse 6 months later. Violence prevention pressure is reminiscent of safety climate (see Chapter 6), a workplace factor found to be related to accident risk.

A Small Corps of Patients and the Context of Assaults

Working in mental hospitals or institutions for the criminally insane poses a risk to nurses. Evidence from Canada (Cooper & Mendonca, 1991; Harris & Varney, 1986; Quinsey & Varney, 1977), Norway (Bjørkly, 1999), and the United Kingdom (Aiken, 1984) indicates that a small number of mental patients is responsible for most assaults. Risk factors for patients acting in an assaultive manner include criminal insanity (Bjørkly, 1999; Harris & Varney, 1986), a history of substance abuse (Flannery et al.,

---

[8] OSHA is the Occupational Safety and Health Administration in the United States.

2001), poor preadmission social functioning (Harris & Varney, 1986), a history of violence (Aiken, 1984; Flannery, Stevens, Juliano, & Walker, 2000), having been victimized by others (Flannery et al., 2000), and younger patient age (Harris & Varney, 1986; Quinsey & Varney, 1977). Assaultive behavior was more likely to occur during periods of containment or restraint than from direct attack (Carmel & Hunter, 1989, 1993; Cooper & Mendonca, 1991; Flannery et al., 2001). Other findings (Chou, Lu, & Chang, 2001) suggest that the locations of assaults are likely to include what are high traffic areas for patients (e.g., bedrooms, dining rooms, corridors). There is some evidence that, in retrospect, victimized staff could have anticipated the attack, on the basis of observing anger or other cues in the patient (Aiken, 1984).

In one respect, psychiatric nursing has something in common with professional football in the United States. The injury rate in the National Football League is about 10% per week in a season that lasts 17 weeks (Halchin, 2008), not counting the high injury rate during the 5-week preseason (Feeley et al., 2008), suggesting an annual injury rate close to 100%. There is evidence that the injury rate may be equally high among psychiatric nurses. Consider that a 14-week London study (Whittington & Wykes, 1994) found that 32% of nurses in a psychiatric hospital were attacked. Extrapolating roughly to the course of a year, one could expect close to 100% of the nurses to be victims. Men and women were equally victimized. The investigators ruled out a victim-proneness hypothesis, finding that nurse personality factors (impulsiveness and venturesomeness, dimensions of risk-taking) were unrelated to victimization. As in other studies, attacks tended to be launched by a small corps of aggressive patients.

Summary of the Nursing Findings

The research suggests that some types of nursing roles (e.g., in psychiatric facilities, ERs) are more vulnerable than others (e.g., surgical care). Risk factors for assault include patients having a history of violence and substance abuse. A relatively small group of patients tends to be responsible for many assaults. There is evidence that assaults are more likely to occur in situations in which nurses have to make impositions on a patient (e.g., administer a medication, apply restraints). In some instances, victimized nurses, in retrospect, have thought that they could have observed cues that would have helped them anticipate violent behavior in a patient. One factor that appears to be related to reduced violence exposure is a commitment by hospital management to not tolerate violence.

Teachers

The first author was once a mathematics teacher in a tough, low-achieving New York City (NYC) public school. One afternoon, during his first year on the job, he was walking into the school after lunch when he was struck in the back by a rock thrown by a student. The injury led to a brief medical leave—he did not quit right then, although he eventually left this dangerous school. It should be stressed that concerns about violence are generally shared by teachers who work in the same school, whether victimized or not, and that these shared concerns are related to poor morale and lower student achievement (Wittmer, Sinclair, Martin, Tucker, & Lang, 2013). Within 10 years, almost the entire staff in the first author's school had turned over.

What Qualitative Research Has to Say

Although our focus has been on quantitatively organized research, sometimes qualitative studies (e.g., Bloch, 1978) open the door to research efforts to identify problems that quantitatively oriented researchers have *not yet* pursued (Schonfeld & Mazzola, 2012). Qualitative studies document a side of teaching that has sometimes been missed in other types of studies. Ginsberg, Schwartz, Olson, and Bennett (1987) found that teachers and students in urban U.S. schools were exposed to violence and its threat, including gang warfare, and vandalism. Problems included unauthorized individuals entering a school building and frequent false fire alarms. Schonfeld and Santiago (1994) found violence and security concerns were a major theme that emerged from NYC teachers' descriptions of their jobs (e.g., a female teacher was attacked by a 16-year-old boy; a female teacher was attacked by a taller, heavier assistant; armed intruders entered a school; male high school students propositioned female teachers). In many instances, administrators did little in response. Terry (1998) found that students in urban secondary schools in the English Midlands directed insolent and abusive behavior at teachers. More than 10% of the teachers were subjected to physical threats.

Smith and Smith (2006) identified unusually violent events affecting teachers in urban U.S. schools (who subsequently quit their jobs). For example, a pregnant teacher was pinned against a blackboard by a large fifth grader. Warring students used whatever weapons they could find (e.g., stakes in the ground supporting newly planted trees, soda bottles) in waging a gang war. Younghusband (2008), in her Newfoundland study, found that teachers were exposed to violence and its threat from both students *and* their parents and that teachers had to be concerned about threatening telephone calls to their homes. She also found evidence of administrator callousness and indifference. Thus, qualitative research indicates that violence against teachers is a significant problem.

Official Data on Assault

One of the obstacles to identifying factors that put teachers at risk is that violence against teachers, like violence against nurses, often goes unreported. Bearing in mind that official records tend to undercount assaults (Schonfeld, 2006), Casteel, Peek-Asa, and Limbos (2007), in their study of reportable assaults victimizing Los Angeles teachers, found that there were 153 assaults in 1 year in the district of 460 schools and 23,000 teachers. Middle school teachers were at the highest risk, and high school teachers, next highest. Consistent with ecological/contextual models of school violence (Schonfeld, 2006), Casteel et al. found that the amount of criminality in the area surrounding a school was related to the risk of in-school assault.

Data Obtained From the Teachers Themselves

In order to understand the dimensions of the problem of violence against teachers, it is important to obtain accurate information. One way to obtain accurate information is to independently survey teachers rather than rely on official reports. Reports from many countries and localities in which teachers were specifically asked about assaults provide a clearer picture of risk. For example, a Minnesota study (Gerberich et al., 2011) found that 8% of teachers reported that they were assaulted in the course of a year; 38% reported that they had been victims of psychological aggression such as sexual harassment. Three percent of a Dutch secondary school teacher sample indicated that they were exposed to pushing and kicking over the course of 6 months and 1%, to severe violence such as beatings (Mooij, 2011). In the United States as a whole, 10% of teachers in city schools reported having been physically attacked or threatened with injury in a year with slightly lower rates in suburban (6%) and rural (5%) schools (Robers, Zhang, & Truman, 2012; Tourkin et al., 2007). About half a Slovakian secondary school sample experienced "harmful student behaviors" such as destruction of personal property, threats of physical harm, or assault in the last month, with teachers at vocational schools at even greater risk (Dzuka & Dalbert, 2007). In a British Columbia teacher sample, 10% reported having been threatened with violence or subjected to attempted violence in the previous 12 months; 5%, having been victims of violence; and 29%, having been subjected to abusive language and gestures (Wilson, Douglas, & Lyon, 2011). In Finland, 2% of the teachers sampled indicated that they were subjected to physical threats and to physical violence almost weekly; 5%, to name-calling; and 9%, to obscene comments (Kauppi & Pörhölä, 2012).

It is also helpful to collect data in real time in order to minimize the risk of forgetting and ascertain events as they occur, as in the next study. Schonfeld and Feinman (2012) followed more than 250 NYC public school teachers every day for 2 weeks. Over the time period, 25% of the teachers observed at least one student physically hurting another, an unsettling statistic if one considers that the duration of the study is only a small fraction of the school year, a finding consistent with Mooij (2011), who documented high rates of exposure to student-on-student fighting in his Netherlands study. Over 2 weeks, students threatened 6% of the NYC teachers with physical harm. As in the nationwide study by Robers et al. (2012), NYC teachers who taught at secondary schools (including middle schools) were at the highest risk. Teaching in low-achieving schools was also a risk factor for threats.

Summary of the Teacher Findings

Teachers are commonly exposed to physical and psychological aggression in two different ways. They are direct victims, and they observe students hurting other students. The types of violence to which teachers are exposed are on a continuum and range from being hit to student-on-student fighting to rock throwing to sexual improprieties to threats of violence. Secondary/middle school teachers are at the highest risk for exposure to aggression, although elementary school teachers are not exempt. Teaching at low-achieving schools is also a risk factor. Violence in neighborhoods in which schools are located can set the stage for aggressive behavior within schools. Administrative indifference has also been a factor in connection to violence exposure.

Bus Drivers

Bus drivers are exposed to the public every day, and with that exposure comes risk. A cross-sectional study (Duffy & McGoldrick, 1990) of more than 370 bus drivers in a city in the United Kingdom found that 30% had been victims of physical assault on the job, although the time frame was not clear. In a small study of 22 London bus drivers who were assaulted, researchers found that assaults most often occurred in the evening and were evenly distributed across all days of the week (Fisher & Jacoby, 1992). Most of the assailants were male. In seven (22%) of the episodes, more than one attacker was involved. About half of the assaults involved disputes over bus fare. A little more than half of the attackers were adults, with the remainder, juveniles. The police were involved in more than 80% of the incidents, but in only five cases were attackers apprehended.

CONSEQUENCES OF VIOLENCE EXPOSURE AT THE WORKPLACE

Although the focal concern of this chapter is the psychological impact of violence exposure, a major consequence of workplace violence is physical injury. For example, Ryan and Poster (1989) followed for 1 year 61 nurses who had been physically assaulted at the California neuropsychiatric hospital in which they worked. Three suffered severe back injuries that collectively contributed to 94 sick days. The most commonly occurring consequences in the mental health worker study by Flannery et al. (2001) were bruises, head injuries, and soft tissue injuries. In Carmel and Hunter's (1989, 1993) study of a large California forensic hospital, head injuries were more common than any other physical consequence of patient violence.

With regard to the psychological consequences of violence exposure, the stress reaction model (Zapf, Dormann, & Frese, 1996) is noteworthy. According to the model, the impact of a stressor on psychological functioning (e.g., distress) is in approximate proportion to exposure time. An alternative but related model holds that the severity and unpredictability of a directly or vicariously experienced violent workplace event is directly related to the seriousness of the psychological and physiological outcomes (Barling, 1996). Fear, negative mood, and distraction are likely candidate variables mediating the relation of the violent event to potential outcomes such as depression, psychosomatic symptoms, and disengagement from work (Barling, 1996). The presence of mediators, however, is difficult to test because ascertaining the timing of each of the mental events within a chain of mental events hypothesized to occur is challenging.

For ease of presentation, the rest of this section is divided into subsections on the basis of study types. A later section examines the consequences of exposure to psychological aggression in the workplace.

Cross-Sectional Research on the Consequences of Exposure to Workplace Violence

While violence in the workplace can lead to physical injury, it can also give rise to psychological injury. Consistent with Barling's (1996) mediational model, cross-sectional evidence (Rogers & Kelloway, 1997) from frontline (e.g., customer service) employees at a Canadian financial institution suggests that the adverse effect of violence exposure (as a victim or observer) on mental health (and turnover intentions) is mediated by fear. There is also evidence that a violent assault is likely to provoke sustained physiological arousal (Eriksen, Bjorvatn, Bruusgaard, & Knardahl, 2008) and psychosomatic symptoms (Yang et al., 2012). Although most of the violence-related injuries to Canadian health care workers were "surface wounds" (e.g., bruises), data from Ontario indicated that 58% of stress-related, that is, psychological, worker compensation claims were linked to exposure to violence (Yassi et al., 2005).

In a study involving ER medical staff in three urban Canadian hospitals, Alden, Regambal, and Laposa (2008) found that, compared with staff who witnessed a patient being subjected to a direct threat, staff who were subjected to a direct threat experienced more fear, arousal, and job dissatisfaction. Duffy and McGoldrick (1990) found that bus drivers who were assaulted on the job, compared with drivers who were not victims, showed more symptoms of depression, anxiety, and so forth. Budd et al. (1996) found that individuals who had been victims of workplace violence or had been threatened with violence in the previous 12 months showed increased distress, job dissatisfaction, and worry about future attacks. Recently victimized or threatened workers were more inclined to bring a weapon to work, potentially sparking a cycle of violence. Data from a study of Canadian health care workers suggest that having been a victim of physical violence increased feelings of fear, which in turn mediated the relation of violence to elevated scores on the GHQ (Schat & Kelloway, 2003—the GHQ is discussed in Chapter 3), a finding consistent with Barling (1996) and Rogers and Kelloway (1997). Organizational support was found to help buffer the impact of violence exposure on emotional well-being, but not on fear of future violence and neglect of job duties (Schat & Kelloway, 2003).

A few cross-sectional studies link exposure to aggression to poor outcomes in teachers. Exposure to aggression is linked to fear, which in turn is linked to job dissatisfaction; job dissatisfaction influences intentions to quit (Sinclair, Martin, & Croll, 2002). A study of U.S. secondary school teachers (Ting, Sanders, & Smith, 2002) found that those working in high-violence schools, compared with teachers in low-violence schools, had significantly more PTSD-like symptoms (e.g., intrusive thoughts, avoidant behaviors), a result consistent with Bloch (1978). In their study of Belgian teachers, Galand, Lecoq, and Philippot (2007) found that their broadly defined measure of school violence (which included psychological aggression) was related to depression, anxiety, and somatization symptoms. Colleague and administrator support was related to improved well-being. Increased symptoms and lower support were related to reduced professional engagement (e.g., having plans to leave teaching). Dzuka and Dalbert (2007) found that Slovakian teachers' exposure to harmful behaviors was related to increased negative affect and reduced life satisfaction. Wilson et al. (2011) found that exposure to violence or its threat was related to increased fear, reduced morale, and increased physical, emotional, and psychosomatic symptoms in British Columbia teachers.

Case-Control Research on the Consequences of Exposure to Workplace Violence

In a case-control study involving more than 14,000 Danish hospital inpatients and outpatients suffering from either an affective (e.g., depression) or anxiety disorder and more than 58,000 demographically matched controls, Wieclaw et al. (2006) found that the cases were significantly more likely to have worked at jobs associated with increased risk for violence exposure. In men, but not in women, jobs associated with high levels of threat were at elevated risk for anxiety disorders. The study has two limitations. First, the selection-based hypothesis that vulnerable individuals select themselves, or are selected by the workplace gatekeepers, into high-exposure jobs cannot be ruled out. Second, because the exposure variable is a proxy, it is not clear if the cases and controls differed in actual exposure to violence or its threat.

Although transport workers are at risk for being victims of violence (Fitzpatrick & Grant, 2012), they have not been extensively studied. In a small case-control study involving London bus crews, Fisher and Jacoby (1992) compared 22 victims of assault with 22 matched nonassaulted controls. Although bruising was the most common injury, some bus drivers were stabbed or suffered fractures. Assault victims lost, on average, more than 90 days of work, with days lost related to severity of the injury. Compared with controls, assault victims showed significantly higher GHQ scores, with more symptoms of avoidance and thought intrusion[9] regardless of whether they were diagnosed for PTSD. Symptom intensity was related to the severity of the assault, consistent with the theories of Barling (1996) and Zapf et al. (1996).

Longitudinal Research on the Consequences of Exposure to Workplace Violence

Compared with longitudinal research on the other psychosocial workplace stressors (e.g., decision latitude) affecting the mental health of workers, longitudinal research on the impact of workplace violence is more difficult to conduct. Researchers have to assess mental health before the occurrence of workplace violence, wait for the seemingly unpredictable exposures to occur while hoping on humanitarian grounds that the exposures will not occur, and then assess mental health afterward, adjusting for preincident mental health. It is important that researchers include in the sample groups of comparable workers who were and were not assaulted. Although such research would help pin down the effects of violence exposure, research along these lines is difficult to implement and, understandably, rarely seen.

Two studies (Wykes & Whittington, 1998; Yang et al., 2012) illustrate these methodological difficulties. Wykes and Whittington were able to include only 10 nurses who were seen pre- and postassault, although the investigators were able to identify 97 consecutive assaults on nurses at a London psychiatric hospital. Yang et al.'s two-wave, 6-month longitudinal study of Florida nurses identified four groups that could be compared: (1) no physical violence during the time periods antedating both waves of data collection; (2) no violence before wave 1 and violence before wave 2; (3) violence before wave 1 but not during the 6 months antedating wave 2; and (4) violence before each time period. Groups 2 and 3, however, were small ($\leq$18).

Longer-Term Longitudinal Studies

Two studies (Bjørkly, 1999; Høgh et al., 2003) examined the long-term consequences of exposure to violence in the workplace. Høgh et al. (2003), in their study of a representative sample of Danish workers, found that violence or its threat at baseline predicted fatigue 5 years later, controlling for a number of covariates including baseline fatigue. The investigators also found that two covariates, lack of support from coworkers and lack of support from managers, also predicted later fatigue. In Bjørkly's (1999) 10-year study of nurses in a secure psychiatric facility in Norway, only about 0.5% of 2,000 incidents resulted in serious injury. Most injuries, however, led to nurses taking days off from work, although there were no data on psychological trauma.

Shorter-Term Longitudinal Studies

Other studies have been concerned with shorter-term consequences of violence exposure. In the 6-month study by Yang et al. (2012), nurses who were exposed to violence at wave 2 but not wave 1 showed a significant increase in somatic

---

[9] Thought intrusion refers to involuntary images or thoughts that, in the case of the assault victims described here, are displeasing and unwelcome.

symptoms over the 6 months when compared with nurses who were not exposed at either wave. Nurses exposed at wave 1 but not wave 2 showed a significant decrease in symptoms over the 6 months compared with nurses who were exposed at both waves. In a 1-year, two-wave study involving more than 2,800 first-year Danish health care assistants, Høgh, Sharipova, and Borg (2008) found that violence and its threat in previous jobs adversely affected later mental health (symptoms of anxiety, depression, etc.) and vitality (fatigue), controlling for baseline mental health. Another short-term, two-wave study yielded a surprising result. Camerino et al. (2008), in their study of more than 13,800 nurses in eight European countries, unexpectedly found that physical violence at baseline was not significantly related to perceived health 1 year later. Baseline violence exposure, however, exerted an adverse effect on later organizational commitment, controlling for baseline commitment. Despite the study's large sample size, and its concomitant statistical power, the lack of effect on perceived health may be partly explained by the loss at follow-up of more than 20,000 nurses seen at baseline, particularly the nurses who were most exposed to violence at baseline.

Wykes and Whittington (1998), in following 39 nurses who were assaulted, found high levels of psychological distress after the assault compared with levels in control nurses. The high symptom levels observed immediately after the assault declined with time, although anger remained high. The 10 control nurses who were subsequently assaulted showed a significant pre- to postassault decrease in their ability to control anger. In Ryan and Poster's (1989) earlier mentioned follow-up of nurses who were assaulted, reactions to assault (e.g., fear of returning to work) diminished over the course of the weeks following the event. Anger was the most common response. About 20% of the nurses continued to experience severe reactions to the assault after 6 months or a year. Consistent with Zapf et al.'s (1996) and Barling's (1996) models, assaults resulting in physical injury were associated with higher levels of psychological symptoms of traumatic stress. Consistent with the two models, victims who, postassault, were placed in more dangerous ward environments showed higher levels of traumatic stress symptoms than comparable nurses who, postassault, were placed in less dangerous wards. A longitudinal component built into Fisher and Jacoby's (1992) earlier mentioned case-control study indicated that in 15 of the 22 transport worker assault victims, many psychological symptoms declined over the 18-month follow-up. By contrast, symptoms of thought intrusion tended to persist.

A study (Beale, Clarke, Cox, Leather, & Lawrence, 1999) of violence occurring in British pubs heralds the idea of "system memory," the investigators' term for the past influencing the future as opposed to each day being unrelated to the previous day. The occurrence of a violent incident at a pub increased the risk of violence reoccurring in the next 6 months, particularly the 7 days following the initial incident. Findings from the British Crime Survey indicate that 43% of victims of workplace crimes are repeat victims (Cookson & Buckley, 2012).

Summing up the Consequences of Violence Exposure

Consequences of workplace violence include physical injury, for example, bruising, head and back injuries, fractures, and soft tissue injuries. Workplace violence engenders psychological consequences, including symptoms of depression and anxiety as well as PTSD-like symptoms. Workplace violence also provokes fear and/or anger in the victim and can produce disengagement from work. In addition, violence exposure tends to predict future violence exposure. There is evidence that the severity of the exposure is related to the severity of the symptom response. Evidence also suggests that organizational support can be helpful to victims. Some problems that arise in the aftermath of an assault are more likely to decline over time (e.g., psychological distress) than others (e.g., fear, anger).

CONSEQUENCES OF WORKPLACE PSYCHOLOGICAL AGGRESSION

Psychological aggression, short of overt violence, also has adverse consequences for the victim. Symptoms of depression, anxiety, and burnout; reduced job satisfaction; and reduced self-esteem are concurrently related to reports of victimization (Aquino & Thau, 2009; Bowling & Beehr, 2006). The theoretical framework known as "stress-as-offense-to-self" (SOS; Semmer, Jacobshagen, Meier, & Elfering, 2007) is relevant to understanding the impact of psychological aggression. According to the SOS framework, an individual's self-esteem is an important personal resource. Self-esteem reflects the individual's sense of his or her own worth, although some have suggested that self-esteem also reflects the confidence the individual has in his or her abilities, particularly abilities in those areas he or she believes to be most personally important (Andrews, 1998).

According to conservation of resources theory, self-esteem is part of an array of interlinked personal resources such as optimism and a sense of mastery of the environment, resources that contribute to stress resistance, and that low levels of one resource are related to low levels of the others (Hobfoll, 2001). Psychologically aggressive behaviors such as bullying constitute an assault on the target's self-esteem. Bowling and Beehr (2006) suggested that job-related bullying or harassment can damage the target's self-image by making the victim very conscious of his or her powerlessness and low status.

SOS theory recognizes that humans have a need to belong to, and be accepted by, a group, such as the group of people with whom the individual works. SOS theory acknowledges that the disrespect dished out to a target by psychologically aggressive coworkers and managers (e.g., workplace bullies) drives the target away from the group and can cause the individual to lose face. Belongingness is closely linked to self-esteem.

The impact of psychological aggression on self-esteem is thus an important component of the SOS framework. Reduced self-esteem is associated with depression, as succinctly explained by one psychologist who remarked that "low self-esteem has been conceptualized as a cause, a result, and a symptom of depression" (M. C. Spett, personal communication, April 2013). Some have advanced the view that low self-esteem can mediate the relation of job stressors to depression (Lee, Joo, & Choi, 2013). An alternative hypothesis, known as the "scar hypothesis," suggests that low self-esteem can be a result of depression (Sowislo & Orth, 2013). Finally, "unrealistic negative evaluations of one's worth" are a symptom of depression (American Psychiatric Association, 2013). Regardless of the connection between low self-esteem and depression, the SOS theory holds that the damage psychological aggression does to the target's self-esteem is dispiriting, and increases the risk of depression.

Although much of the chapter underlines longitudinal research, two pioneering cross-sectional studies stand as landmarks (Cortina et al., 2001; Leymann & Gustafsson, 1996) in research on aggression. An intensive study of 64 Swedish workers who were mobbing victims, and, consequently, undergoing treatment, revealed that more than 90% of the victims met criteria for PTSD (Leymann & Gustafsson, 1996). The consequences of workplace bullying can be severe. In the earlier mentioned study of U.S. court workers, Cortina et al. (2001) found that exposure to incivility, which is not as intense as bullying, was related to lower job satisfaction, reduced intentions to persist at the job, and psychological distress.

Longitudinal Research on the Consequences of Exposure to Workplace Psychological Aggression

While a host of cross-sectional studies involving 66 different samples have linked workplace bullying to a variety of mental health outcomes, including anxiety, depression, psychosomatic, and PTSD symptoms (Nielsen & Einarsen, 2012), rigorously designed longitudinal studies are necessary for establishing the temporal priority of bullying over these outcomes. The following subsections examine longitudinal studies that evaluated the mental health consequences of psychological aggression—mainly in the form of bullying—assessed at a baseline period of measurement, controlling for baseline mental health.

Longitudinal Studies on Distress and Depression With Longer Time Lags

A number of studies (Høgh, Henriksson, & Burr, 2005; Lahelma et al., 2011; Stoetzer et al., 2009) have employed time-1-to-time-2 lags of 3 or more years. In a study involving a representative sample of more than 4,000 Stockholm residents, Stoetzer et al. (2009) found that two forms of bullying, being excluded by superiors and being excluded by coworkers, were related to elevated risk of depression 3 years later, controlling for baseline depression and other confounders. Lahelma et al. (2012), in a study of more than 6,000 Helsinki municipal employees, found that workplace bullying (e.g., isolation, devaluing the target's work) was related to elevated GHQ scores 5 to 7 years later, controlling for baseline GHQ and other confounders (e.g., childhood bullying). In a follow-up of a sample of more than 4,600 Danes, Høgh, Henriksson, and Burr (2005) found that workplace exposure to nasty teasing predicted distress, anxiety, and so forth in both men and women 5 years later, controlling for mental health at baseline; the effect in women, however, became nonsignificant when the investigators controlled for supervisor and colleague support and work conflict.

Longitudinal Studies on Distress and Depression With Shorter Time Lags

Other longitudinal studies have employed lags of 2 years or less. One 18-month study of more than 2,000 Swedish workers (Emdad, Alipour, Hagberg, & Jensen, 2013) focused on the secondary victims of aggression (Barling, 1996), that is, the bystanders, as opposed to the primary or direct victims. Emdad et al. (2013) found that baseline exposure as a bystander to workplace bullying increased the risk of later elevations in depressive symptoms. There was also a study with a null result. Eriksen, Tambs, and Knardahl (2006), who followed more than 4,000 Norwegian nurses' aides over a 15-month period, found that bullying at baseline did not exert effects on psychological distress at follow-up, statistically controlling for baseline covariates such as time-1 distress. In a study of more than 5,600 Danish women working in eldercare, Rugulies et al. (2012) found that exposure to bullying at baseline predicted the occurrence of a major depressive episode 2 years later, controlling for confounding factors.

Bidirectional Effects

Some research has evaluated the occurrence of a reciprocal relation between victimization and psychological distress. Nielsen et al. (2012), who followed a representative sample of 1,775 Norwegian workers for 2 years, found that victimization at baseline predicted later distress, controlling for baseline symptoms. In addition, both baseline distress and baseline bullying predicted victimization 2 years later, underlining both the persistence of bullying and bullies singling out individuals who are already distressed. In another study that examined reverse causality, Finne, Knardahl, and Lau (2011) followed almost 2,000 employees working in 20 public and private Norwegian organizations. The study team found that (a) workplace bullying predicted psychological distress 2 years later, controlling for baseline distress and other confounders (e.g., job demands), and (b) distress predicted bullying 2 years later, controlling for baseline bullying and other confounders. In the earlier mentioned hospital-worker study, Kivimäki et al. (2003) found that having been a victim of workplace bullying at both baseline *and* the 2-year follow-up was related to an almost five-fold increase in risk for incidence of doctor-diagnosed depression (it is not clear if depression at time 2 followed or antedated bullying at time 2). Having been depressed at time 1, however, predicted newly incident cases of bullying at time 2. The evidence is not unequivocal. In the earlier mentioned study by Rugulies et al. (2012), when statistically adjusting for baseline bullying and major depression, only baseline bullying predicted bullying 2 years later. A weakness in their evidence, however, is that the investigators did not use their measures of depression as dimensional scales, which would have provided more statistical power to detect effects.

The evidence suggests that workplace bullying contributes to psychological distress and depression. A review and two-stage meta-analysis (Theorell et al., 2015) involving studies with high scientific quality indicated that there is "moderately strong evidence" that workplace bullying has a significant impact on depressive symptoms. There is also some evidence (Rugulies et al. [2012] is an exception) of reverse causal effects, suggesting that workers who are already feeling distress are at risk for becoming targets of workplace bullies. Consistent with the aforementioned findings, Nielsen and Einarsen (2012), in their two-stage meta-analysis involving 13 large (total $n > 60,000$), mainly Scandinavian samples, found that the relation of bullying and mental health is bidirectional, with bullying adversely affecting mental health and poor mental health eliciting psychological aggression from others.

Outcomes Other Than Distress and Depression

Longitudinal research on workplace bullying has examined outcomes other than psychological distress and depression. These outcomes include fatigue, intentions to quit, actual quitting, sickness absence, fibromyalgia (a functional disorder characterized by musculoskeletal pain, fatigue, and sleep disturbance, which cannot be explained in terms of underlying medical pathology), and, even, cardiovascular disease (CVD). In their Danish sample, Høgh et al. (2005) found that exposure to nasty teasing predicted fatigue 5 years later in women but not in men, controlling for covariates such as fatigue at baseline. In a 3-month study of more than 4,700 Norwegian nurses' aides, Eriksen et al. (2008) found that exposure to threats and violence[10] predicted poor sleep quality. Berthelsen, Skogstad, Lau, and Einarsen (2011), in a study involving the Norwegian sample (2,000 employees) also followed by Finne et al. (2011), found that while controlling for baseline intentions to leave a job, baseline victimization was related to elevated intentions to leave the job 2 years later and actual job-leaving over the course of the follow-up. In a study of more than 5,400 Finnish hospital employees, Kivimäki et al. (2003) found that having been a victim of workplace bullying at both the time 1 baseline *and* the 2-year follow-up was related to a two-fold increase in risk for CVD, adjusting for other risk factors. However, it is not clear if CVD at time 2 followed or antedated bullying at time 2.

In addition, bullying at baseline predicted sick leave taken at follow-up. Clausen, Høgh, and Borg (2011), in a time-series study involving more than 9,500 women working in Danish eldercare facilities, found that exposure to bullying at baseline was related to higher rates of sickness-absence episodes that lasted 8 consecutive weeks or more, over the course of a 1-year follow-up period, controlling for several confounders (e.g., age, smoking, body mass). However, there was no control for past history of extended sickness absence. In a study of a large ($n = 5,655$) Finnish hospital sample that overlapped with the sample employed in other research (Kivimäki et al., 2003), Kivimäki, Elovainio, and Vathera (2000) found that workplace bullying, controlling for baseline sickness absence and other confounders, was related to elevated rates of sickness absence over the course of the 2-year follow-up. In a study involving the same sample, Kivimäki et al. (2004) found that exposure to bullying, controlling for baseline confounders, predicted the occurrence of newly incident cases of fibromyalgia 2 years later.

Coping

The literature on coping with aggression in the workplace has not been promising. Most of the literature is cross-sectional. One of the rare longitudinal studies (Tepper, Duffy, & Shaw, 2001) involving workplace coping examined predictors of coping behaviors but did not evaluate the effectiveness of coping behaviors in mitigating aggression directed by supervisors. The coping response of confronting the perpetrator risks a cycle of retaliation and escalation (Aquino & Thau, 2009). Cross-sectional research suggests that the most effective coping response is transferring to another unit or taking another job (Aquino & Thau, 2009; Zapf & Gross, 2001), a response that is difficult when labor markets are tight. Sometimes a victim can be vigilant enough to avoid or sidestep a perpetrator. A study (Zhou et al., 2015) of first-year nurses, however, holds some promise. The study team found that two of four political skill dimensions, interpersonal influence (e.g., getting people to like one) and apparent sincerity (e.g., trying to show genuine interest in another person), assessed before job entry were related to lower risk of later exposure to physical aggression on the job. No political skills were related to exposure to psychological aggression. Political skills were, however, found to buffer the impact of physical and psychological aggression

---

[10] The question asked was "Have you been exposed to threats or violence at work during the last two years?" (Lindström et al., 2000). It would have been preferable if the survey included a separate item that explicitly asked about "threats of violence" and not lumped threats and violence together. Separate questions about threats of violence and other kinds of threats (e.g., threat of demotion) and being a victim of workplace violence would have been preferable. I thank Violeta Contreras for pointing out the vagueness of the item used in the study.

on anger, job satisfaction, career commitment, and musculoskeletal injury, although in these analyses aggression and the outcomes were assessed contemporaneously.

SUMMARY

A pattern emerges from the bulk of the evidence bearing on the effects of violence and psychological aggression in the workplace. Physical victimization is more common among members of some occupational groups (e.g., bus drivers, nurses, teachers) than others (e.g., workers in the financial sector). Violence, clearly, elevates the risk of physical injury. Although psychological injury is distinctly associated with exposure to physical injury, the unpredictable nature of violent incidents makes it difficult for researchers to design studies assessing the impact of workplace violence that conform to the highest canons of scientific practice (e.g., longitudinal studies having clear before-and-after periods with controls for psychological baseline characteristics before violence occurs). A reasonable conclusion is that no psychological good can come from exposure to violence and that bad outcomes are largely the only outcomes of exposure to violence. The stress reaction (Zapf et al., 1996) and severity models (Barling, 1996) suggest that the psychological outcomes resulting from exposure to violence are in approximate proportion to exposure time and seriousness of the violence. There is some evidence that an antiviolence organizational climate can be helpful in preventing workplace violence.

Psychological aggression is, unfortunately, relatively common in workplaces. Research indicates that psychological aggression at the workplace has clear negative mental health consequences for workers, including bystanders. Although the SOS theoretical framework suggests that the impact of psychological aggression on mental health is mediated by aggression's impact on self-esteem, self-esteem has been conceptualized as a cause, effect, and symptom of depression. Research findings, particularly from the highest quality longitudinal studies, consistently indicate that psychological aggression (e.g., bullying) is related to elevations in distress, depression, and so forth. Research also shows that high levels of distress can act as a magnet for bullying. The research on coping has not been promising except that there is some evidence that changing jobs and political skills may be helpful in reducing exposures to physical and/or psychological aggression.

REFERENCES

Aiken, G. (1984). Assaults on staff in a locked ward: Prediction and consequences. *Medicine, Science, and the Law, 24*(3), 199–207.

Alden, L. E., Regambal, M. J., & Laposa, J. M. (2008). The effects of direct versus witnessed threat on emergency department healthcare workers: Implications for PTSD Criterion A. *Journal of Anxiety Disorders, 22*, 1337–1346. doi:10.1016/j.janxdis.2008.01.013

Andrews, B. (1998). Self-esteem. *The Psychologist, 11*(7), 339–342.

American Psychiatric Association. (2013). *Diagnostic and statistical manual of mental disorders* (5th ed.). Arlington, VA: American Psychiatric Publishing.

Aquino, K., & Thau, S. (2009). Workplace victimization: Aggression from the target's perspective. *Annual Review of Psychology, 60*, 717–741. doi:10.1146/annurev.psych.60.110707.163703

Arnetz, J., & Arnetz, B. (2000). Implementation and evaluation of a practical intervention programme for dealing with violence towards health care workers. *Journal of Advanced Nursing, 31*(3), 668–680.

Bacharach, S. B., Bamberger, P. A., & McKinney, V. M. (2007). Harassing under the influence: The prevalence of male heavy drinking, the embeddedness of permissive workplace drinking norms, and the gender harassment of female coworkers. *Journal of Occupational Health Psychology, 12*, 232–250. doi:10.1037/1076-8998.12.3.232

Barling, J. (1996). The prediction, experience, and consequences of workplace violence. In G. R. VandenBos & E. Q. Bulatao (Eds.), *Violence on the job: Identifying risks and developing solutions* (pp. 29–49). Washington, DC: American Psychological Association. doi:10.1037/10215-001

Beale, D., Clarke, D., Cox, T., Leather, P., & Lawrence, C. (1999). System memory in violent incidents: Evidence from patterns of reoccurrence. *Journal of Occupational Health Psychology, 4*, 233–244. doi:10.1037/1076-8998.4.3.233

Beehr, T. A. (1995). *Psychological stress in the workplace.* New York, NY: Routledge.

Berthelsen, M., Skogstad, A., Lau, B., & Einarsen, S. (2011). Do they stay or do they go? A longitudinal study of intentions to leave and exclusion from working life among targets of workplace bullying. *International Journal of Manpower, 32*, 178–193. doi:10.1108/01437721111130198

Bjørkly, S. (1999). A ten-year prospective study of aggression in a special secure unit for dangerous patients. *Scandinavian Journal of Psychology, 40*(1), 57–63.

Bloch, A. M. (1978). Combat neurosis in inner-city schools. *American Journal of Psychiatry, 135*(10), 1189–1192.

Bowling, N. A., & Beehr, T. A. (2006). Workplace harassment from the victim's perspective: A theoretical model and meta-analysis. *Journal of Applied Psychology, 91*(5), 998–1012. doi:10.1037/0021-9010.91.5.998

Budd, J. W., Arvey, R. D., & Lawless, P. (1996). Correlates and consequences of workplace violence. *Journal of Occupational Health Psychology, 1*, 197–210. doi:10.1037/1076-8998.1.2.197

Bureau of Labor Statistics. (2012, September). *Census of fatal occupational injuries summary, 2011.* Retrieved from www.bls.gov/news.release/cfoi.nr0.htm

Bureau of Labor Statistics. (2013a). *Labor force statistics from the Current Population Survey.* Retrieved from www.bls.gov/webapps/legacy/cpsatab9.htm

Bureau of Labor Statistics. (2013b, January). *Workplace homicides from shootings.* Washington, DC: Author. Retrieved from www.bls.gov/iif/oshwc/cfoi/osar0016.htm

Camerino, D., Estryn-Behar, M., Conway, P., van Der Heijden, B., & Hasselhorn, H. (2008). Work-related factors and violence among nursing staff in the European NEXT study: A longitudinal cohort study. *International Journal of Nursing Studies, 45*(1), 35–50.

Carmel, H., & Hunter, M. (1989). Staff injuries from inpatient violence. *Hospital & Community Psychiatry, 40*(1), 41–46.

Carmel, H., & Hunter, M. (1993). Staff injuries from patient attack: Five years' data. *Bulletin of the American Academy of Psychiatry and the Law, 21*(4), 485–493.

Casteel, C., Peek-Asa, C., & Limbos, M. (2007). Predictors of nonfatal assault injury to public school teachers in Los Angeles City. *American Journal of Industrial Medicine, 50*(12), 932–939.

Chen, W.-C., Sun, Y.-H., Lan, T.-H., & Chiu, H.-J. (2009). Incidence and risk factors of workplace violence on nursing: Staffs caring for chronic psychiatric patients in Taiwan. *International Journal of Environmental Research and Public Health, 6*, 2812–2821. doi:10.3390/ijerph6112812

Chou, K., Lu, R., & Chang, M. (2001). Assaultive behavior by psychiatric in-patients and its related factors. *The Journal of Nursing Research, 9*(5), 139–151.

Clausen, T., Høgh, A., & Borg, V. (2011). Acts of offensive behaviour and risk of long-term sickness absence in the Danish elder-care services: A prospective analysis of register-based outcomes. *International Archives of Occupational and Environmental Health, 85*, 381–387. doi:10.1007/s00420-011-0680-1

Cookson, H., & Buckley, P. (2012). *Violence at work: Findings from the 2010/11 British Crime Survey.* London, England: Health and Safety Executive.

Cooper, A., & Mendonca, J. (1991). A prospective study of patient assaults on nurses in a provincial psychiatric hospital in Canada. *Acta Psychiatrica Scandinavica, 84*(2), 163–166.

Cortina, L. M., Magley, V. J., Williams, J., & Langhout, R. (2001). Incivility in the workplace: Incidence and impact. *Journal of Occupational Health Psychology, 6*, 64–80. doi:10.1037/1076-8998.6.1.64

Crilly, J., Chaboyer, W., & Creedy, D. (2004). Violence towards emergency department nurses by patients. *Accident and Emergency Nursing, 12*(2), 67–73.

Douglas, S. C., & Martinko, M. J. (2001). Exploring the role of individual differences in the prediction of workplace aggression. *Journal of Applied Psychology, 86*, 547–559. doi:10.1037/0021-9010.86.4.547

Duffy, C. A., & McGoldrick, A. E. (1990). Stress and the bus driver in the UK transport industry. *Work & Stress, 4*, 17–27. doi:10.1080/02678379008256961

Dzuka, J., & Dalbert, C. (2007). Student violence against teachers: Teachers' well-being and the belief in a just world. *European Psychologist, 12*, 253–260. doi:10.1027/1016-9040.12.4.253

Emdad, R., Alipour, A., Hagberg, J., & Jensen, I. B. (2013). The impact of bystanding to workplace bullying on symptoms of depression among women and men in industry in Sweden: An empirical and theoretical longitudinal study. *International Archives of Occupational and Environmental Health, 86,* 709–716. doi:10.1007/s00420-012-0813-1

Eriksen, W., Bjorvatn, B., Bruusgaard, D., & Knardahl, S. (2008). Work factors as predictors of poor sleep in nurses' aides. *International Archives of Occupational and Environmental Health, 81*(3), 301–310.

Eriksen, W., Tambs, K., & Knardahl, S. (2006). Work factors and psychological distress in nurses' aides: A prospective cohort study. *BMC Public Health, 6,* 290.

Feeley, B. T., Kennelly, S., Barnes, R. P., Muller, M. S., Kelly, B. T., Rodeo, S. A., & Warren, R. F. (2008). Epidemiology of National Football League training camp injuries from 1998 to 2007. *American Journal of Sports Medicine, 36,* 1597–1603. doi:10.1177/0363546508316021

Finne, L. B., Knardahl, S., & Lau, B. (2011). Workplace bullying and mental distress: A prospective study of Norwegian employees. *Scandinavian Journal of Work, Environment & Health, 37*(4), 276–286.

Fisher, N., & Jacoby, R. (1992). Psychiatric morbidity in bus crews following violent assault: A follow-up study. *Psychological Medicine, 22*(3), 685–693.

Fitzpatrick, A., & Grant, C. (2012). *The 2010/11 British Crime Survey (England and Wales)* (Vol. 1, 2nd ed.). London, England: Home Office.

Flannery, R. B., Stevens, V., Juliano, J., & Walker, A. (2000). Past violence and substance use disorder and subsequent violence towards others: Six year analysis of the Assaulted Staff Action Program (ASAP). *International Journal of Emergency Mental Health, 2*(4), 241–247.

Flannery, R. B., Jr., Stone, P., Rego, S., & Walker, A. P. (2001). Characteristics of the staff victims of patient assault: Ten year analysis of the Assaulted Staff Action Program (ASAP). *Psychiatric Quarterly, 72*(3), 237–248.

Fujita, S., Ito, S., Seto, K., Kitazawa, T., Matsumoto, K., & Hasegawa, T. (2012). Risk factors of workplace violence at hospitals in Japan. *Journal of Hospital Medicine, 7,* 79–84. doi:10.1002/jhm.976

Galand, B., Lecoq, C., & Philippot, P. (2007). School violence and teacher professional disengagement. *British Journal of Educational Psychology, 77,* 465–477. doi:10.1348/000709906X114571

Gerberich, S., Church, T., McGovern, P., Hansen, H., Nachreiner, N., Geisser, M., . . . Jurek, A. (2005). Risk factors for work-related assaults on nurses. *Epidemiology, 16*(5), 704–709.

Gerberich, S., Nachreiner, N., Ryan, A., Church, T., McGovern, P., Geisser, M., . . . Pinder, E. (2011). Violence against educators: A population-based study. *Journal of Occupational and Environmental Medicine, 53,* 294–302. doi:10.1097/JOM.0b013e31820c3fa1

Ginsberg, R., Schwartz, H., Olson, G., & Bennett, A. (1987). Working conditions in urban schools. *The Urban Review, 19,* 3–23. doi:10.1007/BF01108421

Giorgi, G., Ando, M., Arenas, A., Shoss, M. K., & Leon-Perez, J. M. (2013). Exploring personal and organizational determinants of workplace bullying and its prevalence in a Japanese sample. *Psychology of Violence, 3,* 185–197. doi:10.1037/a0028049

Greenberg, L., & Barling, J. (1999). Predicting employee aggression against coworkers, subordinates and supervisors: The roles of person behaviors and perceived workplace factors. *Journal of Organizational Behavior, 20,* 897–913. doi:10.1002/(SICI)1099-1379(199911)20:6<897::AID-JOB975>3.0.CO;2-Z

Halchin, L. E. (2008). *Former NFL players: Disabilities, benefits, and related issues* (Report No. RL34439). Washington, DC: Congressional Research Service, Government and Finance Division.

Harrell, E. (2011). *Workplace violence, 1993-2009.* Report No. NCJ233231. Washington, DC: U.S. Department of Justice, Bureau of Justice Statistics.

Harris, G. T., & Varney, G. W. (1986). A ten-year study of assaults and assaulters on a maximum security psychiatric unit. *Journal of Interpersonal Violence, 1,* 173–191. doi:10.1177/088626086001002003

Hashemi, L., & Webster, B. S. (1998). Non-fatal workplace violence workers' compensation claims (1993–1996). *Journal of Occupational and Environmental Medicine, 40*(12), 561–567.

Hershcovis, M. (2011). "Incivility, social undermining, bullying . . . Oh my!": A call to reconcile constructs within workplace aggression research. *Journal of Organizational Behavior, 32,* 499–519. doi:10.1002/job.689

Hershcovis, M., Turner, N., Barling, J., Arnold, K. A., Dupré, K. E., Inness, M., . . . Sivanathan, N. (2007). Predicting workplace aggression: A meta-analysis. *Journal of Applied Psychology, 92,* 228–238. doi:10.1037/0021-9010.92.1.228

Hobfoll, S. E. (2001). The influence of culture, community, and the nested-self in the stress process: Advancing Conservation of Resources Theory. *Applied Psychology: An International Review, 50*(3), 337–421.

Høgh, A., Borg, V., & Mikkelsen, K. L. (2003). Work-related violence as a predictor of fatigue: A 5-year follow-up of the Danish Work Environment Cohort Study. *Work & Stress, 17,* 182–194. doi:10.1080/0267837031000156876

Høgh, A., Henriksson, M. E., & Burr, H. (2005). A 5-year follow-up study of aggression at work and psychological health. *International Journal of Behavioral Medicine, 12*(4), 256–265.

Høgh, A., Sharipova, M., & Borg, V. (2008). Incidence and recurrent work-related violence towards healthcare workers and subsequent health effects: A one-year follow-up study. *Scandinavian Journal of Public Health, 36*(7), 706–712.

Høgh, A., & Viitasara, E. (2005). A systematic review of longitudinal studies of nonfatal workplace violence. *European Journal of Work and Organizational Psychology, 14*, 291–313. doi:10.1080/13594320500162059

Inness, M., LeBlanc, M., & Barling, J. (2008). Psychosocial predictors of supervisor-, peer-, subordinate-, and service-provider-targeted aggression. *Journal of Applied Psychology, 93*, 1401–1411. doi:10.1037/a0012810

Kauppi, T., & Pörhölä, M. (2012). Teachers bullied by students: Forms of bullying and perpetrator characteristics. *Violence and Victims, 27*, 396–413. doi:10.1891/0886-6708.27.3.396

Kivimäki, M., Elovainio, M., & Vathera, J. (2000). Workplace bullying and sickness absence in hospital staff. *Occupational and Environmental Medicine, 57*(10), 656–660.

Kivimäki, M., Leino-Arjas, P., Virtanen, M., Elovainio, M., Keltikangas-Järvinen, L., Puttonen, S., . . . Vahtera, J. (2004). Work stress and incidence of newly diagnosed fibromyalgia: Prospective cohort study. *Journal Of Psychosomatic Research, 57*, 417–422. doi:10.1016/j.jpsychores.2003.10.013

Kivimäki, M., Virtanen, M., Vartia, M., Elovainio, M., Vahtera, J., & Keltikangas-Järvinen, L. (2003). Workplace bullying and the risk of cardiovascular disease and depression. *Occupational and Environmental Medicine, 60*(10), 779–783.

Lahelma, E., Lallukka, T., Laaksonen, M., Saastamoinen, P., & Rahkonen, O. (2012). Workplace bullying and common mental disorders: A follow-up study. *Journal of Epidemiology and Community Health, 66*, e3, 1–5. doi:10.1136/jech.2010.115212

LaMar, W. J., Gerberich, S. G., Lohman, W. H., & Zaidman, B. (1998). Work-related physical assault. *Journal of Occupational and Environmental Medicine, 40*(4), 317–324.

Lee, J., Joo, E., & Choi, K. (2013). Perceived stress and self-esteem mediate the effects of work-related stress on depression. *Stress and Health, 29*, 75–81. doi:10.1002/smi.2428

Leymann, H. (1990). Mobbing and psychological terror at workplaces. *Violence and Victims, 5*(2), 119–126.

Leymann, H. (1996). The content and development of mobbing at work. *European Journal of Work and Organizational Psychology, 5*, 165–184. doi:10.1080/13594329608414853

Leymann, H., & Gustafsson, A. (1996). Mobbing at work and the development of post-traumatic stress disorders. *European Journal of Work and Organizational Psychology, 5*, 251–275. doi:10.1080/13594329608414858

Lindström, K., Elo, A.-L., Skogstad, A., Dallner, M., Gamberale, F., Hottenen, V., . . . , Ørhede, E. (2000). *User's guide for the QPS NORDIC.* Copenhagen, Denmark: Nordic Council of Ministers.

Lion, J., Snyder, W., & Merrill, G. (1981). Underreporting of assaults on staff in a state hospital. *Hospital & Community Psychiatry, 32*(7), 497–498.

Lorenz, K. (1967). *On aggression* (M. K. Wilson, Trans.). New York, NY: Bantam.

Luksyte, A., Spitzmueller, C., & Maynard, D. C. (2011). Why do overqualified incumbents deviate? Examining multiple mediators. *Journal of Occupational Health Psychology, 16*, 279–296. doi:10.1037/a0022709

Meier, L. L., & Spector, P. E. (2013). Reciprocal effects of work stressors and counterproductive work behavior: A five-wave longitudinal study. *Journal of Applied Psychology, 98*, 529–539. doi:10.1037/a0031732

Milam, A. C., Spitzmueller, C., & Penney, L. M. (2009). Investigating individual differences among targets of workplace incivility. *Journal of Occupational Health Psychology, 14*, 58–69. doi:10.1037/a0012683

Mooij, T. (2011). Secondary school teachers' personal and school characteristics, experience of violence and perceived violence motives. *Teachers and Teaching: Theory and Practice, 17*, 227–253. doi:10.10 80/13540602.2011.539803

Nachreiner, N., Hansen, H., Okano, A., Gerberich, S., Ryan, A., McGovern, P., . . . Watt, G. (2007). Difference in work-related violence by nurse license type. *Journal of Professional Nursing, 23*(5), 290–300.

Nielsen, M. B., & Einarsen, S. (2012). Outcomes of exposure to workplace bullying: A meta-analytic review. *Work & Stress, 26*, 309–332. doi:10.1080/02678373.2012.734709

Nielsen, M. B., Hetland, J., Matthiesen, S. B., & Einarsen, S. (2012). Longitudinal relationships between workplace bullying and psychological distress. *Scandinavian Journal of Work, Environment, & Health, 38*, 38–46. doi:10.5271/sjweh.3178

Peek-Asa, C., Howard, J., Vargas, L., & Kraus, J. F. (1997). Incidence of non-fatal workplace assault injuries determined from employer's reports in California. *Journal of Occupational and Environmental Medicine, 39*(1), 44–50.

Quinsey, V. L., & Varney, G. W. (1977). Characteristics of assaults and assaulters in a maximum security psychiatric unit. *Crime & Justice, 5*(3), 212–220.

Robers, S., Zhang, J., & Truman, J. (2012). *Indicators of school crime and safety: 2011 (NCES 2012-002/NCJ 236021)*. Washington, DC: National Center for Education Statistics, U.S. Department of Education, and Bureau of Justice Statistics, Office of Justice Programs, U.S. Department of Justice.

Rogers, K., & Kelloway, E. (1997). Violence at work: Personal and organizational outcomes. *Journal of Occupational Health Psychology, 2*, 63–71. doi:10.1037/1076-8998.2.1.63

Rugulies, R., Madsen, I. H., Hjarsbech, P. U., Høgh, A., Borg, V., Carneiro, I. G., & Aust, B. (2012). Bullying at work and onset of a major depressive episode among Danish female eldercare workers. *Scandinavian Journal of Work, Environment & Health, 38*, 218–227. doi:10.5271/sjweh.3278

Ryan, J. A., & Poster, E. C. (1989). The assaulted nurse: Short-term and long-term responses. *Archives of Psychiatric Nursing, 3*(6), 323–331.

Salminen, S. (1997). Violence in the workplaces in Finland. *Journal of Safety Research, 28*, 123–131. doi:10.1016/S0022-4375(97)00003-0

Schat, A. H., Frone, M. R., & Kelloway, E. (2006). Prevalence of workplace aggression in the U.S. workforce: Findings from a national study. In E. K. Kelloway, J. Barling, & J. J. Hurrell, Jr. (Eds.), *Handbook of workplace violence* (pp. 47–89). Thousand Oaks, CA: Sage.

Schat, A. H., & Kelloway, E. (2003). Reducing the adverse consequences of workplace aggression and violence: The buffering effects of organizational support. *Journal of Occupational Health Psychology, 8*, 110–122. doi:10.1037/1076-8998.8.2.110

Schonfeld, I. S. (2006). School violence. In E. K. Kelloway, J. Barling, & J. J. Hurrell, Jr. (Eds.), *Handbook of workplace violence* (pp. 169–229). Thousand Oaks, CA: Sage.

Schonfeld, I. S., & Feinman, S. J. (2012). Difficulties of alternatively certified teachers. *Education and Urban Society, 44*, 215–246. doi:10.1177/0013124510392570

Schonfeld, I., & Mazzola, J. J. (2012). Strengths and limitations of qualitative approaches to research in occupational health psychology. In R. R. Sinclair, M. Wang, & L. E. Tetrick (Eds.), *Research methods in occupational health psychology: Measurement, design, and data analysis* (pp. 268–289). New York, NY: Routledge/Taylor & Francis Group.

Schonfeld, I. S., & Santiago, E. A. (1994). Working conditions and psychological distress in first-year women teachers: Qualitative findings. In L.C. Blackman (Ed.), *What works? Synthesizing effective biomedical and psychosocial strategies for healthy families in the 21st century* (pp. 114–121). Indianapolis: University of Indiana Press.

Semmer,, N. K., Jacobshagen, N., Meier, L. L., & Elfering, A. (2007). Occupational stress research: The "stress-as-offense-to-self" perspective. In J. Houmont & S. McIntyre (Eds.), *Occupational health psychology: European perspectives on research, education and practice* (pp. 43–60). Maia, Portugal: ISMAI Publishers.

Sinclair, R. R., Martin, J. E., & Croll, L. W. (2002). A threat-appraisal perspective on employees' fears about antisocial workplace behavior. *Journal of Occupational Health Psychology, 7*, 37–56. doi:10.1037/1076-8998.7.1.37

Smith, D. L., & Smith, B. J. (2006). Perceptions of violence: The views of teachers who left urban schools. *The High School Journal, 89*, 34–42. doi:10.1353/hsj.2006.0004

Sowislo, J., & Orth, U. (2013). Does low self-esteem predict depression and anxiety? A meta-analysis of longitudinal studies. *Psychological Bulletin, 139*, 213–240. doi:10.1037/a0028931

Spector, P. E. (2011). The relationship of personality to counterproductive work behavior (CWB): An integration of perspectives. *Human Resource Management Review, 21*, 342–352. doi:10.1016/j.hrmr.2010.10.002

Spector, P. E., Fox, S., & Domagalski, T. (2006). Emotions, violence, and counterproductive work behavior. In E. K. Kelloway, J. Barling, & J.J. Hurrell, Jr. (Eds.), *Handbook of workplace violence* (pp. 29–46). Thousand Oaks, CA: Sage.

Spector, P. E., Yang, L.-Q., & Zhou, Z. E. (2015). A longitudinal investigation of the role of violence prevention climate in exposure to workplace physical violence and verbal abuse. *Work & Stress, 29*, 325–340. doi:10.1080/02678373.2015.1076537

Spector, P. E., Zhou, Z. E., & Che, X. X. (2014). Nurse exposure to physical and nonphysical violence, bullying, and sexual harassment: A quantitative review. *International Journal of Nursing Studies, 51*, 72–84. doi:10.1016/j.ijnurstu.2013.01.010

Stoetzer, U., Ahlberg, G., Johansson, G., Bergman, P., Hallsten, L., Forsell, Y., & Lundberg, I. (2009). Problematic interpersonal relationships at work and depression: A Swedish prospective cohort study. *Journal of Occupational Health, 51*(2), 144–151.

Ta, M., Marshall, S., Kaufman, J., Loomis, D., Casteel, C., & Land, K. (2009). Area-based socioeconomic characteristics of industries at high risk for violence in the workplace. *American Journal of Community Psychology, 44*, 249–260. doi:10.1007/s10464-009-9263-7

Tepper, B. J., Duffy, M. K., & Shaw, J. D. (2001). Personality moderators of the relationship between abusive supervision and subordinates' resistance. *Journal of Applied Psychology, 86*, 974–983. doi:10.1037/0021-9010.86.5.974

Terry, A. A. (1998). Teachers as targets of bullying by their pupils: A study to investigate incidence. *British Journal of Educational Psychology, 68*, 255–268. doi:10.1111/j.2044-8279.1998.tb01288.x

Theorell, T., Hammarström, A., Aronsson, G., Träskman Bendz, L., Grape, T., Hogstedt, C., . . . Hall, C. (2015). A systematic review including meta-analysis of work environment and depressive symptoms. *BMC Public Health, 15*(738). doi:10.1186/s12889-015-1954-4

Ting, L., Sanders, S., & Smith, P. L. (2002). The teachers' reactions to School Violence Scale: Psychometric properties and scale development. *Educational and Psychological Measurement, 62*, 1006–1019. doi:10.1177/0013164402238087

Tourkin, S. C., Warner, T., Parmer, R., Cole, C., Jackson, B., Zukerberg, A., . . . Soderborg, A. (2007). *Documentation for the 2003–04 Schools and Staffing Survey (NCES 2007–337)*. Washington, DC: U.S. Department of Education, National Center for Education Statistics.

Whittington, R., & Wykes, T. (1994). Violence in psychiatric hospitals: Are certain staff prone to being assaulted? *Journal of Advanced Nursing, 19*, 219–225. doi:10.1111/1365-2648.ep8534655

Wieclaw, J., Agerbo, E., Mortensen, P., Burr, H., Tüchsen, F., & Bonde, J. (2006). Work related violence and threats and the risk of depression and stress disorders. *Journal of Epidemiology and Community Health, 60*(9), 771–775.

Wilson, C. M., Douglas, K. S., & Lyon, D. R. (2011). Violence against teachers: Prevalence and consequences. *Journal of Interpersonal Violence, 26*, 2353–2371. doi:10.1177/0886260510383027

Wittmer, J. S., Sinclair, R. R., Martin, J. E., Tucker, J. S., & Lang, J. (2013). Shared aggression concerns and organizational outcomes: The moderating role of resource constraints. *Journal of Organizational Behavior, 34*, 370–388. doi:10.1002/job.1807

Wykes, T., & Whittington, R. (1998). Prevalence and predictors of early traumatic stress reactions in assaulted psychiatric nurses. *Journal of Forensic Psychiatry, 9*(3), 643.

Yang, L., Spector, P., Chang, C., Gallant-Roman, M., & Powell, J. (2012). Psychosocial precursors and physical consequences of workplace violence towards nurses: A longitudinal examination with naturally occurring groups in hospital settings. *International Journal of Nursing Studies, 49*, 1091–1102. doi:10.1016/j.ijnurstu.2012.03.006

Yassi, A., Gilbert, M., & Cvitkovich, Y. (2005). Trends in injuries, illnesses, and policies in Canadian healthcare workplaces. *Canadian Journal of Public Health, 96*(5), 333–339.

Younghusband, L. J. (2008, March). *Violence in the classroom: The reality of a teacher's workplace*. Paper presented at the Work, Stress, and Health 2008 Conference, Washington, DC.

Zapf, D., Dormann, C., & Frese, M. (1996). Longitudinal studies in organizational stress research: A review of the literature with reference to methodological issues. *Journal of Occupational Health Psychology, 1*, 145–169. doi:10.1037/1076-8998.1.2.145

Zapf, D., & Gross, C. (2001). Conflict escalation and coping with workplace bullying: A replication and extension. *European Journal of Work and Organizational Psychology, 10*, 497–522. doi:10.1080/13594320143000834

Zhou, Z. E., Yang, L., & Spector, P. E. (2015). Political skill: A proactive inhibitor of workplace aggression exposure and an active buffer of the aggression–strain relationship. *Journal of Occupational Health Psychology, 20*(4), 405–419. doi:10.1037/a0039004

SIX

Organizational Climate and Leadership

KEY CONCEPTS AND FINDINGS COVERED IN CHAPTER 6

Organizational climate: A brief history
    Levels of analysis
    Dimensions of organizational climate
Safety climate
    Antecedents of safety climate
    Safety-related outcomes of safety climate
    Other effects of safety climate
Mistreatment climate
Psychosocial safety climate
Other climates relevant to occupational health psychology
Organizational leadership: A brief history
Contemporary leadership theories and occupational health
    Transformational leadership
    Leader–member exchange
    Abusive supervision
Summary

Organizations can be viewed as social systems in which collections of individuals work for a common purpose. Like any other social system, structures and rules exist to guide the functioning of the organization. This chapter focuses on two factors that help define the functioning of organizations—climate and leadership. Coverage of these characteristics is included in a book about occupational health psychology because they have implications for workers' health, safety, and well-being.

ORGANIZATIONAL CLIMATE: A BRIEF HISTORY

The initial work on organizational climate can be traced back to research conducted by Lewin, Lippitt, and White (1939) on boys working under different teachers who displayed different leadership styles. Lewin and his colleagues found that boys whose leader (teacher) adopted a more democratic or participative leadership style acted in a more cooperative manner with each other and with the leader, experienced less stress, and exhibited more positive emotions. In contrast, boys who worked under an authoritarian teacher were more likely to behave in an individualistic manner and experience comparatively more stress and negative affect. Lewin and his colleagues highlighted the fact that the different leaders did not directly tell the boys how to behave or feel. Rather, the boys sensed how they should behave and feel in response to the behaviors of the leader and their peers. Lewin et al. (1939) adopted the term "social climate" to describe the different behavioral and attitudinal patterns that emerged in the context of the different leadership styles. Although Lewin et al. did not directly measure the social climate construct, they introduced the term to describe how different patterns of behaviors and attitudes could be created in different social groups.

The application of the social climate idea to the occupational setting did not occur until the late 1950s and 1960s (Schneider, Ehrhart, & Macey, 2011). Works by Argyris (1957), McGregor (1960), and Likert (1967) discussed how work design and managers' behaviors toward employees can influence employees' work experiences, which in turn shape their behaviors in the workplace. The early research on organizational climate tended to focus on two important themes: distinguishing levels of analysis and identifying dimensions of the workplace that relate to employees' social well-being (Hellriegel & Slocum, 1974). In what follows, we describe these themes and how they inform contemporary approaches to studying climate.

Levels of Analysis

In terms of levels of analysis, early research on organizational climate focused on individual climate perceptions of objective organizational characteristics (e.g., organizational structure; Payne & Pugh, 1976) or personal experiences (e.g., leader support; Forehand & Gilmer, 1964), and examined the relationships between these perceptions and individual outcomes (e.g., sales volume; Schneider & Barlett, 1968). James and Jones (1974), however, explicitly differentiated between psychological and organizational (or unit-level) climate. Psychological climate is assessed at the individual level; it represents the individual worker's perceptions of his or her work environment, including the procedures and practices in the worker's organization or organizational unit. James and Jones (1974) suggested that psychological climate emerges out of the interaction of "perceived organizational attributes and individual characteristics" (p. 110). By contrast, organizational climate is assessed by aggregating numerous individual responses into a single "unit."

Instead of focusing on psychological climate and the individual level of analysis, other scholars (e.g., Ashforth, 1985; Glick, 1985) highlighted the view that climate research should focus on the shared perceptions of members of the same unit and the meanings associated with these perceptions. Although the level of measurement is individual, the level of the construct—organizational climate—resides in the organization (Schneider et al., 2011). As such, the individual perceptions of the organizational characteristics should be aggregated to the organizational level of analysis, and organizational climate is expected to relate to outcomes at the organizational level (Glick, 1985). Because measures of climate are meant to assess organizational functioning (Ostroff, 1993), they are expected to reflect a high level of consensus within organizations and a high level of variance between organizations (Bliese, 2000).

The contemporary approach to climate continues to consider the individual-based, psychological climate as a construct that is distinct from unit-level or organizational climate (James et al., 2008; Schneider et al., 2011). This distinction is important as almost all of the different definitions of organizational climate regard organizational climate as a composite of perceptions shared among organizational members about certain key features of their organizations (Verbeke, Volgering, & Hessels, 1998; Zohar & Hofmann, 2012). In this chapter, we use "psychological climate" to refer to individual employees' perceptions of their workplace characteristics, and "unit-level" or "organizational climate" to refer to the aggregated, shared perceptions among members of the same unit or organization.

In addition to differentiating between psychological and organizational climate constructs, contemporary research on organizational climate has drawn from multilevel theory (Kozlowski & Klein, 2000) and identified important guidelines concerning the aggregation of individual perceptions. First, because measures of organizational climate intend to capture the unit-level attributes, it is important to frame the items for respondents by clearly describing the unit to which the items will be aggregated (e.g., work team; department; organization as a whole; Schneider et al., 2011). For example, Anderson and West's (1998) measure of innovation climate intends to assess the climate at the team level, and the wording of the items consistently refers to the people (e.g., team members) and practices (e.g., keeping each other informed) specifically within the team.

Second, the idea of consensus among members of the same unit is central for meaningful interpretation of the aggregated measure of organizational climate (Schneider et al., 2011; Zohar & Hofmann, 2012). In order for the mean or average of individual members' climate perceptions to reflect the unit climate, researchers should assess the extent to which consensus exists among members' ratings. Consensus is typically established by assessing interrater agreement and interrater reliability (Kozlowski & Hattrup, 1992). Interrater agreement reflects the extent to which raters from the same unit provide similar absolute ratings of the climate. For example, a unit where all five of its members rated an item as 3 indicates high interrater agreement, compared with another unit where five members give a wide range of ratings (e.g., 1, 2, 3, 4, and 5). The most common measure of within-group interrater agreement is $r_{WG(J)}$ (James, Demaree, & Wolf, 1993). Although some scholars have used a cutoff of 0.70 for $r_{WG(J)}$, others have discussed the arbitrary nature of such a cutoff and recommended interrater agreement to be evaluated on a continuum rather than through a dichotomy (e.g., LeBreton & Senter, 2008).

Interrater reliability assesses the extent to which the rank ordering of the ratings is consistent across members within the units (Bliese, 2000). Typical interrater reliability measures also provide information about interrater agreement (LeBreton & Senter, 2008). The most common measure of interrater reliability is the intraclass correlation coefficient, or $ICC_{(1)}$, which represents the ratio of between-unit variance over total variance, and can be interpreted as a percentage of variance accounted for by unit membership (Bliese, 2000). High values of $ICC_{(1)}$ indicate that the variability within units is low (i.e., high interrater agreement) and the variability between units is high. Low values of $ICC_{(1)}$, however, may result from high within-unit variability and/or little between-unit variability. Table 6.1 provides an illustration of how changes in within- and between-unit variability may affect $ICC_{(1)}$. In particular, from scenario A to scenario B, the between-unit variance remains the same, because the four groups have the same means across the four members' ratings. However, the within-unit variability increases in scenario B for groups 2 and 3, resulting in a smaller overall $ICC_{(1)}$. Similarly, from scenario A to scenario C, changes in members' ratings from group 3 results in not only lower between-unit variability (because group 3 now has the same mean as groups 1 and 4), but also higher within-unit variability for group 3. As a result, the $ICC_{(1)}$ also becomes smaller. LaBreton and Senter's (2008) review suggested that a value of 0.10 could be viewed as a median effect size for $ICC_{(1)}$. In addition to

TABLE 6.1	Example of $ICC_{(1)}$ Changes as a Function of Within- and Between-Unit Variability						
		Ratings					
	Group	Member 1	Member 2	Member 3	Member 4	Group Mean	Group Standard Deviation
Scenario A: $ICC_{(1)} = 0.53$	1	4	5	4	5	4.50	0.58
	2	4	4	3	3	3.50	0.58
	3	3	3	3	4	3.25	0.50
	4	4	5	5	4	4.50	0.58
Scenario B: $ICC_{(1)} = 0.04$	1	4	5	4	5	4.50	0.58
	2	5*	5*	2*	2*	3.50	1.73*
	3	2*	4*	2*	5*	3.25	1.50*
	4	4	5	5	4	4.50	0.58
Scenario C: $ICC_{(1)} = 0.33$	1	4	5	4	5	4.50	0.58
	2	4	4	3	3	3.50	0.58
	3	4*	5*	4*	5*	4.50*	0.58*
	4	4	5	5	4	4.50	0.58
*Indicates changes in numbers from Scenario A.							

$ICC_{(1)}$, $ICC_{(2)}$ or $ICC_{(K)}$ is another commonly reported statistic for interrater reliability (LeBreton & Senter, 2008). $ICC_{(2)}$ reflects the reliability of unit means and is related to $ICC_{(1)}$ as a function of group size, such that higher $ICC_{(1)}$ and/or larger units both can yield higher $ICC_{(2)}$ (Bliese, 2000). $ICC_{(2)}$ values are typically interpreted in line with other indicators of reliability, with 0.70 being recommended as a cutoff for adequate interrater reliability (LeBreton & Senter, 2008).

Dimensions of Organizational Climate

The second theme to emerge from the early research on climate is an interest in identifying specific climate dimensions that characterize employees' experiences at work (Schneider et al., 2011). For example, a review on the organizational climate research by Campbell, Dunnette, Lawler, and Weick (1970) identified four climate dimensions: individual autonomy; degree of structure imposed on the situation; reward orientation; and consideration, warmth, and support. Similarly, Locke's (1976) review of climate literature identified four dimensions along which employees evaluate or perceive their organizations (James & McIntyre, 1996): clarity, harmony, and justice; challenge, independence, and responsibility; work facilitation, support, and recognition; and warm and friendly social relations. Later, James and James (1989) continued to emphasize a four-dimensional climate structure, which included role stress and lack of harmony; job challenge and autonomy; leader support and facilitation; and work-group cooperation and friendliness; with three to six subdimensions in each category. More recently, Ostroff (1993) identified three overall climate dimensions—affective, cognitive, and instrumental—with each dimension consisting of four specific facets. For example, the affective climate dimension reflects the employees' involvement in the workplace and the quality of their social interactions, and includes facets such as participation and cooperation.

There are clear overlaps between these different ways of categorizing organizational climate. Most of them include categories for capturing employees' perceptions of the interpersonal or social aspects of their organizations, such as Campbell et al.'s (1970) consideration, warmth, and support dimension; and Ostroff's (1993) affective dimension. The majority of these categorizations also include dimensions for describing how work is organized and how employees are evaluated and rewarded. Differences, however, exist in regard to how these scholars categorize the climate dimensions. These differences can result in difficulties in understanding what these dimensions really mean, whether they fully reflect employees' experiences at work, and how to integrate or reconcile research results that are based on different categorizations of the climate constructs (Burke, Borucki, & Kaufman, 2002).

Interestingly, during the same time when these dimensions of organizational climate were developed, Schneider (1975) proposed a different approach. He suggested that instead of developing a comprehensive taxonomy to encompass all possible dimensions, researchers should focus on organizational climate that is related to one or more strategic outcomes of the organization. A comprehensive list of organizational climate dimensions without a focus is somewhat useless. Rather, identifying an important organizational outcome (e.g., innovation, service quality, or safety) and then focusing on organizational procedures and practices that are closely associated with the focal outcome will not only facilitate theoretical development, but also generate psychometrically sound measures of organizational climate.

Consistent with the idea of climate research based on specific strategic outcomes, work by Schneider and his colleagues (e.g., Schneider, White, & Paul, 1998) showed that customers of bank branches that had a higher service climate perceived higher service quality and reported higher satisfaction with the service. Similarly, in teams with a high innovation climate, individual members engaged in more innovative behaviors, and the teams as a whole performed better in innovation tasks (e.g., generating more patents; Bain, Mann, & Pirola-Merlo, 2001).

In the following sections, we will adopt the strategic climate approach and review organizational climate that pertains to employees' occupational health and safety. We will consider both psychological climate assessed at the individual level and unit-level climate. The antecedents and outcomes of these climate variables will be summarized.

SAFETY CLIMATE

Following the strategic approach to climate proposed by Schneider (1975), Zohar (1980) first developed a target-specific climate that is related to employee safety. "Safety climate" is defined as employees' perceived priority of safety relative to other organizational goals (e.g., reaching production targets; providing high-quality service; Zohar, 2011), and is reflected in employees' perceptions of the policies, procedures, and practices related to safety (Griffin & Neal, 2000). Neal and Griffin (2004) developed a taxonomy that includes eight safety climate dimensions.

Management commitment refers to the extent to which workers perceive that top management values safety within the organization. Human resource management practices capture employees' perceptions about the extent to which other practices such as selection, training, and the compensation system support safety. Safety system perceptions refer to the perceived quality of policy, procedures, and practices designed to improve organizational safety outcomes. Supervisor support reflects the extent to which workers perceive that their immediate supervisors (as opposed to top management) value safety. Internal group processes refer to employees' perceptions of the extent to which their coworkers or work-group members encourage or support safety. Boundary management captures the extent to which the work group communicates effectively with other external stakeholders (e.g., other work groups; safety professionals within the organization) regarding safety issues. Risk refers to employees' perception of whether the work itself is dangerous. Finally, work pressure refers to whether employees experience high levels of workload that prevent them from performing their jobs safely.

Antecedents of Safety Climate

Various contextual characteristics related to the job, role, work group, leadership, and organization have been identified as antecedents to safety climate. Positive job characteristics such as autonomy have been shown to be positively related to employees' safety climate perceptions (e.g., Geller, Roberts, & Gilmore, 1996). A meta-analysis calculated the corrected (for measurement error) correlation between job characteristics (e.g., challenging tasks, autonomy) and individual safety climate perceptions to be 0.42 (Clarke, 2010). However, role stressors such as role ambiguity, conflict, and overload have been shown to negatively predict employees' psychological safety climate perceptions (Clarke, 2010). Clarke (2010) argued that employees who do not perceive a clear role definition, receive conflicting demands from different sources, or have excessive workloads are likely to view production as prioritized over safety in their organization, and as such, their safety climate perceptions suffer.

Work-group characteristics, such as cohesion and coworker support, have been shown to have positive associations with employees' psychological safety climate in the meta-analysis (Clarke, 2010). Both conflict within the work group and uncivil treatment received from coworkers correlated negatively with employees' individual safety climate perceptions (Haines, Stringer, & Duku, 2007). Leaders' safety-specific transformational behaviors, such as expressing their own values and beliefs about the importance of safety, modeling safety behaviors themselves, and encouraging safe behaviors among employees through rewards or recognition relate positively to employees' psychological safety climate perceptions (Clarke, 2010). On the other hand, passive leadership behaviors, such as avoiding making decisions related to employee safety or waiting to take safety-related actions until something goes wrong, are negatively related to safety climate (Kelloway, Mullen, & Francis, 2006). Finally, organizational characteristics, such as open communication, employee participation in safety-related decisions and activities, and perceived organizational support have been shown to correlate positively with safety climate (Clarke, 2010; Wallace, Popp, & Mondore, 2006).

In addition to situational characteristics, personal factors have also been shown to predict employees' psychological safety climate. For example, negative emotions such as depression and frustration are negatively related to safety climate perceptions (Golubovich, Chang, & Eatough, 2014). A meta-analysis shows that personality traits such as agreeableness and conscientiousness are positively related to safety climate perceptions, whereas a negative relationship exists between neuroticism and safety climate (Beus, Dhanani, & McCord, 2015). Finally, research has found a positive relationship between safety climate and individual differences that contribute to employees' personal resources. For example, employees with an internal locus of control, who believe that they control the consequences of their own behaviors, tend to report higher safety climate (e.g., Cigularov, Chen, & Stallones, 2009; Geller et al., 1996). Positive evaluations of one's self, or the level of self-esteem, are also related to enhanced safety climate perceptions (Geller et al., 1996). Finally, psychological hardiness, which refers to a composite personality variable that enhances individuals' ability to manage stressful circumstances, has been shown to be positively related to psychological safety climate (Golubovich et al., 2014; Hystad, & Bye, 2013).

Safety-Related Outcomes of Safety Climate

Researchers have examined both proximal and distal outcomes of psychological and unit-level safety climate. Neal and Griffin (2004) proposed a model relating safety climate to safety outcomes. They argued that safety climate should be directly linked to proximal outcomes such as individual employees' safety motivation and safety knowledge, which in turn relate to safety performance behaviors. These safety behaviors are associated with objective safety outcomes, such as accidents and injuries. Empirical studies have found that employees' psychological safety climate was positively related to their safety knowledge (e.g., Neal, Griffin, & Hart, 2000; Probst, 2004), suggesting that a positive safety climate perception at the individual level is related to increased knowledge concerning how to work safely (e.g., how to handle hazardous materials or use personal protective equipment when necessary). Moreover, both psychological and unit-level safety climate have been shown to predict employees' safety motivation or the value they perceive with regard to workplace safety as well as their willingness to exert effort to perform safely at work (e.g., Neal & Griffin, 2006; Neal et al., 2000; Probst, 2004). Meta-analytic findings have shown strong, positive relationships between safety climate with both safety knowledge and motivation (Christian, Bradley, Wallace, & Burke, 2009), suggesting that when employees perceive their organizations value safety, they are likely to be more informed about workplace safety and motivated to perform safely at work.

The knowledge and motivation, in turn, positively contribute to employees' actual safety performance (Neal & Griffin, 2004). Researchers typically differentiate between two dimensions of safety performance: compliance and participation. Safety compliance refers to performing the core activities needed to maintain workplace safety, such as following safety-oriented work procedures and wearing the required personal protective equipment (Neal & Griffin, 2006). On the other hand, safety participation refers to behaviors that are not required by the organization, but indirectly contribute to workplace safety through developing a psychosocial environment that supports safety. Safety participation includes activities such as volunteering for safety committees and helping coworkers with safety-related issues (Neal & Griffin, 2006). Safety compliance is akin to task performance because compliance is prescribed by the organization and tied to the specific jobs, whereas safety participation is similar to organizational citizenship behaviors (voluntary behaviors that are helpful to the organization), which is more general across different jobs and not required by the organization (Borman & Motowidlo, 1993).

Both individual and unit-level safety climate perceptions have been linked to higher levels of safety compliance and participation (Neal & Griffin, 2006; Neal et al., 2000). Multiple meta-analyses have shown positive relationships between safety climate and safety performance (e.g., Christian et al., 2009; Clarke, 2006, 2010). Research has also been consistent with the view that safety knowledge and motivation mediates the effect of safety climate on safety performance. For example, Neal, Griffin, and Hart (2000) showed that in a sample of 525 hospital employees in Australia, individual safety climate perceptions enhanced employees' safety knowledge and motivation, which in turn were associated with better safety compliance and participation. Similarly, Neal and Griffin (2006), in a rare longitudinal study, showed that unit-level safety climate was predictive of employees' safety motivation and participation over 5 years, controlling for accidents at baseline. Moreover, the positive effect of unit safety climate on safety participation was partially mediated by individuals' safety motivation.

Finally, safety climate has been linked to objective safety outcomes, such as accidents and injuries, through the aforementioned mediators. For example, meta-analyses (e.g., Beus, Payne, Bergman, & Arthur, 2010; Christian et al., 2009) have supported the view that both individual and unit-level safety climate are negatively related to accidents and injuries. In other words, a positive safety climate is associated with lower rates of accidents and injuries. These relationships were stronger when data on accidents and injuries were extracted from objective records (e.g., medical records; records reported to the Occupational Safety and Health Administration) compared with participants' self-report (Christian et al., 2009). Moreover, relationships were stronger when climate was assessed at the unit level (e.g., work group or organization) compared with the individual level (Christian et al., 2009). Finally, support was found for the mediating roles of safety motivation, knowledge, and performance for the relationship between safety climate and accidents and injuries (Christian et al., 2009). In this case, employees who perceive better safety climate are more likely to work safely, which in turn reduces the likelihood of accidents and injuries.

Other studies, however, suggest a reciprocal relationship between safety climate and injuries (Beus et al., 2010). In particular, prior safety climate perceptions negatively predicted subsequent injuries, and prior injuries also predicted lower future safety climate perceptions. Injuries provide strong cues to employees about workplace safety, and may prompt employees to reflect negatively on policies and practices related to safety (Zohar, 2011). In this case, injured workers may have lower safety climate perceptions because they attribute their injuries to the poor safety climate in the workplace. A limitation of much research on the relationship of safety climate to injuries has been a reliance on cross-sectional designs (Leitão & Greiner, 2016). Leitão and Greiner (2016) nevertheless observed that we should "not overlook the favourable and encouraging associations [safety climate] showed with safety indicators" such as accidents and injuries (p. 87).

Other Effects of Safety Climate

In addition to safety-specific outcomes such as accidents and injuries, safety climate has also been linked to other indicators of employee health and well-being. For example, individual employees' psychological safety climate has been shown to have implications for their job satisfaction, affective commitment to the organization, and well-being (Clarke, 2010). For example, positive associations were found between psychological safety climate perceptions and job satisfaction among employees who worked in safety-critical industries such as construction and offshore petroleum sites (Nielsen, Mearns, Matthiesen, & Eid, 2011; Siu, Phillips, & Leung, 2004). Similarly, positive safety climate perceptions are related to stronger organizational commitment (Mearns, Hope, Ford, & Tetrick, 2010). In a study of health care workers in a community-based hospital, psychological safety climate was found to mediate the relationship between injuries and turnover intentions. In particular, health care workers who experienced injuries were likely to perceive poor safety climate, which in turn led to high turnover intentions (McCaughey, DelliFraine, McGhan, & Bruning, 2013). Finally, researchers have found negative associations between psychological safety climate and burnout (Nahrgang, Morgeson, & Hofmann, 2011) and psychological strain (Fogarty, 2005). Interestingly, a study conducted with health care workers showed that although unit-level safety climate was not directly related to individual nurses' occupational strain, it attenuated the positive association between job demands and strain (Chowdhury & Endres, 2010). Taken together, both psychological and unit-level safety climate have important implications beyond safety-related outcomes.

MISTREATMENT CLIMATE

Broadly speaking, "mistreatment climate" refers to employees' perceptions of organizational policies, procedures, and practices that deter interpersonal mistreatment (Yang, Caughlin, Gazica, Truxillo, & Spector, 2014). These negative interpersonal interactions may include incivility, psychological aggression and bullying, and physical violence, initiated by different groups of perpetrators (e.g., clients or customers of the organizations; coworkers) who target employees (see Chapter 5 of this book for a more detailed description). Regardless of the nature, severity, and perpetrator of the mistreatment, employees' perceptions of the mistreatment climate typically involve at least two facets. First, mistreatment climate involves employees' perceptions of the adequacy of formal policies and procedures designed to prevent or curtail mistreatment behaviors. For example, violence prevention climate (e.g., Kessler, Spector, Chang, & Parr, 2008) concerns the extent to which employees view the violence prevention policies in their organizations as adequate and widely communicated. The second facet of mistreatment climate is the perceived workplace norms concerning the level of tolerance for negative interpersonal behaviors. Specifically, coworker and supervisor responses to incidents of mistreatment are often considered indicators of the extent to which such behaviors are acceptable or sanctioned in the workplace (e.g., Inness, LeBlanc, & Barling, 2008). Similarly, reactions to the perpetrators (beyond the incidents) of mistreatment (e.g., Hutchinson, Jackson, Wilkes, & Vickers, 2008) have also been thought to reflect the extent of workplace tolerance for mistreatment.

Virtually all empirical studies on mistreatment climate have focused on its role as a predictor of mistreatment-related outcomes. A meta-analysis categorized outcomes three ways: mistreatment exposure, mistreatment reduction effort, and employee general health and well-being (Yang et al., 2014). Overall, psychological mistreatment climate was negatively related to employees' exposure to mistreatment, suggesting that a more positive mistreatment climate (i.e., a climate that frowns upon employee mistreatment) was associated with fewer incidents of mistreatment (Yang et al., 2014). In addition, mistreatment climate was positively associated with employees' mistreatment reduction efforts (Yang et al., 2014). For example, Chang, Eatough, Spector, and Kessler (2012) found that psychological violence prevention climate was positively related to employees' violence prevention behaviors through reduced emotional strain and increased prevention motivation. Similarly, unit-level violence prevention climate positively predicted individual employees' violence prevention behaviors (Chang & Golubovich, 2012).

Finally, mistreatment climate has been positively linked to employees' general health and well-being (Yang et al., 2014). In particular, positive psychological mistreatment climate was related to higher levels of job satisfaction and organizational commitment, lower levels of emotional and physical strains, and reduced turnover intentions. Interestingly, Yang et al. (2014) found that, compared with an aggression-inhibition climate, a civility climate had a stronger relationship with attitudinal outcomes (e.g., job satisfaction and commitment). This finding suggests that despite its low intensity, workplace incivility may carry significant implications for employee well-being.

Beyond the main effects just described, mistreatment climate may have moderating effects on the three primary outcomes. For example, Chang and Golubovich (2012) found that in a sample of convenience store employees, unit-level mistreatment climate buffered the effects of emotional strain and cognitive failure on individual employees' violence prevention performance. Individual employees' strain and cognitive failure were negatively related to their prevention behaviors. However, these negative relationships were stronger among those working for a branch with low prevention climate compared with those with high prevention climate. These results show that positive mistreatment climate may attenuate the negative effects of employee strains on outcomes.

PSYCHOSOCIAL SAFETY CLIMATE

"Psychosocial safety climate" (PSC), a recently developed construct, is defined as employees' perceptions of policies, practices, and procedures designed to protect their psychological health and safety (Dollard, 2007). Unlike the aforementioned safety climate, which focuses on the prevention of workplace accidents and employees' physical injuries, the focus of PSC is on the prevention of psychological and social risk or harm among employees (Dollard & Bakker, 2010). The PSC of a workplace is driven primarily by top management's priorities (Dollard & Bakker, 2010). A positive PSC is viewed as an upstream organizational resource that may influence other organizational practices, job designs, and interpersonal interactions to promote employee psychosocial well-being (Hall et al., 2010).

Four dimensions of PSC are often discussed (Dollard & Bakker, 2010; Hall, Dollard, & Coward, 2010). The first dimension of PSC indexes senior management's commitment to and support for employee stress prevention and reduction. The second dimension reflects the priority management gives to employee psychological health and well-being over production goals. The third dimension is organizational communication, which encapsulates the degree of openness of communication from management to its employees on issues related to psychosocial health. Finally, the dimension of organizational participation reflects the extent to which employees and other stakeholders (e.g., unions) are consulted on decisions related to employees' psychosocial health and well-being.

Because it is considered an organizational resource originating from senior management priorities (Hall et al., 2010; Dollard & Bakker, 2010), most of the empirical studies involving PSC have treated it either as an antecedent of other organizational contextual characteristics that may promote or hamper employees' psychosocial well-being or as a moderator that may attenuate the negative impact of workplace burdens on well-being. Idris and Dollard (2011) showed that management-level PSC was positively related to job resources (e.g., support from supervisors and coworkers), and negatively related to job demands (e.g., emotional demands, role conflict). Reduced demands, in turn, mediated the relationship between PSC and lower levels of anger and depression, whereas resources mediated the relationship between PSC and higher levels of engagement. Similarly, Bailey, Dollard, and Richards (2015) showed that PSC was directly related to employees' job control 1 year later, and inversely related to subsequent psychological work demands. Employees who reported lower PSC were at a higher risk for developing depression.

Dollard and Bakker (2010) showed that school-level PSC was negatively related to teachers' and administrators' psychological distress and burnout, and positively related to their engagement through reduced job demands (e.g., psychological pressures and emotional demands) and increased resources (e.g., skill discretion). Idris, Dollard, and Yulita (2014) replicated, in a sample of private sector employees, a similar mediational effect, with unit-level PSC leading to reduced job-related emotional demands on employees, which, in turn, led to lower levels of burnout symptoms. Unit-level PSC was negatively related to nurses' subsequent workload, and positively related to their subsequent job control and supervisor support (Dollard et al., 2012). PSC-related reduced workload, in turn, mediated the beneficial relationship between unit-level PSC and nurses' (lower levels of) burnout. PSC-related increased control mediated the inverse relationship between PSC and nurses' psychological distress (Dollard et al., 2012). Finally, school-level PSC attenuated the positive association between emotional demands on educators and burnout symptoms, such that demands had a weaker relationship with burnout for those working in a unit with high PSC (Dollard & Bakker, 2010). Taken together, these results support the idea that PSC affects employee well-being through its impact on job demands and resources.

OTHER CLIMATES RELEVANT TO OCCUPATIONAL HEALTH PSYCHOLOGY

In addition to the climate variables discussed, researchers have also examined other general or specific organizational climate factors that may have implications for employees' health, safety, and general well-being. For example, "diversity climate of the workplace," which is defined as "employee perceptions regarding the extent to which individual diversity is valued, integrated into organizational life, and supported through fair employment practices" (Kaplan, Wiley, & Maertz, 2011, p. 272), has been shown to have implications for employee well-being. Studies have shown that positive diversity climate contributed to higher employee job satisfaction (e.g., Brimhall, Lizano, & Mor Barak, 2014) and organizational attachment (e.g., Brimhall et al., 2014; Kaplan et al., 2011). Other organizational climate variables that are related to the fair treatment of employees (e.g., "justice climate": Whitman, Caleo, Carpenter, Horner, & Bernerth, 2012) have also been shown to relate to lower employee stress and greater well-being (e.g., Whitman et al., 2012). Finally, extending from the literature concerning employees' perceived family-friendliness of their organizations (Allen, 2001), "work and family climate" is defined as employees' perceptions of the extent to which their organizations facilitate employee efforts to balance responsibilities to work and family (see also Thompson, Beauvais, & Lyness, 1999). Work–family climate has been shown to relate to important employee outcomes (e.g., organizational commitment: O'Neill et al., 2009; and work–family conflict: Paustian-Underdahl & Halbesleben, 2014). We will return to this climate construct in Chapter 9 when we look at the work–family interface.

ORGANIZATIONAL LEADERSHIP: A BRIEF HISTORY

"Leadership" is defined as the social process through which a leader exerts influence over his or her followers' psychological processes and behavioral reactions (Levy, 2013). Historically, researchers have taken a variety of approaches to understanding leadership. The first attempt to systematically understand leadership started in the 1930s and focused on identifying the individual characteristics that exemplify good leaders. Studies based on this trait approach to leadership have examined physical characteristics such as gender and appearance, and psychological traits such as intelligence, dominance, and need for power (Levy, 2013). Stogdill (1948) summarized the early empirical research and concluded that overall, results were not supportive of the existence of any universal traits that predicted leadership or leadership effectiveness.

After the seminal review by Stogdill (1948), leadership researchers took a different direction and began to study leader behaviors that could result in effective outcomes. The dominant paradigm that emerged from this behavioral approach to leadership tends to focus on two distinct categories of leader behaviors. The first, initiating structure, refers to task-oriented behaviors that leaders engage in to define roles and clarify expectations for themselves and their followers. The second, consideration, refers to relationship-oriented behaviors that show concern and support for followers (Fleishman & Harris, 1962). According to the behavioral approach, leaders who exhibit high levels of both initiating structure and consideration are the most effective. Empirical studies, however, have not consistently shown positive effects for these behaviors on leadership effectiveness, and scholars have attributed such inconsistencies to, in part, the situations in which leaders operate (Levy, 2013). This led to the third approach to leadership research—the contingency approach.

Moving away from identifying universal traits or behaviors that define effective leadership, contingency theories focused on the match between leader behaviors and situational characteristics, and suggested that the "fit" between the two is the key to effective leadership (Levy, 2013). Different contingency theories have adopted different ways to characterize the situation, focusing on the controllability of the situation (e.g., Fiedler's [1967] contingency theory), followers' values (e.g., path-goal theory; House, 1971), and followers' job-related abilities and efficacious beliefs (e.g., situational theory; Hersey & Blanchard, 1977). Overall, research has provided support for the basic premise of the contingency approach to leadership, such that the linkages between leaders' behaviors and followers' satisfaction and performance are moderated by contextual characteristics (e.g., Sarin & O'Connor, 2009).

More contemporary approaches to leadership have tended to focus on the roles followers play in the leadership processes. For example, transformational leadership theory (Bass, 1985) describes how the leader motivates his or her followers to go beyond their self-interest to achieve high levels of performance. Leader–member exchange theory (Graen & Scandura, 1987) suggests that high-quality, dyadic interactions between the leader and his or her followers are the key to leadership effectiveness. Interestingly, scholars have also started to pay more attention to how leaders may misuse their power and treat their followers poorly. Abusive supervision reflects followers' perceptions of persistent and hostile treatment they receive from a leader (Tepper, 2000). Although it can be viewed as a type of mistreatment in the workplace involving a unique perpetrator (see Chapter 5), abusive supervision is often found to be more detrimental than other types of psychological aggression because of the power differences between leaders and their followers.

CONTEMPORARY LEADERSHIP THEORIES AND OCCUPATIONAL HEALTH

In the following sections, we discuss the three contemporary leadership theories—transformational leadership, leader–member exchange, and abusive supervision—and their linkages with OHP-related topics.

Transformational Leadership

"Transformational leadership" describes a leadership style wherein leaders inspire in followers greater work-related motivation as well as greater commitment to moral purpose compared with what followers could achieve independently (Bass, 1985). Bass (1985, 1997) suggested that transformational leaders may use four strategies to influence followers. Idealized influence refers to leaders showing charisma to attract followers to identify with leaders. Inspirational motivation occurs when leaders articulate an appealing vision for the group and challenge followers with high standards. Transformational leaders use intellectual stimulation to encourage followers to think critically about a problem and to generate creative solutions. Finally, individualized consideration is similar to the consideration dimension of the behavioral approach to leadership, such that transformational leaders show support and provide coaching for followers.

Traditionally, studies of transformational leadership have focused on its effects on follower performance. Indeed, meta-analytic evidence suggests that transformational leadership is positively related to followers' individual task performance, helping behaviors, and proactive behaviors (e.g., Chiaburu, Smith, Wang, & Zimmerman, 2014; Wang, Oh, Courtright, & Colbert, 2011). Moreover, transformational leadership has been linked with higher levels of group and organizational performance (Wang et al., 2011). Beyond effectiveness indicators, research is supportive of the view that transformational leadership benefits follower well-being. For example, meta-analytic results suggest that transformational leadership is positively related to follower job satisfaction (Piccolo et al., 2012).

More recent studies have focused explicitly on linking transformational leadership with employees' occupational stress, well-being, and safety. In particular, transformational leadership has been shown to have both main and moderating effects on employees' stress and well-being. Using experience sampling methodology (a diary method with multiple reports per day for 2 weeks—see Chapter 2), Bono, Foldes,

Vinson, and Muros (2007) showed that supervisors' transformational leadership behavior was associated with followers' positive affective experiences at the end of the workday. Similarly, Liu, Siu, and Shi (2010) showed in a cross-sectional study that transformational leadership had a positive relationship with followers' job satisfaction, and a negative relationship with their perceived stress and psychosomatic symptoms. Moreover, these relationships were mediated by followers' trust in the leader and their efficacy beliefs.

Other studies with different research designs (e.g., multilevel data; longitudinal studies) have also supported the view that trust in the leader and follower self-efficacy are key mechanisms linking transformational leadership with greater well-being and lower stress in followers (e.g., Kelloway, Turner, Barling, & Loughlin, 2012; Nielsen & Munir, 2009). Finally, research has pointed to additional mediators (e.g., innovation climate: Tafvelin, Armelius, & Westerberg, 2011; meaningfulness of work: Arnold, Turner, Barling, Kelloway, & McKee, 2007) that may help explain the effects of transformational leadership on employee stress and well-being.

In terms of a moderating effect, research has generally supported the view that transformational leadership may lessen the impact of workplace stressors or individual employee traits on employees' well-being. For example, Syrek, Apostel, and Antoni (2013) showed that transformational leadership attenuated the relationship of time pressure to exhaustion and work–life imbalance in employees. Time pressure had a weaker effect on employee exhaustion and work–life imbalance when transformational leadership was high versus low. Similarly, Bono et al. (2007) found that transformational leadership attenuated the negative effects of emotional regulation (i.e., concealing negative emotions and faking positive emotions at work) on employees' daily job satisfaction. When transformational leadership was low, emotional regulation was related to reduced job satisfaction; however, when transformational leadership was high, the relationship between emotional regulation and job satisfaction largely disappeared. Finally, De Hoogh and Den Hartog (2009) found that transformational leadership attenuated the relationship between the personality factor external locus of control and employee burnout, such that employees who believed that they had little control over their environment were less likely to experience burnout if their leaders exhibited more transformational leadership behaviors.

In addition to stress and well-being, researchers have linked transformational leadership with safety outcomes. Barling, Loughlin, and Kelloway (2002) first proposed the construct of safety-specific transformational leadership to characterize transformational leadership behaviors that focus specifically on enhancing occupational safety. They suggested that leaders may engage in idealized influence to shift followers' focus away from short-term production goals and toward doing what is morally right—which is the pursuit of long-term, safety-related goals. Leaders may also set challenging, group-based, safety-related goals to motivate followers using inspirational motivation. Intellectual stimulation may be applied to encourage followers to participate in innovative problem solving to address safety-related issues. Finally, leaders may show concern for followers' physical safety with individualized consideration. Barling et al. (2002) demonstrated that safety-specific transformational leadership was positively related to employees' perceived safety climate, which, in turn, was negatively related to accidents and employee injuries. Results from other studies (e.g., Kelloway et al., 2006; Mullen & Kelloway, 2009) have been consistent with the view that the impact of safety-specific transformational leadership on employee accidents and injuries is mediated by safety climate perceptions. Indeed, findings from a recent meta-analysis (Clarke, 2013) are supportive of the idea that safety-specific transformational leadership contributes to safety climate and worker "participation in health and safety activities" (safety participation). Safety climate partly mediated the link between leadership and safety participation.

Empirical studies have also investigated the effects of safety-specific transformational leadership on employee safety performance. For example, safety-specific transformational leadership has been shown to be a positive predictor of employee safety compliance and participation (e.g., Inness, Turner, Barling, & Stride, 2010; Mullen & Kelloway, 2009). Moreover, much like research on transformational leadership and employee stress and well-being, trust in leaders mediates the effect of safety-specific leadership on safety performance (e.g., Conchie, Taylor, & Donald, 2012). Taken together, transformational leadership may promote not only employee and organizational effectiveness, but also the health, well-being, and safety of employees.

Leader–Member Exchange

"Leader–member exchange" (LMX) theory takes a dyadic approach to leadership, and emphasizes that effective leadership involves leaders developing high-quality relationships with individual followers (Graen & Scandura, 1987; Uhl-Bien, 2006). LMX theory describes the stages through which leaders develop favorable relationships with followers. Initially, leaders and their followers may be drawn to each other on the basis of individual traits, such as similarities in demographic characteristics, personal values, and attitudes (Vecchio & Brazil, 2007). Leaders and their followers then establish exchange expectations based on these characteristics. These expectations may be met and reinforced by their exchange partners, resulting in higher quality exchange relationships. Such relationships are characterized by mutual trust, respect, and support from both leaders and their followers (Maslyn & Uhl-Bien, 2001; Uhl-Bien, Graen, & Scandura, 2000). Alternatively, unmet expectations may lead to a lower evaluation of the exchange partner, resulting in low-quality relationships between leaders and followers.

Similar to transformational leadership, high-quality LMX has been positively linked with follower effectiveness. For example, a meta-analysis by Gerstner and Day (1997) found that LMX was positively related to both subjective and objective performance. LMX has also been linked to organizational citizenship behaviors and discretionary behavior such as helping coworkers or advancing the reputation of the organization (Ilies, Nahrgang, & Morgeson, 2007). Researchers have argued that the positive effects of LMX on performance may be explained by at least two mechanisms. First, leaders who have a high-quality relationship with followers are more likely to empower and trust followers, delegate important responsibilities to followers, and allow followers to have more autonomy and control (Brower, Schoorman, & Tan, 2000). Second, high-quality LMX also suggests that leaders are more likely to have open communications with followers, provide followers with constructive feedback, and be more open to follower feedback that prompts leaders to alter behaviors accordingly (Chang & Johnson, 2010; Uhl-Bien, 2003). High-quality leader behaviors provide followers with role clarification and support, which, in turn, promote effective follower performance (Chen, Kirkman, Kanfer, Allen, & Rosen, 2007).

Similar to transformational leadership, LMX has been linked to employee stress, well-being, and safety. Meta-analyses have consistently shown that LMX is positively related to indicators of employee well-being, such as overall job satisfaction, satisfaction with supervisors, and affective organizational commitment (Gerstner & Day, 1997; Dulebohn, Bommer, Liden, Brouer, & Ferris, 2012). LMX quality has been linked to lower levels of burnout and higher levels of job satisfaction because it empowers followers (Laschinger, Finegan, & Wilk, 2011). Moreover, because employees who enjoy high-quality exchange relationships are more likely to receive task instruction and feedback from their leaders, such employees tend to experience fewer role-related stressors (e.g., role ambiguity and role conflict; Gerstner & Day, 1997; Dulebohn et al., 2012), reducing employee stress. Finally, there is research evidence suggesting the importance of LMX for employees' work–life balance. For example, Culbertson, Huffman, and Alden-Anderson (2010) found that high-quality LMX was related to reduced work–family conflict in followers; the relationship was mediated by lower levels of hindrance stress.

Interestingly, other studies have painted a more complex picture of the relationship between high-quality LMX and employee stress. For example, Harris and Kacmar (2006) argued that followers who have high-quality exchange relationships with their leaders are likely to feel obligated to respond to their leaders' task demands. These demands may become too challenging, and the benefits that come with high-quality LMX (i.e., empowerment and support) may not be able to counteract the stress induced by these demands. Indeed, Harris and Kacmar found that LMX had a curvilinear relationship with employee stress, such that employees experience higher stress at low and high levels of LMX, and lower stress at moderate levels of LMX. Kinicki and Vecchio (1994) also found that LMX within the group was positively related to followers' felt time pressure. Relatedly, Ozer, Chang, and Schaubroeck (2014) found that LMX was positively related to challenge stress, but negatively related to hindrance stress. Their findings suggest that, on the one hand, having high-quality relationships with leaders may garner followers more support and reduce the stress-associated demands that impede goal pursuit at work. On the other hand, high-quality LMX may also increase stress because followers may receive more responsibilities that are demanding, but beneficial for their career progress. Taken together, although having high-quality relationships with leaders is typically beneficial for employees' well-being, there may be unintended consequences associated with these exchanges.

In addition to stress and well-being, LMX has also been linked to employees' safety-related outcomes. For example, a positive relationship was found between LMX and employees' safety climate perceptions (e.g., Hofmann, Morgeson, & Gerras, 2003). Moreover, LMX has been linked to more frequent communication concerning safety-related issues (Hofmann & Morgeson, 1999). High-quality exchanges between leaders and followers are likely to lead to followers' sense of obligation to exert efforts to protect themselves, which is likely to enhance their safety performance (Hofmann et al., 2003). Finally, LMX has been negatively related to accidents (e.g., Hofmann & Morgeson, 1999) and injuries (e.g., Michael, Guo, Wiedenbeck, & Ray, 2006). Taken together, LMX may reduce workplace accidents and injuries through its effects on safety climate and employee safety performance.

Abusive Supervision

"Abusive supervision" refers to followers' "perceptions of the extent to which supervisors engage in the sustained display of hostile verbal and nonverbal behaviors, excluding physical contact" (Tepper, 2000, p. 178). Abusive supervision can be viewed as the antithesis of LMX—instead of exchanges that are characterized by mutual trust and respect, followers who perceive high levels of abusive supervision consider the exchanges intimidating and unfair (Tepper, 2000). Unlike the other two contemporary leadership theories just discussed, abusive supervision focuses on the destructive aspect of leader behavior and has been considered a specific type of workplace mistreatment (Tepper, 2007). As such, the early research on abusive supervision tends to focus more on its adverse effects on followers (e.g., stress, ill-being, counterproductive work behavior).

Indeed, abusive supervision has been linked to low levels of job satisfaction, reduced affective commitment, and turnover intentions (Tepper, 2007). Perceived unfairness appears to mediate these relationships (Mackey, Frieder, Brees, & Martinko, in press; Tepper, 2000). Abusive supervision has also been linked to increases in burnout (e.g., Aryee, Chen, Sun, & Debrah, 2007) and psychological distress (e.g., Restubog, Scott, & Zagenczyk, 2011). Tepper (2000) found that abusive supervision was positively related to work–family conflict. Moreover, Hoobler and Brass (2006) found that abusive supervision directed at followers was related to followers acting negatively or aggressively toward family members. In this case, employees who perceive mistreatment from their supervisors may displace their anger and frustration onto family members, thereby creating work-to-family spillover. Beyond work-to-family problems, Bamberger and Bacharach (2006) demonstrated linkages between abusive supervision and workers' problem drinking. Finally, a meta-analysis (Mackey et al., in press) has shown that abusive supervision has consistent, negative implications for employee well-being indicators (e.g., depression, emotional exhaustion, job tension, and reduced job satisfaction). Taken together, abusive supervision can be viewed as a type of leader behavior that has negative implications for follower health and well-being.

In terms of safety-related outcomes, limited research has examined the implications of abusive supervision for employee safety. In a study with poultry plant workers, Grzywacz et al. (2007) found that abusive supervision was negatively related to employees' safety climate perceptions. In addition, abusive supervision was positively related to workers' musculoskeletal injuries and respiratory symptoms. The limited evidence suggests that abusive supervision has negative implications for follower physical safety.

SUMMARY

In this chapter, we cover key climate and leadership variables that are relevant to the occupational health and safety of employees. In particular, safety climate at both the individual and the unit level is an important factor for employees' physical safety, whereas the mistreatment and psychosocial safety climates are more important for their psychosocial health and well-being. Contemporary leadership theories, including transformational leadership and LMX, have also demonstrated that in addition to employee effectiveness, they may also affect employees' safety, health, and well-being. Interestingly, evidence suggests that safety climate may be a key mediator linking these leadership variables with employee safety outcomes. Finally, with regard to abusive supervision, although its effects on employee well-being have been consistently examined and supported, its association with safety-related outcomes is less clear and requires additional investigation.

REFERENCES

Allen, T. D. (2001). Family-supportive work environments: The role of organizational perceptions. *Journal of Vocational Behavior, 58,* 414–435. doi:10.1006/jvbe.2000.1774

Anderson, N. R., & West, M. A. (1998). Measuring climate for work group innovation: Development and validation of the team climate inventory. *Journal of Organizational Behavior, 19,* 235–258. doi:10.1002/(SICI)1099-1379(199805)19:3<235::AID-JOB837>3.0.CO;2-C

Argyris, C. (1957). *Personality and organization.* New York, NY: Harper.

Arnold, K. A., Turner, N., Barling, J., Kelloway, E. K., & McKee, M. C. (2007). Transformational leadership and psychological well-being: The mediating role of meaningful work. *Journal of Occupational Health Psychology, 12,* 193–203. doi:10.1037/1076-8998.12.3.193

Aryee, S., Chen, Z. X., Sun, L.-Y., & Debrah, Y. A. (2007). Antecedents and outcomes of abusive supervision: Test of a trickle-down model. *Journal of Applied Psychology, 92,* 191–201. doi:10.1037/0021-9010.92.1.191

Ashforth, B. (1985). Climate formation: Issues and extensions. *Academy of Management Review, 10,* 837–847. doi:10.2307/258051

Bailey, T. S., Dollard, M. F., & Richards, P. A. M. (2015). A national standard for psychosocial safety climate (PSC): PSC 41 as the benchmark for low risk of job strain and depressive symptoms. *Journal of Occupational Health Psychology, 20,* 15–26. doi:10.1037/a0038166

Bain, P. G., Mann, L., & Pirola-Merlo, A. (2001). The innovation imperative: The relationships between team climate, innovation, and performance in research and development teams. *Small Group Research, 32,* 55–73. doi:10.1177/104649640103200103

Bamberger, P. A., & Bacharach, S. B. (2006). Abusive supervision and subordinate problem drinking: Taking resistance, stress, and subordinate personality into account. *Human Relations, 59,* 723–752. doi:10.1177/0018726706066852

Barling, J., Loughlin, C., & Kelloway, E. K. (2002). Development and test of a model linking safety-specific transformational leadership and occupational safety. *Journal of Applied Psychology, 87,* 488–496. doi:10.1037/0021-9010.87.3.488

Bass, B. M. (1985). *Leadership and performance beyond expectations.* New York, NY: Free Press.

Bass, B. M. (1997). Does the transactional-transformational leadership paradigm transcend organizational and national boundaries? *American Psychologist, 52,* 130–139. doi:10.1037/0003-066X.52.2.130

Beus, J. M., Dhanani, L. Y., & McCord, M. A. (2015). A meta-analysis of personality and workplace safety: Addressing unanswered questions. *Journal of Applied Psychology, 100,* 481–498. doi:10.1037/a0037916

Beus, J. M., Payne, S. C., Bergman, M. E., & Arthur, W., Jr. (2010). Safety climate and injuries: An examination of theoretical and empirical relationships. *Journal of Applied Psychology, 95,* 713–727. doi:10.1037/a0019164

Bliese, P. D. (2000). Within-group agreement, non-independence, and reliability: Implications for data aggregation and analyses. In K. J. Klein & S. W. J. Kozlowski (Eds.), *Multilevel theory, research, and methods in organizations: Foundations, extensions, and new directions* (pp. 349–381). San Francisco, CA: Jossey-Bass.

Bono, J. E., Foldes, H. J., Vinson, G., & Muros, J. P. (2007). Workplace emotions: The role of supervision and leadership. *Journal of Applied Psychology, 92,* 1357–1367. doi:10.1037/0021-9010.92.5.1357

Borman, W. C., & Motowidlo, S. J. (1993). Expanding the criterion domain to include elements of contextual performance. In N. Schmitt & W. C. Borman (Eds.), *Personnel selection in organizations* (pp. 71–98). San Francisco, CA: Jossey-Bass.

Brimhall, K. C., Lizano, E. L., & Mor Barak, M. E. (2014). The mediating role of inclusion: A longitudinal study of the effects of leader-member exchange and diversity climate on job satisfaction and intention to leave among child welfare workers. *Children and Youth Services Review, 40,* 79–88. doi:10.1016/j.childyouth.2014.03.003

Brower, H. H., Schoorman, D. F., & Tan, H. H. (2000). A model of relational leadership: The integration of trust and leader-member exchange. *The Leadership Quarterly, 11,* 227–250. doi:10.1016/S1048-9843(00)00040-0

Burke, M. J., Borucki, C. C., & Kaufman, J. D. (2002). Contemporary perspective on the study of psychological climate: A commentary. *European Journal of Work and Organizational Psychology, 11,* 325–340. doi:10.1080/13594320244000210

Campbell, J. P., Dunnette, M. D., Lawler, E. E., III, & Weick, K. E. (1970). *Managerial behavior, performance, and effectiveness.* New York, NY: McGraw-Hill.

Chang, C.-H., Eatough, E. M., Spector, P. E., & Kessler, S. R. (2012). Violence-prevention climate, exposure to violence and aggression, and prevention behavior: A mediation model. *Journal of Organizational Behavior, 33,* 657–677. doi:10.1002/job.776

Chang, C.-H., & Golubovich, J. (2012, August). Strain, cognitive failure, and prevention behaviors: Violence prevention climate as a moderator. In D. E. Caughlin, L. Q. Yang, & C. H. Chang (Chairs), *Employee and organizational consequences of aggression prevention climate.* Symposium conducted at the meeting of Academy of Management, Boston, MA.

Chang, C.-H., & Johnson, R. E. (2010). Not all leader-member exchanges are created equal: Importance of leader relational identity. *The Leadership Quarterly, 21,* 797–808. doi:10.1016/j.leaqua.2010.07.008

Chen, G., Kirkman, B. L., Kanfer, R., Allen, D., & Rosen, B. (2007). A multilevel study of leadership, empowerment, and performance in teams. *Journal of Applied Psychology, 92,* 331–346. doi:10.1037/0021-9010.92.2.331

Chiaburu, D. S., Smith, T. A., Wang, J., & Zimmerman, R. D. (2014). Relative importance of leader influences for subordinates' proactive behaviors, prosocial behaviors, and task performance: A meta-analysis. *Journal of Personnel Psychology, 13,* 70–86. doi:10.1027/1866-5888/a000105

Chowdhury, S. K., & Endres, M. L. (2010). The impact of client variability on nurses' occupational strain and injury: Cross-level moderation by safety climate. *Academy of Management Journal, 53,* 182–198. doi:10.5465/AMJ.2010.48037720

Christian, M. S., Bradley, J. C., Wallace, J. C., & Burke, M. J. (2009). Workplace safety: A meta-analysis of the roles of person and situation factors. *Journal of Applied Psychology, 94,* 1103–1127. doi:10.1037/a0016172

Cigularov, K. P., Chen, P. Y., & Stallones, L. (2009). Error communication in young farm workers: Its relationship to safety climate and safety locus of control. *Work & Stress, 23,* 297–312. doi:10.1080/02678370903416679

Clarke, S. (2006). The relationship between safety climate and safety performance: A meta-analytic review. *Journal of Occupational Health Psychology, 11,* 315–327. doi:10.1037/1076-8998.11.4.315

Clarke, S. (2010). An integrative model of safety climate: Linking psychological climate and work attitudes to individual safety outcomes using meta-analysis. *Journal of Occupational and Organizational Psychology, 83,* 553–578. doi:10.1348/096317909X452122

Clarke, S. (2013). Safety leadership: A meta-analytic review of transformational and transactional leadership styles as antecedents of safety behaviours. *Journal of Occupational and Organizational Psychology, 86,* 22–49. doi:10.1111/j.2044-8325.2012.02064.x

Conchie, S. M., Taylor, P. J., & Donald, I. J. (2012). Promoting safety voice with safety-specific transformational leadership: The mediating role of two dimensions of trust. *Journal of Occupational Health Psychology, 17,* 105–115. doi:10.1037/a0025101

Culbertson, S. S., Huffman, A. H., & Alden-Anderson, R. (2010). Leader-member exchange and work-family interactions: The mediating role of self-reported challenge- and hindrance-related stress. *Journal of Psychology, 144,* 15–36. doi:10.1080/00223980903356040

De Hoogh, A. H. B., & Den Hartog, D. N. (2009). Neuroticism and locus of control as moderators of the relationships of charismatic and autocratic leadership with burnout. *Journal of Applied Psychology, 94,* 1058–1067. doi:10.1037/a0016253

Dollard, M. F. (2007). *Psychosocial safety culture and climate: Definition of a new construct.* Adelaide, Australia: Work and Stress Research Group, University of South Australia.

Dollard, M. F., & Bakker, A. B. (2010). Psychosocial safety climate as a precursor to conducive work environments, psychological health problems, and employee engagement. *Journal of Occupational and Organizational Psychology, 83,* 579–599. doi:10.1348/096317909X470690

Dollard, M. F., Opie, T., Lenthall, S., Wakerman, J., Knight, S., Dunn, S., . . . MacLeod, M. (2012). Psychosocial safety climate as an antecedent of work characteristics and psychological strain: A multilevel model. *Work & Stress, 26,* 385–404. doi:10.1080/02678373.2012.734154

Dulebohn, J. H., Bommer, W. H., Liden, R. C., Brouer, R. L., & Ferris, G. R. (2012). A meta-analysis of antecedents and consequences of leader-member exchange: Integrating the past with an eye toward the future. *Journal of Management, 38,* 1715–1759. doi:10.1177/0149206311415280

Fiedler, F. E. (1967). *A theory of leadership effectiveness.* New York, NY: McGraw-Hill.

Fleishman, E. A., & Harris, E. F. (1962). Patterns of leadership behavior related to employee grievances and turnover. *Personnel Psychology, 15,* 43–56. doi:10.1111/j.1744-6570.1962.tb01845.x

Forehand, G. A., & Gilmer, B. H. (1964). Environmental variation in studies of organizational behavior. *Psychological Bulletin, 62,* 361–382. doi:10.1037/h0045960

Fogarty, G. (2005). Psychological strain mediates the impact of safety climate on maintenance errors. *International Journal of Applied Aviation Studies, 5*(1), 53–64.

Geller, E. S., Roberts, D. S., & Gilmore, M. R. (1996). Predicting propensity to actively care for occupational safety. *Journal of Safety Research, 27*, 1–8. doi:10.1016/0022-4375(95)00024-0

Gerstner, C. R., & Day, D. V. (1997). Meta-analytic review of leader–member exchange theory: Correlates and construct issues. *Journal of Applied Psychology, 82*, 827–844. doi:10.1037/0021-9010.82.6.827

Glick, W. H. (1985). Conceptualizing and measuring organizational and psychological climate: Pitfalls in multilevel research. *Academy of Management Review, 10*, 601–616. doi:10.2307/258140

Golubovich, J., Chang, C.-H., & Eatough, E. M. (2014). Safety climate, hardiness, and musculoskeletal complaints: A mediated moderation model. *Applied Ergonomics, 45*, 757–766. doi:10.1016/j.apergo.2013.10.008

Graen, G. B., & Scandura, T. (1987). Toward a psychology of dyadic organizing. In B. Staw & L. L. Cummings (Eds.), *Research in organizational behavior* (Vol. 9, pp. 175–208). Greenwich, CT: JAI Press.

Griffin, M. A., & Neal, A. (2000). Perceptions of safety at work: A framework for linking safety climate to safety performance, knowledge, and motivation. *Journal of Occupational Health Psychology, 5*, 347–358. doi:10.1037/1076-8998.5.3.347

Grzywacz, J. G., Arcury, T. A., Marin, A., Carrillo, L., Coates, M. L., Burke, B., & Quandt, S. A. (2007). The organization of work: Implications for injury and illness among immigrant Latino poultry-processing workers. *Archives of Environmental & Occupational Health, 62*, 19–26, doi:10.3200/AEOH.62.1.19-26

Haines, T., Stringer, B., & Duku, E. (2007). Workplace safety climate and incivility among British Columbia and Ontario operating room nurses: A preliminary investigation. *Canadian Journal of Community Mental Health, 26*(2), 141–152.

Hall, G. B., Dollard, M. F., & Coward, J. (2010). Psychosocial safety climate: Development of the PSC-12. *International Journal of Stress Management, 17*, 353–383. doi:10.1037/a0021320

Harris, K. J., & Kacmar, K. M. (2006). Too much of a good thing: The curvilinear effect of leader-member exchange on stress. *Journal of Social Psychology, 146*, 65–84. doi:10.3200/SOCP.146.1.65-84

Hellriegel, D., & Slocum, S. W., Jr. (1974). Organizational climate: Measures, research, and contingencies. *Academy of Management Journal, 17*, 255–280. doi:10.2307/254979

Hersey, P., & Blanchard, K. H. (1977). *The management of organizational behavior* (3rd ed.). Englewood Cliffs, NJ: Prentice Hall.

Hofmann, D. A., & Morgeson, F. P. (1999). Safety-related behavior as a social exchange: The role of perceived organizational support and leader-member exchange. *Journal of Applied Psychology, 84*, 286–296. doi:10.1037/0021-9010.84.2.286

Hofmann, D. A., Morgeson, F. P., & Gerras, S. J. (2003). Climate as a moderator of the relationship between leader-member exchange and content specific citizenship: Safety climate as an exemplar. *Journal of Applied Psychology, 88*, 170–178. doi:10.1037/0021-9010.88.1.170

Hoobler, J. M., & Brass, D. J. (2006). Abusive supervision and family undermining as displaced aggression. *Journal of Applied Psychology. 91*, 1125–1133. doi:10.1037/0021-9010.91.5.1125

House, R. J. (1971). A path-goal theory of leader effectiveness. *Administrative Science Quarterly, 16*, 321–338. doi:10.2307/2391905

Hutchinson, M., Jackson, D., Wilkes, L., & Vickers, M. H. (2008). A new model of bullying in the nursing workplace: Organizational characteristics as critical antecedents. *Advances in Nursing Science, 31*, E60–E71. doi:10.1097/01.ANS.0000319572.37373.0c

Hystad, S. W., & Bye, H. H. (2013). Safety behaviours at sea: The role of personal values and personality hardiness. *Safety Science, 57*, 19–26. doi:10.1016/j.ssci.2013.01.018

Idris, M. A., & Dollard, M. F. (2011). Psychosocial safety climate, work conditions, and emotions in the workplace: A Malaysian population-based work stress study. *International Journal of Stress Management, 18*, 324–347. doi:10.1037/a0024849

Idris, M. A., Dollard, M. F., & Yulita (2014). Psychosocial safety climate, emotional demands, burnout, and depression: A longitudinal multilevel study in the Malaysian private sector. *Journal of Occupational Health Psychology, 19*(3), 291–302.

Ilies, R., Nahrgang, J. D., & Morgeson, F. P. (2007). Leader-member exchange and citizenship behaviors: A meta-analysis. *Journal of Applied Psychology, 92*, 269–277. doi:10.1037/0021-9010.92.1.269

Inness, M., LeBlanc, M. M., & Barling, J. (2008). Psychosocial predictors of supervisor-, peer-, subordinate-, and service-provider-targeted aggression. *Journal of Applied Psychology, 93*, 1401–1411. doi:10.1037/a0012810

Inness, M., Turner, N., Barling, J., & Stride, C. B. (2010). Transformational leadership and employee safety performance: A within-person, between jobs design. *Journal of Occupational Health Psychology, 15*, 279–290. doi:10.1037/a0019380

James, L. A., & James, L. R. (1989). Integrating work environment perceptions: Explorations in the measurement of meaning. *Journal of Applied Psychology, 69,* 85–98. doi:10.1037/0021-9010.74.5.739

James, L. R., Choi, C. C., Ko, C. H. E., McNeil, P. K., Minton, M. K., Wright, M. A., & Kim, K. (2008). Organizational and psychological climate: A review of theory and research. *European Journal of Work and Organizational Psychology, 17,* 5–32. doi:10.1080/13594320701662550

James, L. R., Demaree, R. G., & Wolf, G. (1993). r_{WG}: An assessment of within-group interrater agreement. *Journal of Applied Psychology, 78,* 306–309. doi:10.1037/0021-9010.78.2.306

James, L. R., & Jones, A. P. (1974). Organizational climate: A review of theory and research. *Psychological Bulletin, 81,* 1096–1112. doi:10.1037/h0037511

James, L. R., & McIntyre, M. D. (1996). Perceptions of organizational climate. In K. R. Murphy (Ed.), *Individual differences and behavior in organizations* (pp. 416–450). San Francisco, CA: Jossey-Bass.

Kaplan, D. M., Wiley, J. W., & Maertz, C. P., Jr. (2011). The role of calculative attachment in the relationship between diversity climate and retention. *Human Resource Management, 50,* 271–287. doi:10.1002/hrm.20413

Kelloway, E. K., Mullen, J., & Francis, L. (2006). Divergent effects of transformational and passive leadership on employee safety. *Journal of Occupational Health Psychology, 11,* 76–86. doi:10.1037/1076-8998.11.1.76

Kelloway, E. K., Turner, N., Barling, J., & Loughlin, C. (2012). Transformational leadership and employee psychological well-being: The mediating role of employee trust in leadership. *Work & Stress, 26,* 39–55. doi:10.1080/02678373.2012.660774

Kessler, S. R., Spector, P. E., Chang, C. H., & Parr, A. D. (2008). Organizational violence and aggression: Development of the three-factor Violence Climate Survey. *Work & Stress, 22,* 108–124. doi:10.1080/02678370802187926

Kinicki, A. J., & Vecchio, R. P. (1994). Influences on the quality of supervisor-subordinate relations: The role of time-pressure, organizational commitment, and locus of control. *Journal of Organizational Behavior, 15,* 75–82. doi:10.1002/job.4030150108

Kozlowski, S. W. J., & Hattrup, K. (1992). A disagreement about within-group agreement: Disentangling issues of consistency versus consensus. *Journal of Applied Psychology, 77,* 161–167. doi:10.1037/0021-9010.77.2.161

Kozlowski, S. W. J., & Klein, K. J. (2000). A multilevel approach to theory and research in organizations: Contextual, temporal, and emergent processes. In K. J. Klein & S. W. J. Kozlowski (Eds.), *Multilevel theory, research, and methods in organizations: Foundations, extensions, and new directions* (pp. 3–90). San Francisco, CA: Jossey-Bass.

Laschinger, H. K. S., Finegan, J., & Wilk, P. (2011). Situational and dispositional influences on nurses' workplace well-being. *Nursing Research, 60,* 124–131. doi:10.1097/NNR.0b013e318209782e

LeBreton, J. M., & Senter, J. L. (2008). Answers to twenty questions about interrater reliability and interrater agreement. *Organizational Research Methods, 11,* 815–852. doi:10.1177/1094428106296642

Leitão, S., & Greiner, B. A. (2016). Organisational safety climate and occupational accidents and injuries: An epidemiology-based systematic review. *Work & Stress, 30,* 71–90. doi:10.1080/02678373.2015.1102176

Levy, P. E. (2013). *Industrial/organizational psychology: Understanding the workplace* (4th ed.). New York, NY: Palgrave Macmillan.

Lewin, K., Lippitt, R., & White, R. K. (1939). Patterns of aggressive behavior in experimentally created "social climates." *Journal of Social Psychology, 10,* 271–299. doi:10.1037/10319-008

Likert, R. (1967). *The human organization.* New York, NY: McGraw-Hill.

Liu, J., Siu, O.-L., & Shi, K. (2010). Transformational leadership and employee well-being: The mediating role of trust in the leader and self-efficacy. *Applied Psychology: An International Review, 59,* 454–479. doi:10.1111/j.1464-0597.2009.00407.x

Locke, E. A. (1976). The nature and causes of job satisfaction. In M. D. Dunnette (Ed.), *Handbook of industrial and organizational psychology* (pp. 1297–1343). Chicago, IL: Rand McNally.

Mackey, J. D., Frieder, R. E., Brees, J. R., & Martinko, M. J. (in press). Abusive supervision: A meta-analysis and empirical review. *Journal of Management.* doi:10.1177/0149206315573997

Maslyn, J. M., & Uhl-Bien, M. (2001). Leader–member exchange and its dimensions: Effects of self-effort and other's effort on relationship quality. *Journal of Applied Psychology, 86,* 697–708. doi:10.1037/0021-9010.86.4.69

McCaughey, D., DelliFraine, J. L., McGhan, G., & Bruning, N. S. (2013). The negative effects of workplace injury and illness on workplace safety climate perceptions and health care worker outcomes. *Safety Science, 51,* 138–147. doi:10.1016/j.ssci.2012.06.004

McGregor, D. M. (1960). *The human side of enterprise.* New York, NY: McGraw-Hill.

Mearns, K., Hope, L., Ford, M. T., & Tetrick, L. E. (2010). Investment in workforce health: Exploring the implications for workforce safety climate and commitment. *Accident Analysis and Prevention, 42,* 1445–1454. doi:10.1016/j.aap.2009.08.009

Michael, J. H., Guo, Z. G., Wiedenbeck, J. K., & Ray, C. D. (2006). Production supervisor impacts on subordinates' safety outcomes: An investigation of leader-member exchange and safety communication. *Journal of Safety Research, 37,* 469–477. doi:10.1016/j.jsr.2006.06.004

Mullen, J. E., & Kelloway, E. K. (2009). Safety leadership: A longitudinal study of the effects of transformational leadership on safety outcomes. *Journal of Occupational and Organizational Psychology, 82,* 253–272. doi:10.1348/096317908X325313

Nahrgang, J. D., Morgeson, F. P., & Hofmann, D. A. (2011). Safety at work: A meta-analytic investigation of the link between job demands, job resources, burnout, engagement, and safety outcomes. *Journal of Applied Psychology, 96,* 71–94. doi:10.1037/a0021484

Neal, A., & Griffin, M. A. (2004). Safety climate and safety at work. In M. R. Frone & J. Barling (Eds.), *The psychology of workplace safety* (pp. 15–34). Washington, DC: American Psychological Association. doi:10.1037/10662-002

Neal, A., & Griffin, M. A. (2006). A study of the lagged relationships among safety climate, safety motivation, safety behavior, and accidents at the individual and group levels. *Journal of Applied Psychology, 91,* 946–953. doi:10.1037/0021-9010.91.4.946

Neal, A., Griffin, M. A., & Hart, P. M. (2000). The impact of organizational climate on safety climate and individual behavior. *Safety Science, 34,* 99–109. doi:10.1016/S0925-7535(00)00008-4

Nielsen, K., & Munir, F. (2009). How do transformational leaders influence followers' affective well-being? Exploring the mediating role of self-efficacy. *Work & Stress, 23,* 313–329. doi:10.1080/02678370903385106

Nielsen, M. B., Mearns, K., Matthiesen, S. B., & Eid, J. (2011). Using the job demands-resources model to investigate risk perception, safety climate and job satisfaction in safety critical organizations. *Scandinavian Journal of Psychology, 52,* 465–475. doi:10.1111/j.1467-9450.2011.00885.x

O'Neill, J. W., Harrison, M. M., Cleveland, J., Almeida, D., Stawski, R., & Crouter, A. C. (2009). Work-family climate, organizational commitment, and turnover: Multilevel contagion effects of leaders. *Journal of Vocational Behavior, 74,* 18–29. doi:10.1016/j.jvb.2008.10.004

Ostroff, C. (1993). The effects of climate and personal influences on individual behavior and attitudes in organizations. *Organizational Behavior and Human Decision Processes, 56,* 56–90. doi:10.1006/obhd.1993.1045

Ozer, M., Chang, C.-H., & Schaubroeck, J. M. (2014). Contextual moderators of the relationship between organizational citizenship behaviours and challenge and hindrance stress. *Journal of Occupational and Organizational Psychology, 87,* 557–578. doi:10.1111/joop.12063

Paustian-Underdahl, S. C., & Halbesleben, J. R. B. (2014). Examining the influence of climate, supervisor guidance, and behavioral integrity on work-family conflict: A demands and resources approach. *Journal of Organizational Behavior, 35,* 447–463. doi:10.1002/job.1883

Payne, R. L., & Pugh, D. S. (1976). Organizational structure and climate. In M. D. Dunnette (Ed.), *Handbook of industrial and organizational psychology* (pp. 1125–1173). Chicago, IL: Rand McNally.

Piccolo, R. F., Bono, J. E., Heinitz, K., Rowold, J., Duehr, E., & Judge, T. A. (2012). The relative impact of complementary leader behaviors: Which matter most? *The Leadership Quarterly, 23,* 567–581. doi:10.1016/j.leaqua.2011.12.008

Probst, T. M. (2004). Safety and insecurity: Exploring the moderating effect of organizational safety climate. *Journal of Occupational Health Psychology, 9,* 3–10. doi:10.1037/1076-8998.9.1.3

Restubog, S. L. D., Scott, K. L., & Zagenczyk, T. J. (2011). When distress hits home: The role of contextual factors and psychological distress in predicting employees' responses to abusive supervision. *Journal of Applied Psychology, 96,* 713–729. doi:10.1037/a0021593

Sarin, S., & O'Connor, G. C. (2009). First among equals: The effect of team leader characteristics on the internal dynamics of cross-functional produce development teams. *Journal of Product Innovation Management, 26,* 188–205. doi:10.1111/j.1540-5885.2009.00345.x

Schneider, B. (1975). Organizational climates: An essay. *Personnel Psychology, 28,* 447–479. doi:10.1111/j.1744-6570.1975.tb01386.x

Schneider, B., & Barlett, C. J. (1968). Individual differences and organizational climate: I. The research plan and questionnaire development. *Personnel Psychology, 21,* 323–333. doi:10.1111/j.1744-6570.1968.tb02033.x

Schneider, B., Ehrhart, M. G., & Macey, W. H. (2011). Perspectives on organizational climate and culture. In S. Zedeck (Ed.), *APA handbook of industrial and organizational psychology* (Vol. 1: Building and developing the organization, pp. 373–414). Washington, DC: American Psychological Association. doi:10.1037/12169-012

Schneider, B., White, S. S., & Paul, M. (1998). Linking service climate and customer perceptions of service quality: Test of a causal model. *Journal of Applied Psychology, 83,* 150–163. doi:10.1037/0021-9010.83.2.150

Siu, O.-L., Phillips, D. R., & Leung, T.-W. (2004). Safety climate and safety performance among construction workers in Hong Kong: The role of psychological strains as mediators. *Accident Analysis and Prevention, 36,* 359–366. doi:10.1016/S0001-4575(03)00016-2

Stogdill, R. M. (1948). Personal factors associated with leadership: A survey of the literature. *Journal of Psychology, 25,* 35–71. doi:10.1080/00223980.1948.9917362

Syrek, C. J., Apostel, E., & Antoni, C. H. (2013). Stress in highly demanding IT jobs: Transformational leadership moderates the impact of time pressure on exhaustion and work-life balance. *Journal of Occupational Health Psychology, 18,* 252–261. doi:10.1037/a0033085

Tafvelin, S., Armelius, K., & Westerberg, K. (2011). Toward understanding the direct and indirect effects of transformational leadership on well-being: A longitudinal study. *Journal of Leadership & Organizational Studies, 18,* 480–492. doi:10.1177/1548051811418342

Tepper, B. J. (2000). Consequences of abusive supervision. *Academy of Management Journal, 43,* 178–190. doi:10.2307/1556375

Tepper, B. J. (2007). Abusive supervision in work organizations: Review synthesis, and research agenda. *Journal of Management, 33,* 261–289. doi:10.1177/0149206307300812

Thompson, C. A., Beauvais, L. L., & Lyness, K. S. (1999). When work–family benefits are not enough: The influence of work–family culture on benefit utilization, organizational attachment, and work–family conflict. *Journal of Vocational Behavior, 54,* 392–415. doi:10.1006/jvbe.1998.1681

Uhl-Bien, M. (2003). Relationship development as a key ingredient for leadership development. In S. Murphy & R. Riggio (Eds.), *The future of leadership development* (pp. 129–147). Mahwah, NJ: Erlbaum.

Uhl-Bien, M. (2006). Relational leadership theory: Exploring the social processes of leadership and organizing. *The Leadership Quarterly, 17,* 654–676. doi:10.1016/j.leaqua.2006.10.007

Uhl-Bien, M., Graen, G., & Scandura, T. (2000). Implications of leader–member exchange (LMX) for strategic human resource management systems: Relationships as social capital for competitive advantage. In G. R. Ferris (Ed.), *Research in personnel and human resources management* (Vol. 18, pp. 137–185). Greenwich, CT: JAI Press.

Vecchio, R. P., & Brazil, D. M. (2007). Leadership and sex-similarity: A comparison in a military setting. *Personnel Psychology, 60,* 303–335. doi:10.1111/j.1744-6570.2007.00075.x

Verbeke, W., Volgering, M., & Hessels, M. (1998). Exploring the conceptual expansion within the field of organizational behavior: Organizational climate and organizational culture. *Journal of Management Studies, 35,* 303–329.

Wallace, J. C., Popp, E., & Mondore, S. (2006). Safety climate as a mediator between foundation climates and occupational accidents: A group-level investigation. *Journal of Applied Psychology, 91,* 681–688. doi:10.1037/0021-9010.91.3.681

Wang, G., Oh, I.-S., Courtright, S. H., & Colbert, A. E. (2011). Transformational leadership and performance across criteria and levels: A meta-analytic review of 25 years of research. *Group & Organization Management, 36,* 223–270. doi:10.1177/1059601111401017

Whitman, D. S., Caleo, S., Carpenter, N. C., Horner, M. T., & Bernerth, J. B. (2012). Fairness at the collective level: A meta-analytic examination of the consequences and boundary conditions of organizational justice climate. *Journal of Applied Psychology, 97,* 776–791. doi:10.1037/a0028021

Yang, L.-Q., Caughlin, D. E., Gazica, M. W., Truxillo, D. M., & Spector, P. E. (2014). Workplace mistreatment climate and potential employee and organizational outcomes: A meta-analytic review from the target's perspective. *Journal of Occupational Health Psychology, 19,* 315–335. doi:10.1037/a0036905

Zohar, D. (1980). Safety climate in industrial organizations: Theoretical and applied implications. *Journal of Applied Psychology, 65,* 96–102. doi:10.1037/0021-9010.65.1.96

Zohar, D. (2011). Safety climate: Conceptual and measurement issues. In J. C. Quick & L. E. Tetrick (Eds.), *Handbook of occupational health psychology* (2nd ed., pp. 141–164). Washington, DC: American Psychological Association. doi:10.1037/10474-006

Zohar, D., & Hofmann, D. A. (2012). Organizational culture and climate. In S. W. J. Kozlowski (Ed.), The *Oxford handbook of industrial and organizational psychology* (Vol. 1, pp. 643–666). New York, NY: Oxford University Press.

SEVEN

OHP Research on Specific Occupations

KEY CONCEPTS AND FINDINGS COVERED IN CHAPTER 7

In contrast to the earlier chapters, which were largely devoted to research that cuts across occupations, this chapter examines research concerning specific occupations. The purpose of the chapter is to give readers a look at specific jobs that employ large numbers of people. The chapter covers research on teachers, nurses, combat soldiers, first responders, construction workers, and agricultural workers. Each occupation has specific challenges that can potentially affect health, although sometimes the challenges are common to many occupations. Job-specific challenges can be missed in research that covers a wide cross-section of jobs because such research must rely on measures that apply across occupations. For example, research that cuts across occupations cannot tell us about the impact of undercover police work in comparison to more standard police work. Research that cuts across occupations cannot home in on the impact of student-initiated violence on teachers. The occupations were selected on the basis of the authors' academic and personal interests.

Where possible, the chapter focuses on longitudinal studies, although some cross-sectional research is examined. The coverage is not exhaustive. Because the literature is vast, the chapter can survey only a relatively small number of studies.

Some other considerations should be borne in mind when discussing research on occupations. First, the diagnostic criteria for stress-related disorders such as post-traumatic stress disorder (PTSD) have changed somewhat from *DSM-III* to *DSM-5*, complicating cross-era comparisons. Second, diagnoses of depression, PTSD, alcohol abuse, and the like should be made by a clinician (e.g., clinical psychologist, psychiatrist) employing valid diagnostic criteria. Many research teams have not had resources needed to underwrite the cost of clinician-administered interviews and, instead, have relied on self-report questionnaires and checklists (e.g., Chiu et al., 2011) that yield, if not a diagnosis per se, a likely classification such as "probable depression" or "probable PTSD." Third, some studies (e.g., Eaton, Anthony, Mandel, & Garrison, 1990) employed trained laypersons to administer highly structured interviews, with the diagnoses derived algorithmically. Fourth, other studies have *not* sought to diagnose mental disorders in job incumbents; instead, the studies have treated psychological functioning as a continuous factor (see Chapter 3 for a discussion of these measures) to reflect the amount of psychological distress experienced. Fifth, some studies have used either disease or biological endpoints (e.g., heart attack) or continuous measures of functioning (e.g., blood pressure) as outcomes.

TEACHERS

For 6 years, the first author was a mathematics teacher in a dangerous public school located in a high-crime, Brooklyn neighborhood. During his first year on the job, he taught a particularly troublesome class during the eighth—and the last—period of the school day. Most students in the class were ill-mannered and, at times, ill-tempered. A student named Derrick sometimes brought drum sticks to class and drummed on his desktop while the first author was trying to teach. Another student, Richard, was a muscular lad who was quick to anger over imagined slights—the slights were mostly imagined because most students (and some teachers) were afraid of him. From the beginning of September, the first author liked to get to his eighth-period classroom early, well before the end of the seventh period. On the walk to his eighth-period classroom, he peeked into Mr. Shepherd's science classroom by looking through the window built into Mr. Shepherd's classroom door. During the seventh period Mr. Shepherd taught the same students the first author would teach during the eighth. Although Mr. Shepherd was a veteran teacher, his classroom was in chaos. Students ran helter-skelter around the room ignoring him. By November, the author observed that Mr. Shepherd was no longer in the room. A few days later, while doing paperwork in the teachers' lounge, the author put his pen down and asked a colleague about Mr. Shepherd. The colleague whispered that Mr. Shepherd suffered "a nervous breakdown."

Schoolteachers constitute a large occupational group; in the United States, teachers make up about 3% of the civilian employee workforce (Bureau of Labor Statistics [BLS], 2015c). Ingersoll (2001) observed that there are about twice as many teachers as there are registered nurses and teachers outnumber lawyers or professors by a ratio of 5 to 1. Teachers are well educated; they ordinarily earn baccalaureate degrees and often hold advanced degrees. Education is related to good health. Because teachers' interactions with students can spark intellectual and emotional growth in the young, teaching has intrinsic rewards. All told, teaching should be a satisfying occupation.

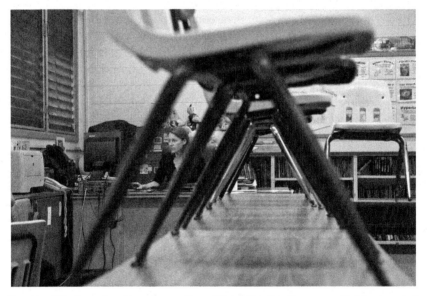

Teacher. (Photographer Doug Leany. From Flickr, Creative Commons. Public domain.)

Among occupations in which incumbents are college graduates, teaching has one of the highest turnover rates (higher than that of nurses but less than that of corrections officers; Ingersoll, 2013). Turnover rates can be considered a proxy variable reflecting the stressfulness of working conditions. Ingersoll (2001) and Ingersoll and May (2012) showed that unsatisfactory working conditions (e.g., student discipline problems, lack of autonomy) are important factors driving turnover (not retirement). A study that followed in real time more than 250 New York City (NYC) teachers found that they frequently contend with student-on-student confrontations, classroom disruptions, student-on-student violence, and wrongful accusations of malfeasance (Schonfeld & Feinman, 2012). Objective and self-report data indicate that, compared with members of other occupational groups, teachers are more likely to be victims of workplace violence (Schonfeld, 2006). Teachers, particularly those in urban schools, often face difficult working conditions.

Mental Disorder, Suicide, and Physical Disorder

A number of studies have estimated the rates with which mental disorders are found in a variety of occupations. Eaton et al. (1990), using cross-sectional data collected in the United States in the Epidemiologic Catchment Area (ECA) study, found that, controlling for sociodemographic factors, individuals classified as "other teachers" (pre-k and special education) and counselors experienced high rates of depression. The rate of depression in elementary school teachers, however, was not different from the average rate. Depression was extremely rare in secondary school teachers. The ECA data also indicated that alcohol abuse was rare in women teachers, but more prevalent in their male counterparts, although the number of male teachers sampled was small (Mandell, Eaton, Anthony, & Garrison, 1992). More recent research is consistent with this finding (Wulsin, Alterman, Bushnell, Li, & Shen, 2014).

Research from the United Kingdom (Travers & Cooper, 1993) and Australia (Finlay-Jones, 1986) suggests that, compared with members of other occupational groups, teachers experience higher levels of psychological distress. Cropley, Steptoe, and Joekes (1999) found that while London teachers in high-strain jobs experienced more psychopathology than did teachers in low-strain jobs, teachers in both high- and low-strain jobs experienced more psychopathology than did a U.K. reference group, controlling for educational and occupational levels. Herloff and Jarvholm (1989) advanced the view that if teaching is a stressful occupation, the stressful-ness of the job would translate into elevated rates of cardiovascular (CV) mortality. They found that Swedish teachers, particularly female teachers, experienced low rates of CV mortality compared with general population rates. They also found that the rates of suicide and accidents in female teachers were not significantly different from those of the general population; the rates for male teachers were significantly lower than the average rates. In a study conducted in Denmark, Agerbo, Gunnell, Bonde, Mortensen, and Nordentoft (2007) found that teaching was not a risk factor for suicide.

Thus, the results that compare rates of morbidity in teaching with the rates in other occupations are somewhat mixed, with some research suggesting that teach-ers are at greater risk for psychological distress but not at greater risk for suicide or cardiovascular disease (CVD).

Within-Occupation Research

Within-occupation research on teachers cannot reveal whether teachers are more or less at risk than are members of other occupational groups; such research, however, can shed light on the risk and protective factors within the profession. A two-stage meta-analysis (Montgomery & Rupp, 2005) that grouped longitudinal and cross-sectional findings indicated that the correlation of adverse working conditions with burnout and other strains (e.g., depressive symptoms) averaged between $r = 0.25$ and 0.27.

Well-controlled longitudinal research better documents some of the impact of working conditions on teacher well-being. In a 7-month study of Israeli teachers,

Shirom, Oliver, and Stein (2009) found that stressors (e.g., having to discipline students) predicted later somatic complaints, controlling for initial complaints. There was no evidence supporting a reverse-causal explanation. A study conducted in Spain (Llorens-Gumbau & Salanova-Soria, 2014) revealed that students' negative attitudes and lack of discipline at baseline predicted high levels of burnout (exhaustion and cynicism combined) and cynicism (individually) 8 months later, controlling for baseline levels of the dependent variables. Another Spanish study (González-Morales, Rodríguez, & Peiró, 2010) also shed light on stressor–strain relations in teachers. Because the stressor–strain analyses in the report were not straightforward, one of us extracted the data from the publication[1] in order to construct a regression analysis. It was found that controlling for time 1 exhaustion and sociodemographic factors, time 1 stressors (e.g., student misbehavior) predicted exhaustion 6 to 9 months later.

Schonfeld (2001) conducted a three-wave, 1-year study involving more than 180 first-year NYC women teachers. Because he initiated the study just after the teachers graduated from college, but before they entered the workforce, he was able to measure and statistically adjust for baseline preemployment strain variables such as depressive symptoms. He found that the frequency of job stressors (student fighting, cursing, etc.) predicted increased depressive symptoms (CES-D), reduced self-esteem, reduced job satisfaction, and lower motivation to continue in the profession. A reverse-causal explanation of the findings was ruled out. Schonfeld (2000) also found that although the most and least exposed teachers did not differ on preemployment depressive symptom levels, by the spring term, the teachers who were most exposed to job stressors had symptom levels high enough to put many in the "clinical range" of the CES-D. By contrast, the least exposed teachers showed a significant drop in symptoms below preemployment levels, underlining the idea that getting a good job is good for one's emotional life. Colleague and supervisor support predicted increased job satisfaction and support from friends and family, and reduced symptoms.

Summary

There is consensus among the strongest within-occupation longitudinal studies of teachers that job conditions that include facing unruly and aggressive students, vandalism, and the like harm the well-being of teachers. Schonfeld and Farrell (2010) advanced the view that these kinds of disruptive and dangerous events are normatively stressful to teachers. There is evidence that mitigating factors include supportive supervisors and colleagues and supportive individuals outside of work.

NURSES

Nursing, like teaching, is a "helping profession," the members of which are well educated. The intrinsic satisfactions associated with nursing include helping individuals regain their health after illness or an accident (Heim, 1991). Nursing, on the other

---

[1] The data were extracted from the correlation matrix in Table 1 of the report and were used to construct a multiple linear regression analysis.

hand, has abundant job-related stressors including patient death and high, unpredictable workloads (Schonfeld & Farrell, 2010; Zangaro & Soeken, 2007). Additional job-related stressors include understaffing and lack of resources (Mazzola, Schonfeld, & Spector, 2011), lack of autonomy (Landsbergis, 1988), intense emotional work (Büssing & Glaser, 1999), and problematic nurse–physician collaboration (Zangaro & Soeken, 2007). As indicated in Chapter 5, nurses are at risk for being victims of assault (e.g., Camerino, Estryn-Beharc, Conway, van Der Heijdend, & Hasselhorng, 2008; Chen, Sun, Lan, & Chiu, 2009; Fujita et al., 2012) by patients or their relatives.

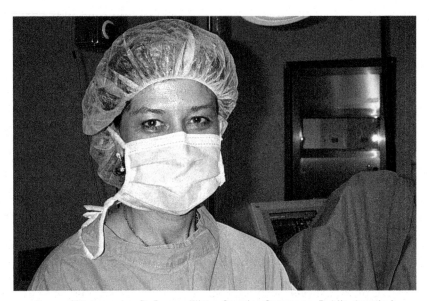

Nurse. (Photographer R. Duran. Flickr, Creative Commons. Public domain.)

Mental Disorder and Suicide

Mandell et al. (1992) and Trinkoff, Eaton, and Anthony (1991) found that, in the ECA sample, the prevalence of alcohol and substance abuse in registered nurses (RNs) was no different from that of the general population. Eaton and colleagues (1990; Trinkoff et al., 1991) found that the risk of major depression in RNs was also no different from that of the general population.

In a review of the literature on suicide in nurses, Hawton and Vislisel (1999) found that the risk of suicide in female nurses was higher than that of the general population. Insufficient data were available to draw conclusions about male nurses. Consistent with Hawton and Vislisel, Agerbo et al. (2007) found that the rate of suicide in Danish nurses was double that of the study's reference group, controlling for income, marital status, and history of hospital admission for psychiatric illness. When Agerbo et al. (2007) limited comparisons with individuals who had never been psychiatric admissions, nurses were at 3.5 times higher risk of suicide than the reference group. Kelly, Charlton, and Jenkins (1995) also found elevated rates of suicide in female nurses in England and Wales. Stack (2001) found that, controlling for gender, age, and marital status, U.S. nurses were significantly more likely to die by suicide than were members of the general population. Kelly et al. (1995) found that the proportion of suicides by overdose in female nurses (56%) was modestly higher than that for women in general (47%). It is plausible that the elevated suicide rates for nurses are at least partly related to their readier access to means of suicide (e.g., potent drugs), a finding consistent with the elevated suicide risk in medical doctors. Moreover, members of occupational groups with access to other lethal means of suicide, firearms in the case of police officers and farmers (Tiesman et al., 2015), tend to employ those means when taking their own lives.

Within-Occupation Research

To be clear, not all nursing positions are equally stressful. In a U.K. study, Payne (2001), surprisingly, found that nurses working at hospices had lower levels of emotional exhaustion than levels found in data obtained by researchers examining samples containing nurses in other positions. Perhaps the finding was the result of successful coping with death and dying. Perhaps the finding reflected self-selection. Longitudinal studies may be able to shed more light on factors that affect the health and psychological well-being of nurses.

A number of researchers examined the relation of nurses' working conditions to CVD or its risk factors. In a 1-year follow-up of Dutch nurses, Riese, Van Doornen, Houtman, and De Geus (2004) found that decision latitude, psychological workload, and support failed to predict ambulatory blood pressure, heart rate, and heart-rate variability. A counterintuitive finding also emerged, namely, that high psychological demands predicted higher blood pressure only when decision latitude was high (rather than, as was expected, when it was low). Lee, Colditz, Berkman, and Kawachi (2002), in a prospective study described in Chapter 4, were unable to link decision latitude, psychological workload, and social support to fatal heart attack and nonfatal coronary disease. In other analyses, the same authors (Lee, Colditz, Berkman & Kawachi, 2004) found that job insecurity was related to later nonfatal heart attack over the initial 2 years of follow-up, controlling for other risk factors (e.g., smoking, body mass), but not over the entire 4-year span. The results suggest that job insecurity is related to a short-term spike in risk.

The aforementioned studies employed general measures of workplace stressors (the Job Content Questionnaire; Karasek, Pieper, Schwartz, Fry, & Schier, 1985), measures that could be used with a great many occupations. Although the studies did not reveal much evidence in terms of an effect of these stressors on CV health, one characteristic of the nursing profession separates it from many other occupations, namely, shift work. Because nurses often have to work day and night shifts, Kubo et al. (2011) compared 36 Japanese nurses on coronary flow reserve (the maximum that the flow of blood through the coronary arteries can increase above the volume of flow when resting) during a day shift and after a night shift. The investigators, referring to blood flow in the small vessels—arterioles, capillaries, and venules—in the heart, found that "coronary microcirculation was impaired after nightshift work" (Kubo et al., 2011, p. 1667), underlining the adverse effect of shift work on health (also see Chapter 4).

Some longitudinal studies have linked particular stressors to psychological outcomes in nurses. An 18-month study (Bourbonnais, Comeau, & Vezina, 1999) found that among female Québec nurses, the combination of high workload and low decision latitude at both time 1 and time 2 was related to the persistence of high levels of psychological distress. Workplace support was contemporaneously related to lower distress. A 3-year panel study (Gelsema et al., 2006) of Dutch nurses found that increments in decision authority from time 1 to time 2 were related to parallel increments in job satisfaction and decrements in psychological distress. Increments in supervisor support were related to increments in satisfaction. A limitation of the studies by Bourbonnais et al. (1999) and Gelsema et al. (2006) is that, although they were technically longitudinal, they were change–change studies that do not provide unambiguous information on the temporal priority of working conditions and putative outcomes. Although the suicide rate for U.S. nurses is about the same as the national rate controlling for age and gender, a longitudinal study that followed more than 90,000 female nurses for up to 14 years found that the combination of severe work stress and severe home stress (these were 1-item measures) was related to future suicide (Feskanich et al., 2002).

A number of better controlled studies linked nurses' working conditions to mental and physical health. In Chapter 1, we saw that Parkes (1982) found that stressful working conditions (affective demands) adversely affected levels of depressive symptoms and work satisfaction in student nurses. Spence Laschinger and Finegan (2008), in a 1-year study of nurse managers in Ontario, found that effort–reward imbalance (ERI) at time 1 predicted emotional exhaustion at time 2, controlling for emotional exhaustion at time 1. In a cohort study of female Danish nurses, Allesøe, Andersen Hundrup, Frølund Thomsen, and Osler (2010) found that excessive work pressure at the outset of the study predicted heart disease over the course of the next 15 years, controlling for health at time 1. The finding held particularly for nurses who were under age 51 when the study began. Influence over the job, however, was not predictive. Because each psychosocial working condition was measured by a single item (with its implications for unreliability), it is surprising that any significant result was obtained.

Summary

Nurses are subject to a number of stressful working conditions including affective demands and unexpected violence (see Chapter 5). There is some evidence that shift work adversely affects physical health, while excessive work pressure adversely affects CV health. Moreover, psychosocial conditions such as high affective demands, low latitude, high workload, and ERI adversely affect mental health.

COMBAT SOLDIERS

He was reluctant to tell. Finally he said, "I've told my wife, because she demanded to know why I sobbed in my sleep." (Rader, 1993, p. 5)

An enlisted man of 17, Charles Durning was a member of a unit in which 70 men survived the first wave of the Allied landing on the beaches of Normandy. A short while later he was the lone survivor of his unit after a machine-gun ambush. He killed seven of the enemy but suffered machine-gun and shrapnel wounds (Brennan, 1994; Rader, 1993). Quick to recover, he was soon out of the hospital and part of the Allies' advance through France but was wounded by a mine, and rehospitalized. After discharge from the military hospital, he joined the campaign in the Ardennes (Berkvist, 2012). A German soldier—a boy of 14 or 15 really—charged at him with a bayonet. Charles told an interviewer, "I didn't see a soldier. I saw a boy. Even though he was coming at me, I couldn't shoot" (Rader, 1993, p. 5). In the hand-to-hand combat that ensued, Charles was stabbed multiple times. Ultimately, he bludgeoned the boy to death with a stone (Berkvist, 2012; Rader, 1993). He was hospitalized and then released in time to participate in the Battle of the Bulge. The Germans captured his company and marched them through the Belgium forest at Malmédy. Charles was fortunate to have escaped during the march. An SS unit ordered the captives into an open field, and then with machine guns opened fire, killing most of the prisoners. A small number managed to run from the field, and hide in a café; the Germans, however, set the café on fire (Gilbert, 1989). Charles was ordered to return to Malmédy, and identify the bodies (Rader, 1993). At the end of the war, Charles was awarded the Silver Star for bravery and three Purple Hearts. He was hospitalized on and off for 4 years after the war, treated for psychological and physical trauma.

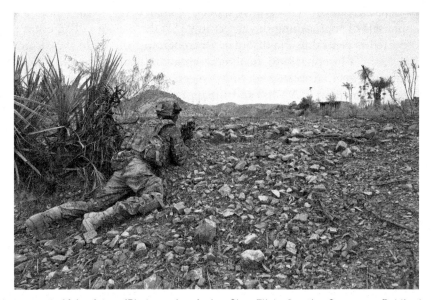

U.S. Army scout, Afghanistan. (Photographer Amber Clay. Flickr Creative Commons. Public domain.)

Goodwin et al. (2015) wrote that "unlike other occupations in which the risk of stressful events may be similar on a day-to-day basis, in the military the frequency and intensity of stressful events experienced by personnel deployed on operations is without comparison" (p. 1881). The evidence cited in Chapter 1, particularly evidence from World War II (Stouffer et al., 1949; Swank, 1949), indicates that exposure to combat can provoke psychopathology in otherwise normal soldiers. Swank found that soldiers who served in units that had sustained casualty rates of 65% or greater were at high risk for "combat exhaustion," the term used in World War II that roughly translates to the contemporary term "PTSD." Stouffer et al. (1949) observed that high rates of psychoneurotic symptoms can occur in soldiers from the Regular Army, that is, soldiers who had been inducted before the U.S. entry into the war, "a group selected under higher physical and psychiatric standards than were ever used again during the war" (p. 438). These historical findings have contemporary relevance. Data collected in the United Kingdom between 2003 and 2008, during the wars in

Iraq and Afghanistan, indicate that, controlling for social demographic factors, the rate of elevated scores on the GHQ (see Chapter 3) in the military (19%) was about twice as high as the rate in the general population (Goodwin et al., 2015).

Posttraumatic Stress Disorder

A section on soldiers is an apt place in which to discuss PTSD,[2] a disorder caused by exposure to an event that is physically or emotionally traumatic. The symptoms of the disorder include reexperiencing the event, avoidance of things that are associated with the event, undesirable changes in thinking or mood, and increased levels of arousal. It is often related to elevated risk for comorbid depression, anxiety disorders, substance abuse, and suicidality. PTSD is a particularly burdensome disorder. It undermines the functioning of the individual as a family member and a worker (Kessler, 2000). Ehlers and Clark (2000) observed that PTSD posed a puzzle when it was classified as an anxiety disorder. Cognitive models of anxiety regard the emotion as reflecting appraisals of approaching threat, yet in PTSD the memory of an event that already occurred is central to the disorder. One cognitive theory of the disorder (Brewin, Dalgleish, & Joseph, 1996), dual representation theory, advances a model involving traumatic experiences engendering two general types of memories, namely, verbally accessible memories (VAMs) and situationally accessible memories (SAMs). VAMs contain some of the perceived features of the trauma and the emotional and physical reactions to it. VAMs are autobiographical, and a person can mentally manipulate them. SAMs are not necessarily tied to "verbally retrievable meanings" (Brewin et al., 1996, p. 676). SAMs include intrusive flashbacks that are precipitated by encounters with stimuli that have some "analogical" link to the original trauma. The eruption of SAMs is thought to reflect the impact of hormonal changes precipitated by the trauma, changes that in turn affect neural activity in such a way as to weaken neural structures serving conscious control and strengthen structures serving "nonconscious perceptual and memory processes" (Brewin et al., 1996, p. 676).

Biological changes in brain function are implicated in PTSD (Kolb, 1987). In one model, a traumatic event is thought to constitute an unconditioned stimulus that provokes the release of powerful stress hormones that contribute to "the formation of a robust and enduring memory of the trauma" (Alberini, 2011, p. 6). Stimuli (conditioned stimuli) that prompt the recall of the event fuel another episode of the release of stress hormones that can further consolidate the traumatic memory (Alberini, 2011). Difficulties, however, exist in identifying neural factors that play a role in the development of PTSD. It is often unclear whether differences between individuals suffering from a psychiatric disorder such as PTSD and comparison samples without the disorder represent the causes or the effects of the disorder in question. Moreover, prospective studies on the impact of trauma have been rare, as has been in the case in research on the impact of exposure to violence (see Chapter 5). Ideally, prospective research must assess individuals before the occurrence of trauma and include individuals who are not exposed, and then assess both groups multiple times after the occurrence of exposures in the index group. Moreover, disentangling

---

[2] PTSD was previously classified as an anxiety disorder but in the *DSM-5* it was not. The *DSM-5* classifies PTSD as part of a separate family of trauma- and stressor-related disorders. The definition of the disorder evolved over time.

neural factors that predispose toward PTSD from factors that are acquired as a result of trauma is important to understanding the emergence of the disorder (Admon, Milad, & Hendler, 2013b).

Although the chapter can only review a small portion of the research, it is notable that with the help of imaging studies that have employed a variety of research designs (twin and genetic studies, studies of environmental influences, and even the rare prospective study), researchers have made progress in sketching models of the neural basis of PTSD. The research has implicated a component of the limbic system, the amygdala, a group of nuclei located in the left and right temporal lobes that plays a role in emotional processing. Abnormalities in the amygdala that heighten responsivity to emotional stimuli can predispose individuals to developing PTSD in reaction to trauma (Admon et al., 2013b). The cingulate cortex, also part of the limbic system, is important in the formation of emotions and memories. Increased activity in the dorsal section of the anterior cingulate cortex is another predisposing factor (Admon et al., 2013b).

The following are two examples of prospective research on the neural impact of combat-related trauma. First, Admon et al. (2009) followed a sample of 10 civilian controls and 37 young soldiers (about half were women) who served as combat paramedics in the Israel Defense Forces (IDF). Both groups were seen before the paramedics were trained (and thus before they were exposed to severe trauma) and 18 months later, after the paramedics were exposed to "one or more highly stressful experience[s] accompanied by intense negative emotions" (Admon et al., 2009, p. 14121). The findings suggested that exposure to trauma leads to reductions in the fibers connecting the amygdala and the ventromedial portion of the prefrontal cortex. While the prefrontal cortex is involved in planning, social behavior, and personality, the ventromedial portion is implicated in the suppression of emotions in response to adverse stimuli. The findings from the second prospective study (Admon et al., 2013a), this one involving 24 IDF paramedics (half were male; there was no control group), indicate that exposure to traumatic stress results in a reduced response to reward in the nucleus accumbens and an increased response to risk in the amygdala. The nucleus accumbens, which is located in the basal forebrain, plays a role in the experience of pleasure.[3]

Mental Disorder and Brain Injury

Critics questioned the high estimates of PTSD diagnoses among U.S. Vietnam War veterans because estimates (a) were based on diagnostic interviews thought to be subject to recall bias and (b) exceeded the percentage of soldiers who were combat troops (about 15%), the estimates necessarily including support troops (Dohrenwend et al., 2006). Dohrenwend et al. (2006), however, documented that veterans' self-reports of exposure to traumatic events were reliable and matched with both military histories and contemporaneous newspaper accounts. Furthermore, the research team found that support troops, like combat troops, were exposed to traumatic war-related events in this "war without a front." The estimated lifetime prevalence of PTSD among U.S. Vietnam War veterans was about 22%.

Studying a clinical sample of U.S. veterans of World War II, Korea, and Vietnam, Fontana and Rosenheck (1994) found that the extent of exposure to traumatic events

---

[3] Additional research on the biological basis of PTSD in the military can be found in Chapter 11.

was related to PTSD symptoms as well as general psychiatric symptoms. In a study of more than 6,000 U.S. Army soldiers and Marines, Hoge et al. (2004) found that the prevalence of probable PTSD (12% to 13% using strict criteria) among those returning from Iraq was significantly higher than that found in a predeployment Army comparison group (5%), adjusting for sociodemographic factors. Among soldiers and Marines deployed to Iraq and Afghanistan, Hoge et al. (2004) found that the risk of PTSD was linearly related to the number of firefights in which a soldier or Marine was involved. The authors also identified disquiet about stigmatization as a barrier to help-seeking. Soldiers called up from reserve units were especially at risk. Among U.S. Army soldiers returning from the Iraq War ($n > 80,000$) the rates for positive screens for PTSD, depression, and alcohol and substance misuse were double in soldiers called up from National Guard and Army Reserve units ($\approx$42%) compared with active-duty soldiers ($\approx$20%; Milliken, Auchterlonie, & Hoge, 2007).

In a study (Tanielian & Jaycox, 2008) involving more than 1,900 personnel (12% female) from all branches of the military who were previously deployed in Iraq and Afghanistan, 14% of the sample met criteria for probable PTSD, 14% for probable major depressive disorder (MDD), and 19.5% for probable traumatic brain injury (TBI); 31% of the sample met criteria for one or more of the diagnoses. PTSD was associated with increased risk for comorbid disorders, particularly alcohol and substance use disorders. Vasterling et al. (2010) obtained pre- and postdeployment data on more than 1,000 male and female members of the U.S. Army and activated National Guard between 2003 and 2006, with about 70% of the troops deploying to Iraq (most of the nondeploying troops deployed after the study concluded). Deploying soldiers, when compared with nondeployed soldiers, showed significant pre- to postdeployment increases in PTSD symptom severity. Controlling for predeployment symptoms, factors such as the intensity of combat exposure and postdeployment and home-front stressors (e.g., family concerns) were related to increases in PTSD symptoms.

Leadership

A component of research on job stress is the identification of factors that either reduce the number or intensity of stressors or buffer their impact. In the military, leadership plays a central role. Recall from Chapter 1 that Spiegel (1944) identified the contribution of leaders to good morale in U.S. Army troops during the Tunisian campaign. Britt, Davison, Bliese, and Castro (2004) reviewed a series of studies on the influence of leadership on the stress process in the U.S. military. Two important findings emerged: (a) the supportiveness of military leaders can reduce the number of stressors affecting soldiers and (b) leaders who clarify goals and guidelines governing efforts to attain goals can buffer the impact of stressors on strain. An example of how leadership may affect the stress process comes from Bliese and Halverson (2002) who found that the supportiveness of leaders (e.g., "concern about a soldier's personal welfare") was related to a reduction in the number of stressors (e.g., intragroup hostility) in a unit. By contrast, when leaders were unsupportive, more hostility was evident in units.

Sexual Harassment

The sexual harassment of women in the U.S. armed forces has been a serious problem. The U.S. military surveyed more than 28,000 service members, 79% of whom were women (Hay & Elig, 1999). Approximately 37% of the women indicated that they were subject to often hostile and "unwanted sexual overtures" in the 12 months before the survey (Fitzgerald, Magley, Drasgow, & Waldo, 1999). The frequency with which they were subject to sexual harassment was related to diminished psychological well-being, increased emotional problems, and decreased satisfaction with supervisors, coworkers, and work itself (Magley, Waldo, Drasgow, & Fitzgerald, 1999). Men in the sample "rarely experienced unwanted sexual attention" (Magley et al., 1999, p. 298).

Suicide

Suicides occurring among military personnel have been documented since the Crimean War (Smith, Masuhara, & Frueh, 2014) and the U.S. Civil War (Frueh & Smith, 2012). During the conflicts in Iraq and Afghanistan, the problem of a growing trend in suicide among U.S. troops emerged (Bachynski et al., 2012). Rates of completed suicide among members of the U.S. military were increasing. The problem, however, antedated those wars. The U.S. Department of Labor found that between 1992 and 2001, the unadjusted rate of suicide among on-duty military was more than five times that of the average workplace suicide rate in the United States (Pegula, 2004). Kaplan, Huguet, McFarland, and Newsom (2007), in a 12-year study involving a representative sample of more than 300,000 U.S. veterans who served during the 1980s and 1990s, found that compared with nonveterans, veterans, were more than twice as likely to die by suicide, controlling for sociodemographic factors. Each of the three disorders (PTSD, MDD, and TBI) Tanielian and Jaycox (2008) identified is a risk factor for suicide. Likewise, Allen, Cross, and Swanner (2005) found psychiatric problems such as alcohol abuse to be a risk factor for suicide in the military (and nonmilitary).

In 2004, there were 64 suicides in the U.S. Army; 4 years later, the number rose to 128 (Kuehn, 2009). Kuehn found that in 2008, the suicide rate among active-duty Army personnel was 20.2 per 100,000, which exceeded the rate in the demographically matched civilian population, 19.5 per 100,000. Availability of means is a factor in suicide; in the military, firearms are widely available (Mahon, Tobin, Cusack, Kelleher, & Malone, 2005). Allen et al. (2005) found that in 2002, 72% of suicides in the U.S. Army involved firearms, which exceeds the 52% the CDC found in the civilian population in the 16 states the CDC followed (Karch, Logan, & Patel, 2011). In their 12-year study, Kaplan et al. (2007) found that compared with nonveteran suicides, veteran suicides were more likely to involve firearms. Of course, it would be helpful if soldiers experiencing suicidal ideation were to seek care. A barrier to help-seeking is stigmatization (Genderson, Schonfeld, Kaplan, & Lyons, 2009).

A previous suicide attempt is itself an important predictor of completed suicide; it is thus imperative to identify risk factors for attempts. Ursano et al. (2015), in a retrospective cohort study (see Chapter 2) involving almost 200,000 U.S. soldiers, identified a number of risk factors for attempted suicide. These risk factors included being an enlisted soldier, being on one's first tour of duty (especially early in the tour), having met criteria for a mental disorder before enlistment, and preenlistment suicidal ideation.

Summary

The men and women in the armed forces are subject to hazardous, maiming, and life-threatening events. Although most soldiers return from the battlefield, research dating back to World Wars I and II tells us that the battlefield can exert adverse medical and psychological effects on soldiers. The length and intensity of the exposures increase risk. Research conducted during World War II indicates that units suffering very high casualty rates put surviving soldiers at risk. Battlefield effects include PTSD along with changes in neural functioning, MDD, TBI, and suicide. High-quality leadership can be important in easing the stress process. Stigmatization is a barrier to seeking help. Women in the military have been subject to sexual harassment.

Postscript

This section began with a short biographical sketch of Charles Durning, who, after having endured so much during the Second World War, was treated for psychological and physical trauma for 4 years following the war. The story of his life, however, does not conclude with the postwar hospitalizations. It should be underlined for readers that there are prospects for resilience despite the terrible conditions to which soldiers have been, and continue to be, exposed. In a sign of resilience, Charles Durning, despite the psychological trauma and physical wounds, went on to get married, father children, and have a long career. He became a successful actor on Broadway and in Hollywood.

FIRST RESPONDERS

When the first author was a boy, he spent an afternoon with some relatives. One of the people he met for the first time was Artie Lasky, his cousins' uncle. Artie, a police detective, told a number of stories about his work. The story the author most vividly remembers began with the detective learning of a horrific traffic accident from his police radio. Because he was nearby, Artie wanted to help. He drove to the scene. Uniformed police officers and ambulances had already arrived. One uniformed officer had picked up a severed arm that lay on the road and wrapped it in a blanket. The officer then stood on the street, with both hands outstretched holding the arm. The officer's feet remained in place as he rocked back and forth. Each time the officer rocked forward, "he puked in the gutter." The term was not known then, but the officer was a first responder.

The U.S. government (The White House, 2003) defines first responders as

> those individuals who in the early stages of an incident are responsible for the protection and preservation of life, property, evidence, and the environment, including emergency response providers as defined in section 2 of the Homeland Security Act of 2002 (6 U.S.C. 101), as well as emergency management, public health, clinical care, public works, and other skilled support personnel (such as equipment operators) that provide immediate support services during prevention, response, and recovery operations.

The term "first responder" embraces police officers, firefighters, public health workers, hospital workers, emergency medical personnel, sanitation workers, construction and iron workers, mental health experts, transportation workers, volunteers, and others.

Police Officers

Police work can be dangerous. In the United States between 1996 and 2010, the Federal Bureau of Investigation database indicated that there were 782 homicides of law enforcement officers; 92% were firearms related (Swedler, Simmons, Dominici, & Hemenway, 2015). In 2014, 51 U.S. law enforcement officers were "feloniously killed in the line of duty" (Federal Bureau of Investigation [FBI], 2015). Each year between 1980 and 2014, on average, 64 U.S. law enforcement officers were feloniously killed. Table 7.1 indicates the context in which those deaths occurred. In 46 of the 51 deaths, the FBI reported that the offenders employed firearms.

By contrast, in the United Kingdom, where there are strict controls on the availability of firearms, in 2014 no police officers were killed in the line of duty (Police Roll of Honour Trust, 2015). In the United States, homicide rates are about three times higher in states with high levels of firearms ownership than in states with low levels (Swedler et al., 2015). The firearms data underline the view that the ease with which individuals in the United States can obtain firearms is a risk factor for police officer fatalities. At the time of the writing of this chapter, it was not clear that fatalities among U.S. law enforcement officers would motivate the U.S. Congress and state legislatures to take steps to curtail the availability of firearms.

Table 7.2 shows that 44 officers were accidentally killed in the line of duty in 2014. There were approximately 1.1 million city, state, and county law enforcement officers in the United States in 2008 (Reaves, 2011). Unfortunately, more recent data from the U.S. Bureau of Justice Statistics census of law enforcement officers were not available as of the writing of this book (B. A. Reaves, personal communication,

TABLE 7.1 Law Enforcement Officers Feloniously Killed in 2014	
Context	**No. Officers Feloniously Killed**
Answering disturbance calls	11
Traffic pursuits/stops	9
Ambush	7
Investigating suspicious person/activity	7
Performance of investigative duties	5
Engaged in tactical situations	4
Handling a mentally ill person	3
Unprovoked attack	1
Attempting to make an arrest	4
Total	51
Firearms-related deaths	46
Handguns	33
Rifles	10
Shotguns	3
Hands, fists as weapons	1
Vehicles used as weapons	4
Total	51
Source: FBI (2015).	

TABLE 7.2 U.S. Law Enforcement Officers Accidentally Killed in 2014	
Context	**No. Officers Accidentally Killed**
Automobile accidents	28
Motorcycle accidents	6
Struck by vehicles	5
Accidental shootings	2
Drowning	1
Trauma	1
Smoke inhalation	1
Total	44
Source: FBI (2015).	

September 2015). However, if one tentatively assumes that there was approximately the same number of officers in the United States in 2014 as there were in 2008, the 1-year homicide rate for law enforcement officers was 4.64 per 100,000 and the 1-year accident fatality rate was 4.00 per 100,000. In the United Kingdom, no officers were killed in accidents occurring in the line of duty although there were three non-duty-related deaths (two resulting from commuting accidents and one, from a heart attack occurring while cycling to work; Police Roll of Honour Trust, 2015). In Scotland, no police officer was killed in the line of duty between 1994 (by a stabbing) and December 2015 (Baker, 2015).

Although police officers must ensure the safety of the public, officers have psychological burdens as well. For example, Roberts and Lee (1993), capitalizing on the national ECA data, found that the lifetime prevalence rates of alcohol abuse or dependence among individuals employed in "protective services" exceeded the national average. In the ECA, protective services referred to police officers, firefighters, and their supervisors. The rates of depression and drug abuse or dependence, however, were low compared with national rates. Because police and firefighters, in many localities, face mandatory drug testing, they experience pressure to desist from illegal drugs. They are more likely to resort to a legally available drug, such as alcohol, as a way to express or discharge psychological distress.

Violanti, Vena, and Petralla (1998) hypothesized that chronic stress and traumatic events associated with police work contribute to the development of a number of disorders. Evidence from a study (Robinson, Sigman, & Wilson, 1997) of male police officers in suburban Cleveland indicates that job-related exposure to death (e.g., suicide) was concurrently related to PTSD symptoms. Violanti et al. (1998), by examining mortality in a virtually all-male cohort of Buffalo police officers, found that officers had a higher-than-average all-cause mortality rate. The mortality rate for atherosclerosis for Buffalo officers who served 10 to 19 years was higher than average. By contrast, a 10-year study of male law enforcement officers in Iowa failed to show that the risk of coronary heart disease differed from that of a reference group (Franke, Cox, Schultz, & Anderson, 1997) although, arguably, police work in Buffalo is, on average, more stressful than police work in Iowa. The Buffalo study found that mortality rates were elevated for a variety of conditions, including malignant neoplasms, cirrhosis of the liver, and suicide.

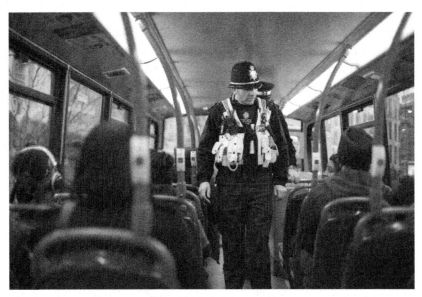

Safer Travel Police on Birmingham buses, 2012. (Photographer unknown. Courtesy of West Midlands Police, U.K.)

Because police officers are often exposed to traumatic events, PTSD is the suspected link between accumulated traumatic stress over years of police work and suicide (O'Hara, 2011). Evidence from a 1-year study (Carlier, Lamberts, & Gersons, 1997) of more than 250 male and female Dutch police officers, all of whom experienced a traumatic event at baseline, indicates that a number of factors predict PTSD symptomatology both 3 and 12 months after the event. These factors include emotional exhaustion at the time of the event, introversion, job insecurity, and the employer not providing sufficient postincident time to come to terms with the event. Evidence also suggests that trauma severity plays a role in PTSD risk. Maguen et al. (2009) followed 180 U.S. police academy trainees (13% women) who would become officers in several different departments. The study team found that at the end of 1 year of police work, negative events in the officer's personal life, personally threatening events in the line of duty, and a stressful work environment (e.g., conflict with peers) predicted elevations in PTSD symptoms.

Using death certificate data collected by NIOSH from 28 states, Violanti (2011) found elevated rates of police suicide between 1984 and 1998. By contrast, Marzuk, Nock, Leon, Portera, and Tardiff (2002) found that the suicide rate among NYC police officers between 1977 and 1996 was comparable with the rate of the general population of NYC, adjusting for demographic factors although female officers were at greater risk than women in the general population. A U.S. Department of Labor study (Pegula, 2004) of suicides that occurred *at* workplaces found that between 1992 and 2001 the unadjusted rate of suicide among police officers was more than five times the national average. Research on suicide risk in police officers has been inconclusive because population comparisons have often not controlled for age, gender, and marital status (Stack, 2001; Stuart, 2008). A review (Hem, Berg, & Ekeberg, 2001) and meta-analysis (Loo, 2003) suggest that suicide risk in police is not greater than the risk in demographically similar reference groups, particularly for federal and municipal forces. Regional police forces may be the exception (Loo, 2003).

Violanti, Robinson, and Shen (2013), using a proxy[4] for mortality rates, found that law enforcement officers working in 23 U.S. states were at higher risk for suicide than were members of other occupational groups. The risk of suicide in officers is likely abetted by the availability of firearms; firearms are overwhelmingly the means used by officers who take their own lives (Marzuk et al., 2002; Stuart, 2008).

It should be stressed that not all police assignments are equally stressful. In a qualitative study of police stress, Arter (2008) examined male officers in metropolitan areas in the southern United States, comparing three groups of officers, namely, those who worked undercover (the most stressful assignment), formerly worked undercover, and never worked undercover. The undercover officers were the most involved in deviant behavior (e.g., excessive alcohol consumption, failure to enforce certain laws); the officers who never worked undercover were least involved. We return to a discussion of police officers in the section devoted to 9/11 responders.

Summary

The job of the police officer entails exposure to traumatic stressors including homicide, rape, suicide, and traffic accidents as well as danger to self and the death of a fellow officer. O'Hara (2011) advanced the view, reporting that over time, these exposures can, cumulatively, exert a heavy psychological toll on an officer and put the officer at risk for excessive alcohol use and PTSD. There is evidence of excess suicide risk in police officers.

Firefighters

Firefighters can be paid employees of localities, work for the national government (e.g., the U.S. Forest Service), or can be volunteers. In the United States in 2013, there were 1,140,750 firefighters, including 354,600 career and 786,150 volunteer firefighters (U.S. Fire Administration, 2015).

Firefighting is an inherently dangerous occupation. During 2013, 106 U.S. firefighters died while on duty (U.S. Fire Administration, 2015), or 9.29 per 100,000. Table 7.3 enumerates the circumstances in which those deaths occurred. About half of the fatalities occurred as a result of the activities in which firefighters were engaged at the scene of a fire. About one-third died as a result of a heart attack. A firefighter who suffers a fatal heart attack or other fatal injury (a) when home but preparing to respond to an emergency or (b) arriving home after responding to an emergency is considered an on-duty fatality (U.S. Fire Administration, 2014). Fourteen died *en route* to an emergency incident or returning from one.

In England, in 2010–2011 (the most up-to-date figures at the time of the writing of this book), there were 41,202 firefighters (Department for Communities and Local Government, 2011). There were two fatal injuries during that period. The work-related fatality rate in England during that period was thus 4.85 per 100,000, approximately half the rate found in the United States. The difference in rates was not a 1-year aberration. The rates in England have been generally lower than the U.S. rates in the preceding years. Why there was a difference is unclear but worth further investigation.

---

[4] Violanti et al. used the proportionate mortality ratio, a statistic that indexes, for any one occupational category, the proportion of deaths due to a specific cause such as suicide. Mortality rates could not be directly calculated because the denominators could not be accurately estimated (Violanti, personal communication, May 2015).

TABLE 7.3 U.S. Firefighter Fatalities, 2013	
Firefighters Died	**No.**
As a result of activities related to an emergency incident	77
As a result of activities at the scene of a fire	55
Heart attacks	36
Responding to or returning from an emergency	14
Vehicle crashes	9
Total	106

Note: A firefighter fatality could belong to more than one category.
Source: U.S. Fire Administration (2015).

The danger associated with the job of the firefighter has psychological implications. After a catastrophic series of brush fires ravaged South Australia (Reuters, 1983), McFarlane (1988) found that delayed psychiatric morbidity was common. He found that firefighters who suffered recurrent disorder tended to have been the most intensely exposed to the brush fires. Chronic sufferers were also likely to be affected by television reminders of the fire. North et al. (2002) followed male firefighters who served as rescue workers in the aftermath of the 1995 Oklahoma City bombing and male primary victims. The study team found that PTSD was diagnosed at a lower rate in the firefighters (13%) than in the primary civilian victims (23%). The rates of any disorder were about the same in the two groups (38% vs. 34%). Firefighters were more likely to be diagnosed with alcohol use disorders than were civilian victims (24% vs. 10%), and civilian victims were more likely to be diagnosed with depression than were firefighters (8% vs. 13%).

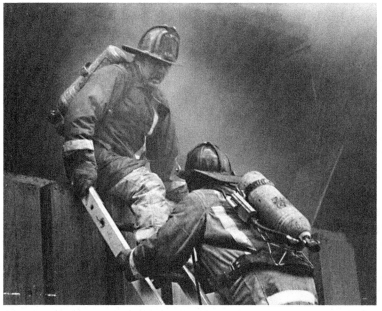

Two firefighters in a three-alarm building fire at Voss & Bergoyne, District 69 (Houston, Texas) in 1986.
(Reprinted from the Digital Library of the University of Houston and the Wikipedia Commons. Public domain. Photographer Jo L. Keener.)

Murphy, Beaton, Pike, and Johnson (1999) observed that "a relatively unique organizational aspect of firefighting includes the 24-hour shift, which is often sleep-disrupted, characterized by uncertainty and potential danger, and is sometimes uneventful and boring" (p. 180). Beaton, Murphy, Johnson, Pike, and Corneil (1998) examined the rates at which firefighters in two urban locations in the northwestern United States experienced seriously stressful events over a 6-month period. At least 10% of the sample witnessed a sudden infant death, 8% were exposed to hazardous chemicals, 26% rendered aid to a seriously injured child, and 27% were at the scene of a multivehicle accident in which one or more individuals were killed. During the 6-month look-back, 2% of the firefighters experienced the death of a firefighter coworker, one of the most stressful job-related events. Murphy et al. (1999) showed that firefighters' exposure to traumatic events is a persistent feature of the job.

Corneil, Beaton, Murphy, Johnson, and Pike (1999) found that 22% of the firefighters in the aforementioned study met criteria for (probable) PTSD; the rate for firefighters working in a comparison Canadian city (100% male) was 17%, comparable with rates found in wounded U.S. Vietnam veterans. Exposure to traumatic incidents (e.g., suicides, gunshot wounds, fire-related fatalities) documented by fire department records over the prior year was associated with increased risk for PTSD. Other factors associated with increased risk of PTSD in the Canadian and U.S. firefighter samples included workplace demands and prior help-seeking behavior (which is likely bound up with need for help). Factors that were related to lower PTSD risk in both samples included work and family support. Wagner, Heinrichs, and Ehlert (1998) found that, controlling for social desirability bias, the prevalence rate for what was essentially probable PTSD in a sample of male German firefighters was about 18%, although the prevalence for any of a number of probable mental disorders (e.g., depression) was greater than 25%, as reflected in elevated scores on a symptom screening scale. Among firefighters with PTSD, there was considerable comorbidity with other disorders (e.g., probable depression, substance abuse). Another German study (Heinrichs et al., 2005), although small ($n = 43$), was innovative because, unlike most of the research on firefighters, data collection began during "the period before exposure to trauma" (p. 2277) and continued for 2 years. The study team found that two baseline personality factors, level of hostility and low levels of self-efficacy, accounted for almost half the variance in PTSD symptoms at follow-up although we do not know about the exposures that occurred over the course of 2 years and how the exposures may have interacted with the personality factors. We return to a discussion of firefighters later in the section devoted to 9/11 responders.

Summary

The role of firefighter often requires exposure to traumatic events, including danger to self and the death of a fellow firefighter. The impact of exposure to a traumatic event can last months, or even years, after the event. As with police officers, these exposures are related to increased risk for PTSD and comorbid disorders. There is preliminary evidence that personality factors increase vulnerability to PTSD symptoms.

9/11

This special section is devoted to the individuals who responded to the call to duty on September 11, 2001, in recognition of the distinguished role of all rescue and recovery workers on that day. However, because there is considerably more research, particularly longitudinal research, on the aftermath of the attack on the World Trade Center (WTC) than on the aftermath of the attack on the Pentagon or the tragic airplane crash in Shanksville, Pennsylvania, the central focus of this section is the first responders in NYC.

In a 5- to 6-year follow-up that included more than 21,000 WTC rescue and recovery workers (firefighters, police officers, emergency medical service personnel, construction workers, engineers, sanitation workers, FEMA workers, and volunteers) and more than 24,000 others (residents, office workers, and passersby) exposed to the events, Brackbill and his colleagues (2009; Farfel et al., 2008) obtained retrospective data on whether individuals experienced PTSD or depression before the events of 9/11 and excluded from analyses those with prior disorder. Brackbill et al. (2009) observed that compared with others (e.g., residents), rescue and recovery workers were more likely to experience delayed-onset probable PTSD; in other words, among those who did not meet criteria for PTSD at wave 1 of data collection, responders were more likely than others in the area to meet criteria at wave 2. In analyses that adjusted for a preevent diagnosis of depression (with prior PTSD cases excluded), the researchers found that the number of days spent at ground zero—including exposure to the dust cloud—and early arrival time predicted PTSD in rescue and recovery workers at wave 2. The authors also found that PTSD and asthma commonly co-occurred. Both acute and prolonged exposures precipitated posttraumatic stress symptoms and asthma. Postevent job loss increased risk, and support from others reduced risk.

Although the prevalence of PTSD in first responders is usually lower than that of the general population, Galea, Nandi, and Vlahov (2005) found that this was not the case in the aftermath of the attack. The rates for any PTSD were similar for first responders (23%), residents (21%), office workers (25%), and passersby (29%; also see Brackbill et al., 2009, Table 7).

9/11 First Responders Who Were Police Officers

Widespread symptomatology was observed in rescue and recovery workers who did *not* meet criteria for probable PTSD (Stellman et al., 2008). In a study confined to male police officers (*n* = 8,400) involved in 9/11 rescue operations and seen about 4 years (range: 2–7 years) after the attack, Pietrzak et al. (2012) found that although about 5% experienced full-blown PTSD, another 15% experienced "subsyndromal PTSD," which refers to officers meeting some but not all the criteria for a diagnosis. The importance of identifying subsyndromal PTSD is twofold. First, many of the risk factors for the full-blown disorder are the same for subsyndromal PTSD. Second, as with the full-blown disorder, a number of comorbid problems accompany the subsyndromal PTSD (e.g., depression, alcohol abuse, suicidal ideation).

In more than 9,600 police officers exposed to the WTC tragedy and seen over the next 9 years, the cumulative incidence of probable PTSD was 9%; probable depression, 7%; and probable panic disorder, 8% (Wisnivesky et al., 2011). These rates were lower than rates observed in other rescue and recovery workers (construction workers, electrical workers): PTSD, 32%; depression, 27.5%; and panic, 21%. It is not clear why police officers were at lower risk, although reasons hypothesized include training, self-selection, and past experience with traumatic stressors. Nevertheless, Pietrzak et al. (2012) found that more officers were also at risk for subsyndromal PTSD than the full-blown disorder. Additional research on 2,940 police responders (86% male) indicates that between a period of 2 to 3 years post-9/11 and a period of

5 to 6 years post-9/11, the prevalence of probable PTSD doubled from 8% to more than 16% (Bowler et al., 2012). Risk factors for PTSD in police officers included number of traumatic events witnessed, losing one's job after 9/11, female sex, older age at 9/11, and smaller size and density of the officer's social network. It is also of note that there was considerable comorbidity of PTSD with physical disorders including airway injury, asthma, and reflux disease (Wisnivesky et al., 2011).

9/11 First Responders Who Were Firefighters

Berninger et al. (2010) focused exclusively on more than 5,600 male firefighters with WTC experience. At baseline, which was between 1 and 6 months post-9/11, approximately 50% of the sample experienced excessive arousal, one of the criteria for PTSD; reexperiencing the event, another criterion, was reported in 38% of the sample; and about 15% reported experiencing numbing, which is reflective of the negative mood criterion. Almost 9% of firefighters met all criteria for probable PTSD at baseline; about 3 years later 11% met criteria. Almost half (44.5%) of the cases at follow-up were delayed-onset cases. Risk factors for delayed-onset PTSD included arrival during the morning of 9/11 on the heels of the attack, duration of work at the site, and subthreshold PTSD at baseline. PTSD in the firefighters was accompanied by difficulties such as increased alcohol use and impaired functioning at work or home.

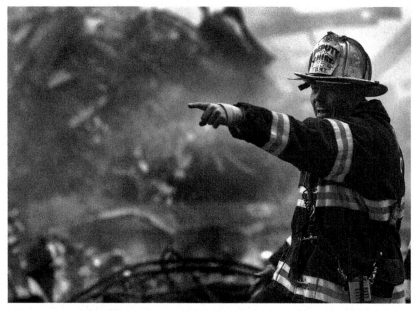

New York City firefighter in the rubble after the 9/11 attack on the World Trade Center. (Photographer is David Mark. Public domain.)

Soo et al. (2011) extended the study by Berninger et al. (2010), examining more than 11,000 NYC firefighters in serial cross-sectional analyses that involved data collection every 18 months until 2010, and a longitudinal study that continued to 9 years post-9/11. Among firefighters who developed PTSD, those in the earliest arrival group were the least likely to recover. Comorbid aerodigestive symptoms (e.g., gastroesophageal reflux) and increased alcohol consumption since 9/11 were also related to a reduced likelihood of recovery. In a study of more than 1,900 firefighters who were exposed to 9/11 but retired by July 25, 2002, Chiu et al. (2011) found that 78% reported the collapse of the Trade Center to be "the most emotionally terrible, frightening, or horrible event they had ever experienced" (p. 204). In 2005, the rates of probable PTSD and probable depression were 22% and 23%, respectively; in 16% of the retirees, the disorders were comorbid. Chiu et al. found that early arrival at the WTC site was a risk factor for PTSD, and PTSD mediated the link between early arrival and depression (but not vice versa).

Children of 9/11 First Responders

Children of 9/11 first responders were also affected by the attack. Hoven et al. (2009) found evidence for the transmission of probable PTSD and other forms of psychopathology to the children of first responders. Stellman et al. (2008) adduced evidence that the children of first responders showed more withdrawal and more aggressive behavior between the months before (these were retrospective data) and the months after 9/11. Duarte et al. (2006) found that children of emergency medical technicians (EMTs) were at higher risk for psychopathology than were children of police officers and firefighters. The investigators suggested that the greater vulnerability of EMTs' children may be related to their greater social disadvantage. It is also possible that because ambulance personnel, compared with other rescue workers, tend to be at higher risk for PTSD (Berger et al., 2012), the likelihood of distress contagion in families of ambulance personnel is greater.

Summary

Exposure to 9/11 placed a great burden on rescue and recovery workers. There is consensus that the intensity and duration of exposure are related to PTSD risk and risk of subsyndromal disorder. Moreover, there was considerable comorbidity with other mental (e.g., depression) and physical disorders (e.g., asthma). The impact of exposure to the trauma, as was found in research on firefighters in South Australia (McFarlane, 1988) and Oklahoma City (North et al., 2002), could last years. The studies by Brackbill et al. (2009; Berninger et al., 2010), and Wisnivesky et al. (2011) suggest that the prevalence of PTSD in firefighters, police, and other rescue and recovery workers tended to increase over time. By contrast, Cukor et al. (2011) found that in a sample of 2,960 disaster recovery utility workers, the prevalence of probable PTSD declined between 2002 and 2008. Considering the nature of the smoky pile to which first responders were exposed, PTSD was comorbid with aerodigestive problems. Mental health problems also emerged in the children of 9/11 first responders.

CONSTRUCTION WORKERS

Construction workers (CWs) build, repair, renovate, and maintain physical infrastructure such as roads and buildings (National Institute for Occupational Safety and Health [NIOSH], 2015a). Construction is one of the most dangerous industries. For example, in the United States in 2013, there were 828 on-the-job fatalities in the construction industry, more than in any other industry. These fatalities comprised 18% of all work-related deaths in the United States that year (BLS, 2015a). In the

European Union, there were 869 fatalities among CWs in 2012 (Eurostat, 2015). The fatality rate is about 9.7 cases per 100,000 full-time equivalent workers in the United States (BLS, 2015a), and 6.4 cases per 100,000 full-time equivalent workers in the European Union (Eurostat, 2015). The fatality rate in the United States slightly exceeds the combined fatality rate (feloniously *and* accidentally killed) for U.S. police officers (see the section on police officers), a job that is known for its inherent dangers.

In addition to fatalities, CWs also suffered high rates of injuries and illnesses owing to work-related exposures. In 2013, there were 203,000 cases of occupational injuries and illnesses reported in construction, accounting for almost 7% of the total number of cases of occupational injuries and illnesses in the United States (BLS, 2015a). The injury and illness rate is about 3.8 cases per 100 full-time equivalent workers in the United States (BLS, 2015a). In 2012, there were 418,414 cases of nonfatal accidents among CWs in the European Union; the incidence rate (3.1 cases per 100 full-time equivalent workers; Eurostat, 2015) is comparable to the rate in the United States. More than half of these cases resulted in days away from work, job transfers, or restrictions from regular job duties, indicating that these illnesses and injuries were severe and impaired employees' ability to attend to their regular responsibilities (BLS, 2015a).

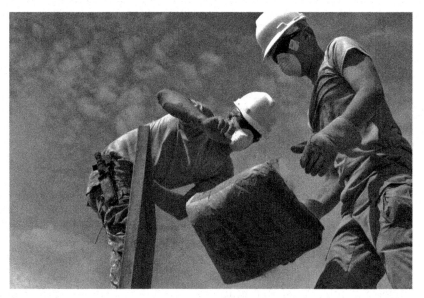

Cement work at a construction site. (Photographer unknown. Public domain.)

Occupational Stress and Safety

Because CWs tend to suffer higher rates of occupational fatalities, illnesses, and injuries, research has focused on identifying psychological mechanisms that may help explain the effects of construction site characteristics on worker safety-related outcomes. Abbe, Harvey, Ikuma, and Aghazadeh (2011) found that workplace factors were associated with increased stress and reduced engagement, which in turn were related to more accidents and injuries among CWs in the United States. In particular, the results showed that skill underutilization and high levels of job demands were associated with psychological strains such as anger, anxiety, and sadness among CWs. Adequate training and support, on the other hand, were negatively related to psychosomatic symptoms (e.g., stomach disorders, headaches). Adequate training was also related to lower rates of self-reported injuries, the more serious, OSHA-recordable injuries, and days lost due to injuries (another indicator of injury seriousness). Importantly, anxiety at work was found to be a predictor of OSHA-recordable injuries, suggesting that negative emotions induced by stressors at work may have implications for worksite accidents and injuries.

Unlike Abbe et al. (2011), Goldenhar, Williams, and Swanson (2003) found that skill utilization, rather than underutilization, was positively related to psychological distress. However, high levels of support and job certainty were associated with lower levels of distress and psychosomatic symptoms. Finally, consistent with Abbe et al.'s (2011) findings, both psychological distress and psychosomatic symptoms were associated with safety-related outcomes, including near-misses and self-reported injuries.

Other research underlines the relationship of psychological stress and uncertainty to injury risk. In a study conducted in Hong Kong, Leung, Chan, and Yu (2012) found that the lack of goal setting was related to injury risk, suggesting that when CWs do not know work-related priorities, they are more likely to experience injuries. In addition, the lack of proper safety equipment was associated with increased emotional distress and psychosomatic symptoms. Although neither emotional distress nor psychosomatic symptoms were directly related to injuries, these stress symptoms were associated with workers more frequently engaging in unsafe behaviors at work. Meliá and Bercerril (2009) showed that among Spanish workers, perceived safety climate (see Chapter 6) was inversely related to microaccidents (e.g., bumps and bruises); a positive climate's effect was mediated by reduced tension at work. Similarly, Siu, Phillips, and Leung (2004) found that in Hong Kong, CWs' safety climate perceptions were related to lower accident rates; the relationship was mediated by lower levels of psychological distress. Finally, Abbe et al. (2011) found that poor safety climate was associated with increased anxiety at work, which in turn was related to more injuries among U.S. CWs.

Given that stress-based psychological processes appear to play a mediating role linking the effects of worksite characteristics to workers' safety-related outcomes, some researchers have conducted studies that focused specifically on these stress-related processes among CWs. Janssen, Bakker, and de Jong (2001) explored the classic demand-control-support model (see Chapter 3) of occupational stress in construction work. They found that contrary to expectations, physical demands did not have the weakest relationship with burnout symptoms when *both* perceived control and support were high. Rather, either high control or high support attenuated the positive relationship between demands and burnout, and the two buffers appeared to be compensatory. Similarly, Lingard and Francis (2006) found that support from different sources, including coworkers, supervisors, and the organization in general, buffered the impact of work–family conflict (see Chapter 9) on burnout in CWs, such that the relationship between work–family conflict and burnout was weaker when workers perceived a more supportive work environment.

Other investigators explored the mediators through which stressors may lead to burnout or other stress symptoms, or the linkages between psychological distress and injuries. CWs who had irregular work hours experienced more work-related interference with their parenting role, personal leisure, and home management, which in turn led to higher levels of burnout symptoms (Lingard & Francis, 2005). Workers who experienced stressors such as receiving competing or conflicting work demands from different sources or having been victims of workplace aggression reported more tension at work, which in turn was associated with burnout symptoms (Meliá & Bercerril, 2007). Jacobsen et al. (2013) found mental distress was associated with work-related injuries and musculoskeletal pain.

Finally, while most of the aforementioned studies were based on self-reported, quantitative survey data, it should be noted that researchers have used other methods to examine the interplay between occupational stress and workplace safety. For example, Choudhry and Fang (2008), who conducted in-depth interviews with CWs and supervisors, found that general safety policies and management practices, as well as the specific onsite safety-related procedures, encouraged safe behaviors. In addition, workers felt more comfortable and less distressed when they perceived that their supervisors cared about their safety, and this psychological comfort increased their willingness to perform their tasks safely. On the other hand, competing goals such as performance pressure or tight deadlines tended to influence CWs to ignore safety procedures.

Occupational Health Issues Unique to Construction Workers

In addition to understanding stress as the key to the psychological processes linking workplace characteristics with CWs' safety-related outcomes, there are two OHP-related issues unique to CWs. The first issue concerns the risk of PTSD. Because major construction accidents often result in severe injuries and fatalities, those who survive or witness these accidents may suffer from PTSD. Peck (1984) reported that about 30% of the survivors of a workplace accident suffered from PTSD. Hu, Liang, Hu, Long, and Ge (2000) found that in a sample of 41 Chinese CWs who witnessed an accident during which three workers fell from the scaffold that was 10 m above the ground, 11 workers (27%) met the diagnostic criteria for PTSD 1 month after the accident. Out of the 11 workers, two left their jobs, five remained but experienced persistent PTSD symptoms, and four recovered and no longer met the diagnostic criteria at a 4-month follow-up. In addition, compared with a control group comprising workers who did not witness the accident, those who were exposed to the accident reported more symptoms of depression, anxiety, psychosomatic problems, and insomnia.

By contrast, Boschman, van der Molen, Sluiter, and Fring-Dresen (2013) found that exposure to construction accidents was not predictive of PTSD or depression in a large-scale, cross-sectional survey conducted in The Netherlands. Two reasons may explain these different findings. First, it is possible that the research method employed by Boschman et al. (2013) was not sufficiently sensitive to detect the effect of CWs' exposure to accidents on PTSD. For example, the characteristics of the exposure (e.g., proximity to death; severity of trauma; time between exposure and assessment of PTSD symptoms; Bryant & Harvey, 1995) were not assessed in Boschman et al.'s study. It is also possible that different contextual factors may explain the discrepant findings. These two research contexts are different in a number of ways, including the cultural values of the participants, national policies regarding workplace safety, and local worksite characteristics. More research is necessary to explore the effect of exposure to accidents on CWs' mental health and well-being.

The second issue concerns the fact that CWs are overwhelmingly male. In the United States, males, Whites, and Hispanics are overrepresented in relation to the general worker population (BLS, 2015b). Given the gender imbalance and concerns about ethnic diversity among CWs, female and minority CWs may be vulnerable to workplace harassment. Surprisingly, little research is available to estimate the extent to which female or minority CWs are victims of workplace harassment and how such negative treatment may affect the health and well-being of the victims. One exception is the work by Goldenhar and colleagues (e.g., Goldenhar, Swanson, Hurrell, Ruder, & Deddens, 1998; Goldenhar et al., 2003). Goldenhar and colleagues (1998) found that about 51% of the female CWs in the United States reported experiencing some form of sexual harassment or discrimination, originating from coworkers or supervisors in the past year. In another study of both male and female CWs, Goldenhar et al. (2003) found that about 23% of the participants reported some form of harassment or discrimination in the past year. Harassment and discrimination were strong predictors of lower job satisfaction in women (Goldenhar et al., 1998) and greater psychological distress and psychosomatic symptoms for both women and men (Goldenhar et al., 1998; Goldenhar et al., 2003). Finally, in a study of intimate partner violence among CWs, Cunradi, Ames, and Moore (2008) assessed workers' reports of racial and ethnic discrimination at work. The investigators found that workers who experienced workplace discrimination were more likely to not only engage in hazardous drinking, but also perpetrate physical violence against their intimate partners. Taken together, the existing research suggests that perceived harassment or discrimination has negative effects on CWs' health and well-being.

Summary

Much of the research suggests that stressful working conditions lead to psychological strains in CWs. Strains such as distress, psychosomatic symptoms, and burnout pave the way to compromised safety and injury. It should, however, be noted that the aforementioned findings are tentative because most of these results were based on studies with cross-sectional designs. Longitudinal research is needed to better model the stress process in CWs. In that vein, one massive ($n > 75,000$ male CWs) prospective study (Schiöler, Söderberg, Rosengren, Järvholm, & Torén, 2015) conducted in Sweden found that the psychosocial stressor job demands were modestly but significantly related to coronary heart disease although job control and strain were not.

AGRICULTURAL WORKERS

Agriculture employs workers who are involved in crop or animal production. It is one of the most hazardous industries (NIOSH, 2015b). In the United States in 2013, there were 360 on-the-job fatalities among workers in the agricultural sector, which accounted for 8% of all work-related deaths in the United States that year (BLS, 2015a). In 2012, there were a total of 395 fatalities among agricultural workers (AWs) in the 28 countries that made up the European Union, accounting for 10.1% of the total work-related deaths (Eurostat, 2015). In the United States, the fatality rate was 22.9 cases per 100,000 full-time equivalent workers for crop production workers and 15.6 cases per 100,000 full-time equivalent workers for animal production workers

(BLS, 2015a). The fatality rate in the United States exceeds by a factor of two the fatality rate for U.S. police officers (feloniously *and* accidentally killed combined) and firefighters (see the section on first responders), further underlining the danger of this type of work in the United States. Tractor overturns were the leading cause of fatalities among U.S. AWs. The fatality rate was 3.8 cases per 100,000 full-time equivalent workers in the European Union (Eurostat, 2015), which was one-fourth to one-fifth the U.S. rate.

Similar to CWs, AWs also suffered high rates of injuries and illnesses due to work-related exposures. In 2013 in the United States, there were around 52,000 cases of occupational injuries and illnesses (BLS, 2015a). The injury and illness rate was 5.5 cases per 100 full-time equivalent crop production workers and 6.2 cases per 100 full-time equivalent workers for animal production workers in the United States. The incidence rate, based on 2012 data, for nonfatal accidents among AWs in the European Union was 1.2 cases per 100 full-time equivalent workers (Eurostat, 2015), much lower than the rate in the United States. More than half of the cases in the United States resulted in serious impairment to workers' ability to perform their regular responsibilities (BLS, 2015a).

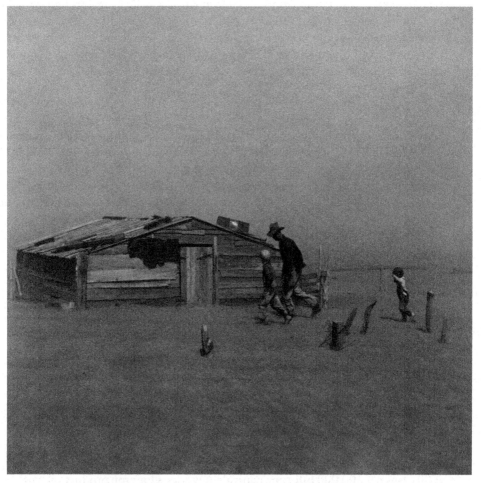

A farmer and his two sons during a dust storm in Cimarron County, Oklahoma, 1936. (Photographer is Arthur Rothstein for the U.S. Farm Security Administration. Public domain.)

Occupational Stress

Research on occupational stress in the agricultural context has focused on identifying the unique stressors faced by AWs. Early reviews of stressors unique to AWs often center on financial concerns and the unpredictability associated with agricultural work (e.g., weather concerns; Olson & Schellenberg, 1986; Schulman & Armstrong, 1990). Among AWs, economic constraints, such as low income, poverty, and high debt, have been linked to poor mental health, including increased depressive symptoms and psychological distress (Rathge, Ekstrom, & Leistritz, 1988; Simmons, Braun, Charnigo, Havens, & Wright, 2008). Simmons et al. (2008), using three waves of panel data over 2 years, found that for rural women, economic status at time 1 was predictive of later depressive symptoms controlling for time 1 symptoms. The findings support a social causation model that maintains the view that the stress of poor economic conditions is a contributing cause of depression in rural women. The research team found that a social selection model, that is, a model that holds that an innate propensity toward mental disorder leads to poor job performance and downward mobility, was incompatible with the findings.

Financial concerns remain a primary stressor for AWs in other studies. Kearney, Rafferty, Hendricks, Allen, and Tutor-Marcom (2014) showed that farmers in North Carolina were most concerned about the weather, followed by market prices for crops/livestock, and taxes and health care costs. LaBrash et al. (2008) found that Canadian AWs who reported worries about daily cash flow had higher rates of sleep loss and sleep deprivation, especially during the peak season (i.e., April through November) versus nonpeak season (December through March). Similarly, Lima, Rossini, and Reimão (2010) found that rural laborers in Brazil who worked as coffee harvesters were more likely to suffer from poor sleep quality and anxiety symptoms compared with those who had fixed employment. Lima et al. attributed the between-group differences in stress symptoms to the job insecurity and long periods of unemployment between harvest seasons, conditions that are unique to the coffee harvest work. Taken together, research has pointed to the financial concerns as a significant stressor among AWs.

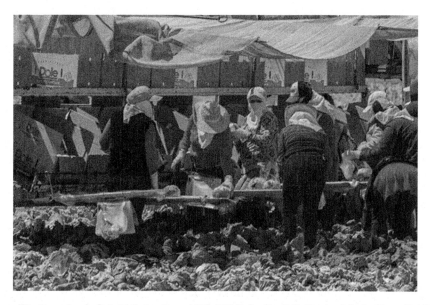

Farmworkers. (Photographer is Bob Nichols, August 27, 2013, for the U.S. Dept. of Agriculture. Public domain.)

In addition to identifying unique stressors, research has also focused on examining buffers that help protect AWs. In particular, social support and relationship networks appear to be a consistent stress buffer for AWs. Schulman and Armstrong (1990) found that adequate social support was associated with lower stress symptoms in AWs. Similarly, Hiott, Grzywacz, Davis, Quandt, and Arcury (2008) found that isolation from family and friends was positively related to anxiety and depression in Latino AWs in the United States. Berkowitz and Perkins (1984) found that among dairy farm women in upstate New York, husband support had a beneficial effect and conflict between the demands of farm and home, a negative effect on stress symptoms (e.g., trouble sleeping, worries).

Interestingly, a finer-grained analysis revealed that the benefit of social support may not be the equivalent for male versus female AWs. McClure and colleagues (2015) found that for female Mexican immigrant AWs working in Oregon, social support from family was related to lower physiological stress symptoms (e.g., immune function, blood pressure), and this effect was more pronounced if they lived in a predominantly White community. On the other hand, family support was unrelated to male AWs' physiological stress symptoms, regardless of their community. These findings suggest that family support may be particularly important for female immigrant AWs who are isolated from their larger community.

Occupational Safety

Researchers have focused on establishing how stress may contribute to AWs' safety-related outcomes. Financial concerns have been linked to AWs' safety-related outcomes, such as safety climate perceptions, safety behaviors, and accidents, injuries, and occupation-related illnesses. For example, Arcury, Summers, et al. (2015) found that perceived job insecurity and high levels of work stress were related to lower safety climate perceptions among legal immigrant AWs in North Carolina. Beseler and Stallones (2006) found that financial concerns were positively related to AWs' depressive symptoms, which in turn were associated with poorer safety behaviors in a sample of Colorado farmworkers. Glasscock, Rasmussen, Carstensen, and Hansen (2006) found that economic concerns were related to increased accidents and injuries over a 12-month period for AWs in Denmark. Moreover, AWs' psychological distress interacted with their safety behaviors in predicting accidents and injuries. In particular, AWs were more likely to suffer from accidents and injuries if they reported higher levels of psychological distress and did not perform regular safety checks on their farm equipment. Overall, as an occupational stressor, AWs' financial concerns have implications for not only their psychological well-being, but also their physical safety.

In addition to establishing the linkage between stress and safety among AWs, researchers have also examined the effects of other psychosocial characteristics of the worksite on AWs' safety-related outcomes. Consistent with the existing literature (see also Chapter 6), AWs' safety climate perceptions were directly related to safety performance and inversely related to occupational injuries (e.g., musculoskeletal disorders [MSDs]) and illnesses (e.g., respiratory symptoms; Arcury et al., 2012, 2013; Grzywacz et al., 2007). Unfortunately, studies on the association between other workplace characteristics and AWs' injuries have yielded more equivocal results. For example, while some research (e.g., Grzywacz et al., 2007) found that AWs' MSD symptoms were positively predicted by high psychological workload and low perceived control, other studies (e.g., Rosenbaum, Mora, Arcury, Chen, & Quandt, 2014) found no relationship between job demands and control, on the one hand, and MSD symptoms, on the other. Some studies (e.g., Mora et al., 2016) even found that Latino immigrant AWs had lower rates of MSD injuries compared with Latino immigrants who worked in other sectors (e.g., food preparation and service, construction) after controlling for symptoms assessed 1 year earlier.

Finally, research has also explored postinjury recovery and rehabilitation among AWs. For example, research has shown that positive safety climate was related to a lower likelihood to work while injured or ill (Arcury et al., 2012); desistance from work when injured is expected to contribute to better recovery. In a study in China, Wang et al. (2010) found that AWs who suffered from an injury in the past 12 months were more likely to consume alcohol in general and to drink during breakfast or lunch, a finding that suggests that some injured AWs may use maladaptive coping strategies that inhibit their recovery.

Occupational Health Issues Unique to Agricultural Workers

Finally, we discuss two OHP-related issues that are unique to the context of agricultural work. First, in the United States, a large proportion of AWs are youth (i.e., workers under 20 years old) compared with the proportions in other industries. According to NIOSH (2015b), almost 1 million youth lived on farms in 2012, with an estimated 472,000 youth performing farmwork. An estimated 259,000 youth in addition to those who lived on farms were employed to work on farms in the United States in 2012. Young AWs in North Carolina perceived high levels of job insecurity, received minimum safety training, and reported poor safety climate in farm practices (Arcury, Kearney, Rodriguez, Arcury, & Quandt, 2015). However, owing to the low base rate, Arcury, Kearney, et al. (2015) did not find a significant relationship between poor safety climate and injuries in young AWs. Other research indicated that compared with young female AWs, young male AWs were more likely to be subject to safety risks, such as pesticide exposure, performing dusty jobs, or overturning tractors (Arcury, Rodriguez, Kearney, Arcury, & Quandt, 2014; Reed, Browning, Westneat, & Kidd, 2006). Compared with young female AWs, young male AWs were less likely to wear personal protective equipment (e.g., gloves, masks; Arcury et al., 2014; Reed et al., 2006). These findings suggest that young AWs in the United States do not receive adequate protection from exposure to occupational hazards, and more attention needs to be paid to this particular segment of AWs.

A second unique issue related to AWs in the United States reflects acculturation-related concerns. A large proportion of AWs in the United States are Latino immigrants with varying immigration statuses. This population faces various challenges as they assimilate into the mainstream U.S. society. For example, Hiott et al. (2008) showed that Latino AWs often faced racial and ethnic harassment and discrimination at work, and these negative experiences were related to increased anxiety and depression. Hovey and Magaña (2002) found that in addition to occupational stressors, acculturative stressors, such as problems with English-as-a-second-language and isolation from family and friends back in countries of origin, were associated with increased anxiety and depression. Arcury, Trejo, et al. (2015) found that Latina mothers who belonged to migrant farm families (i.e., relocating the family to pursue farmwork) reported worse personal health and greater family conflict compared with those who had stable farmwork.

Finally, similar to the effects of social support, Latino male and female AWs had different reactions toward racial and ethnic discrimination and showed different acculturation-related response patterns (McClure et al., 2010). Male AWs who perceived discrimination had higher systolic blood pressure, whereas female AWs' blood pressure was unrelated to perceived discrimination. However, among women workers greater facility with the English language and more years in the United States were associated with higher blood pressure. McClure et al. (2010) suggested that while acculturation contributed to higher stress among female AWs, it had the opposite effect on stress for male AWs.

Summary

Similar to CWs, AWs suffer high rates of occupational injuries and illnesses, and much of the research on AWs suggests that financial stress may contribute to poor psychological well-being and reduced physical safety. Moreover, the unique demographics of AWs (i.e., high proportion of immigrant workers and young workers who are under 20 years of age) may add challenges to interventions designed to address the exposure risks and occupational injuries and illnesses among AWs. Finally, the majority of studies involving AWs were cross-sectional, which limits our ability to draw conclusions about causality.

REFERENCES

Abbe, O. O., Harvey, C. M., Ikuma, L. H., & Aghazadeh, F. (2011). Modeling the relationship between occupational stressors, psychosocial/physical symptoms and injuries in the construction industry. *International Journal of Industrial Ergonomics, 11*, 106–117. doi:10.1016/j.ergon.2010.12.002

Admon, R., Lubin, G., Rosenblatt, J. D., Stern, O., Kahn, I., Assaf, M., & Hendler, T. (2013a). Imbalanced neural responsivity to risk and reward indicates stress vulnerability in humans. *Cerebral Cortex, 23*, 28–35. doi:10.1093/cercor/bhr369

Admon, R., Lubin, G., Stern, O., Rosenberg, K., Sela, L., Ben-Ami, H., & Hendler, T. (2009). Human vulnerability to stress depends on amygdala's predisposition and hippocampal plasticity. *Proceedings of the National Academy of Sciences of the United States of America, 106*, 14120–14125. doi:10.1073/pnas.0903183106

Admon, R., Milad, M., & Hendler, T. (2013b). A causal model of post-traumatic stress disorder: Disentangling predisposed from acquired neural abnormalities. *Trends in Cognitive Sciences, 17*, 337–347. doi:10.1016/j.tics.2013.05.005

Agerbo, E., Gunnell, D., Bonde, J. P., Mortensen, P. B., & Nordentoft, M. (2007). Suicide and occupation: The impact of socioeconomic, demographic and psychiatric differences. *Psychological Medicine, 37*, 1131–1140. doi:10.1017/S0033291707000487

Alberini, C. M. (2011). The role of reconsolidation and the dynamic process of long-term memory formation and storage. *Frontiers in Behavioral Neuroscience, 5*, 1–10. doi:10.3389/fnbeh.2011.00012

Allen, J. P., Cross, G., & Swanner, J. (2005). Suicide in the army: A review of current information. *Military Medicine, 170*(7), 580.

Allesøe, K., Andersen Hundrup, Y., Frølund Thomsen, J., & Osler, M. (2010). Psychosocial work environment and risk of ischaemic heart disease in women: The Danish Nurse Cohort Study. *Occupational and Environmental Medicine, 67*, 318–322. doi:10.1136/oem.2008.043091

Arcury, T. A., Grzywacz, J. G., Anderson, A. M., Mora, D. C., Carrillo, L., Chen, H., & Quandt, S. A. (2013). Employer, use of personal protective equipment, and work safety climate: Latino poultry processing workers. *American Journal of Industrial Medicine, 56*, 180–188. doi:10.1002/ajim.22101

Arcury, T. A., Kearney, G. D., Rodriguez, G., Arcury, J., & Quandt, S. A. (2015). Work safety culture of youth farmworkers in North Carolina: A pilot study. *American Journal of Public Health, 105*, 344–350. doi:10.2105/AJPH.2014.302254

Arcury, T. A., O'Hara, H., Grzywacz, J. G., Isom, S., Chen, H., & Quandt, S. A. (2012). Work safety climate, musculoskeletal discomfort, working while injured, and depression among migrant farmworkers in North Carolina. *American Journal of Public Health, 102,* S272–S278. doi:10.2105/AJPH.2011.300597

Arcury, T. A., Rodriguez, G., Kearney, G. D., Arcury, J. T., & Quandt, S. A. (2014). Safety and injury characteristics of youth farmworkers in North Carolina: A pilot study. *Journal of Agromedicine, 19,* 354–363. doi:10.1080/1059924X.2014.945712

Arcury, T. A., Summers, P., Talton, J. W., Nguyen, H. T., Chen, H., & Quandt, S. A. (2015). Job characteristics and work safety climate among North Carolina farmworkers with H-2A visas. *Journal of Agromedicine, 20,* 64–76. doi:10.1080/1059924X.2014.976732

Arcury, T. A., Trejo, G., Suerken, C. K., Grzywacz, J. G., Ip, E. H., & Quandt, S. A. (2015). Work and health among Latina mothers in farmworker families. *Journal of Occupational and Environmental Medicine, 57,* 292–299. doi:10.1097/JOM.0000000000000351

Arter, M. L. (2008). Stress and deviance in policing. *Deviant Behavior, 29,* 43–69. doi:10.1080/01639620701457774

Bachynski, K. E., Canham-Chervak, M., Black, S. A., Dada, E. O., Millikan, A. M., & Jones, B. H. (2012). Mental health risk factors for suicides in the US Army, 2007–8. *Injury Prevention, 18,* 405–412. doi:10.1136/injuryprev-2011-040112

Baker, A. (2015, December 12). A trip abroad to study policing without guns. *The New York Times,* pp. A1, A15.

Beaton, R., Murphy, S., Johnson, C., Pike, K., & Corneil, W. (1998). Exposure to duty-related incident stressors in urban firefighters and paramedics. *Journal of Traumatic Stress, 11,* 821–828. doi:0894-9867/98/1000-0821$15.00

Berger, W., Coutinho, E. F., Figueira, I., Marques-Portella, C., Luz, M. P., Neylan, T. C., . . . Mendlowicz, M. V. (2012). Rescuers at risk: A systematic review and meta-regression analysis of the worldwide current prevalence and correlates of PTSD in rescue workers. *Social Psychiatry and Psychiatric Epidemiology, 47,* 1001–1011. doi:10.1007/s00127-011-0408-2

Berkowitz, A. D., & Perkins, H. W. (1984). Stress among farm women: Work and family as interacting systems. *Journal of Marriage and Family, 46,* 161–166.

Berkvist, R. (2012, December 26). Charles Durning: Prolific character actor (from Nazi to priest), dies at 89. *The New York Times,* p. 23.

Berninger, A., Webber, M. P., Niles, J. K., Jackson, G., Lee, R., Cohen, H. W., . . . Prezant, D. J. (2010). Longitudinal study of probable post-traumatic stress disorder in firefighters exposed to the World Trade Center Disaster. *American Journal of Industrial Medicine, 53,* 1177–1185.

Beseler, C. L., & Stallones, L. (2006). Structural equation modeling of the relationships between pesticide poisoning, depressive symptoms and safety behaviors among Colorado farm residents. *Journal of Agromedicine, 11,* 35–46. doi:10.1300/J096v11n03_05

Bliese, P. D., & Halverson, R. R. (2002). Using Random Group Resampling in multilevel research: An example of the buffering effects of leadership climate. *The Leadership Quarterly, 13,* 53–68.

Boschman, J. S., van der Molen, H. F., Sluiter, J. K., & Fring-Dresen, M. H. W. (2013). Psychosocial work environment and mental health among construction workers. *Applied Ergonomics, 44,* 748–755. doi:10.1016/j.apergo.2013.01.004

Bourbonnais, R., Comeau, M., & Vezina, M. (1999). Job strain and evolution of mental health among nurses. *Journal of Occupational Health Psychology, 4,* 95–107. doi:10.1037/1076-8998.4.2.95

Bowler, R. M., Harris, M., Li, J., Gocheva, V., Stellman, S. D., Wilson, K., . . . Cone, J. E. (2012). Longitudinal mental health impact among police responders to the 9/11 terrorist attack. *American Journal of Industrial Medicine, 55,* 297–312. doi:10.1002/ajim.22000

Brackbill, R. M., Hadler, J. L., DiGrande, L., Ekenga, C. C., Farfel, M. R., Friedman, S., . . . Thorpe, L. E. (2009). Asthma and posttraumatic stress symptoms 5 to 6 years following exposure to the World Trade Center terrorist attack. *Journal of the American Medical Association, 302,* 502–516. doi:10.1001/jama.2009.1121

Brennan, P. (1994, May 29). Charles Durning: Healing the wounds of Normandy. *The Washington Post.*

Brewin, C. R., Dalgleish, T., & Joseph, S. (1996). A dual representation theory of posttraumatic stress disorder. *Psychological Review, 103,* 670–686. doi:10.1037/0033-295X.103.4.670

Britt, T. W., Davison, J., Bliese, P. D., & Castro, C. A. (2004). How leaders can influence the impact that stressors have on soldiers. *Military Medicine, 169*(7), 541–545.

Bryant, R. A., & Harvey, A. G. (1995). Posttraumatic stress in volunteer firefighters: Predictors of distress. *Journal of Nervous and Mental Disease, 183*(4), 267–271.

Bureau of Labor Statistics. (2015a). *Census of fatal occupational injuries (CFOI): Current and revised data.* Washington, DC: U.S. Department of Labor.

Bureau of Labor Statistics. (2015b). *Labor force statistics from the current population survey.* Washington, DC: U.S. Department of Labor.

Bureau of Labor Statistics. (2015c). *Occupational employment statistics. May 2014 national occupational employment and wage estimates.* Washington, DC: U.S. Department of Labor.

Büssing, A., & Glaser, J. (1999). Work stressors in nursing in the course of redesign: Implications for burnout and interactional stress. *European Journal of Work and Organizational Psychology, 8,* 401–426. doi:10.1080/135943299398249

Camerino, D., Estryn-Beharc, M., Conway, P. M., van Der Heijdend, B. I. J. M., & Hasselhorng, H.-M. (2008). Work-related factors and violence among nursing staff in the European NEXT study: A longitudinal cohort study. *International Journal of Nursing Studies, 45,* 35–50. doi:10.1016/j.ijnurstu.2007.01.013

Carlier, I. E., Lamberts, R. D., & Gersons, B. R. (1997). Risk factors for posttraumatic stress symptomatology in police officers: A prospective analysis. *Journal of Nervous and Mental Disease, 185,* 498–506. doi:10.1097/00005053-199708000-00004

Chen, W.-C., Sun, Y.-H., Lan, T.-H., & Chiu, H.-J. (2009). Incidence and risk factors of workplace violence on nursing: Staffs caring for chronic psychiatric patients in Taiwan. *International Journal of Environmental Research and Public Health, 6,* 2812–2821; doi:10.3390/ijerph6112812

Chiu, S., Niles, J. K., Webber, M. P., Zeig-Owens, J., Gustave, J., Lee, R., . . . Prezant, D. J. (2011). Evaluating risk factors and possible mediation effects in posttraumatic depression and posttraumatic stress disorder comorbidity. *Public Health Reports, 126*(2), 201–209.

Choudhry, R. M., & Fang, D. (2008). Why operatives engage in unsafe work behavior: Investigating factors on construction sites. *Safety Science, 46,* 566–584. doi:10.1016/j.ssci.2007.06.027

Corneil, W., Beaton, R., Murphy, S., Johnson, C., & Pike, K. (1999). Exposure to traumatic incidents and prevalence of posttraumatic stress symptomatology in urban firefighters in two countries. *Journal of Occupational Health Psychology, 4,* 131–141. doi:10.1037/1076-8998.4.2.131

Cropley, M., Steptoe, A., & Joekes, K. (1999). Job strain and psychiatric morbidity. *Psychological Medicine, 29,* 1411–1416. doi:10.1017/S003329179900121X

Cukor, J., Wyka, K., Mello, B., Olden, M., Jayasinghe, N., Roberts, J., . . . Difede, J. (2011). The longitudinal course of PTSD among disaster workers deployed to the World Trade Center following the attacks of September 11th. *Journal of Traumatic Stress, 24,* 506–514. doi:10.1002/jts.20672

Cunradi, C. B., Ames, G. M., & Moore, R. S. (2008). Prevalence and correlates of intimate partner violence among a sample of construction industry workers. *Journal of Family Violence, 23,* 101–112. doi:10.1007/s10896-007-9131-x

Department for Communities and Local Government. (2011). *Fire and rescue service operational statistics bulletin for England 2010–11.* London, UK: Author.

Dohrenwend, B. P., Turner, J. B., Turse, N. A., Adams, B. G., Koenen, K. C., & Marshall, R. (2006). The psychological risks of Vietnam for U.S. veterans: A revisit with new data and methods. *Science, 313*(5789), 979–982. doi:10.1002/jts.20296

Duarte, C. S., Hoven, C. W., Wu, P., Bin, F., Cotel, S., Mandell, D. J., et al. (2006). Posttraumatic stress in children with first responders in their families. *Journal of Traumatic Stress, 19,* 301–306. doi:10.1002/jtd.20120

Eaton, W. W., Anthony, J. C., Mandel, W., & Garrison, R. (1990). Occupations and the prevalence of major depressive disorder. *Journal of Occupational Medicine, 32*(11), 1079–1087.

Ehlers, A., & Clark, D. (2000). A cognitive model of posttraumatic stress disorder. *Behaviour Research and Therapy, 38,* 319–345. doi:10.1016/S0005-7967(99)00123-0

Eurostat. (2015, June). *Accident at work statistics.* Retrieved from http://ec.europa.eu/eurostat/statistics-explained/index.php/Accidents_at_work_statistics

Farfel, M., DiGrande, L., Brackbill, R., Prann, A., Cone, J., Friedman, S., . . . Thorpe, L. (2008). An overview of 9/11 experiences and respiratory and mental health conditions among World Trade Center Health Registry enrollees. *Journal of Urban Health: Bulletin of the New York Academy of Medicine, 85,* 880–909. doi:10.1007/s11524-008-9317-4

Federal Bureau of Investigation. (2015). *FBI releases 2014 statistics for law enforcement officers killed and assaulted.* Washington, DC: Author. Retrieved from https://www.fbi.gov/news/pressrel/press-releases/fbi-releases-2014-statistics-on-law-enforcement-officers-killed-and-assaulted

Feskanich, D., Hastrup, J., Marshall, J., Colditz, G., Stampfer, M., Willett, W., & Kawachi, I. (2002). Stress and suicide in the Nurses' Health Study. *Journal of Epidemiology and Community Health, 56,* 95–98. doi:10.1136/jech.56.2.95

Finlay-Jones, R. (1986). Factors in the teaching environment associated with severe psychological distress among school teachers. *Australia and New Zealand Journal of Psychiatry, 20*, 304–313. doi:10.3109/00048678609158878

Fitzgerald, L. F., Magley, V. J., Drasgow, F., & Waldo, C. R. (1999). Measuring sexual harassment in the military: The Sexual Experiences Questionnaire (SEQ-DoD). *Military Psychology, 3*, 243–263. doi:10.1207/s15327876mp1103_3

Fontana, A., & Rosenheck, R. (1994). Traumatic war stressors and psychiatric symptoms among World War II, Korean, and Vietnam War veterans. *Psychology and Aging, 9*, 27–33. doi:10.1037/0882-7974.9.1.27

Franke, W. D., Cox, D. F., Schultz, D. P., & Anderson, D. F. (1997). Coronary heart disease risk factors in employees of Iowa's Department of Public Safety compared to a cohort of the general population. *American Journal of Industrial Medicine, 31*(6), 733–737.

Frueh, B. C., & Smith, J. A. (2012). Suicide, alcoholism, and psychiatric illness among union forces during the U.S. Civil War. *Journal of Anxiety Disorders, 26*, 769–775. doi:10.1016/j.janxdis.2012.06.006

Fujita, S., Ito, S., Seto, K., Kitazawa, T., Matsumoto, K., & Hasegawa, T. (2012). Risk factors of workplace violence at hospitals in Japan. *Journal of Hospital Medicine, 7*, 79–84. doi:10.1002/jhm.976

Galea, S., Nandi, A., & Vlahov, D. (2005). The epidemiology of post-traumatic stress disorder after disasters. *Epidemiologic Reviews, 27*, 78–91. doi:10.1093/epirev/mxi1003

Gelsema, T. I., Van Der Doef, M., Maes, S., Janssen, M., Akerboom, S., & Verhoeven, C. (2006). A longitudinal study of job stress in the nursing profession: Causes and consequences. *Journal of Nursing Management, 14*, 289–299. doi:10.1111/j.1365-2934.2006.00635.x

Genderson, M. R., Schonfeld, I. S., Kaplan, M. S., & Lyons, M. J. (2009). Suicide associated with military service. *Newsletter of the Society for Occupational Health Psychology, 6*, 5–7. Retrieved from www .sohp-online.org/NewsletterDownloads/SOHPNewsletterV6May2009.pdf

Gilbert, M. (1989). *The Second World War: A complete history*. New York, NY: Holt.

Glasscock, D. J., Rasmussen, K., Carstensen, O., & Hansen, O. N. (2006). Psychosocial factors and safety behaviour as predictors of accidental work injuries in farming. *Work & Stress, 20*, 173–189. doi:10.1080/02678370600879724

Goldenhar, L. M., Swanson, N. G., Hurrell, J. J., Jr., Ruder, A., & Deddens, J. (1998). Stressors and adverse outcomes for female construction workers. *Journal of Occupational Health Psychology, 3*, 19–32. doi:10.1037/1076-8998.3.1.19

Goldenhar, L. M., Williams, L. J., & Swanson, N. G. (2003). Modelling relationships between job stressors and injury and near-miss outcomes for construction labourers. *Work & Stress, 17*, 218–240. doi:10 .1080/02678370310001616144

González-Morales, M. G., Rodríguez, I., & Peiró, J. M. (2010). A longitudinal study of coping and gender in a female-dominated occupation: Predicting teachers' burnout. *Journal of Occupational Health Psychology, 15*, 29–44. doi:10.1037/a0018232

Goodwin, L., Wessely, S., Hotopf, M., Jones, M., Greenberg, N., Rona, R. J., . . . Fear, N. T. (2015). Are common mental disorders more prevalent in the UK serving military compared to the general working population? *Psychological Medicine, 45*, 1881–1891. doi:10.1017/S0033291714002980

Grzywacz, J. G., Arcury, T. A., Marin, A., Carrillo, L., Coates, M. L., Burke, B., & Quandt, S. A. (2007). The organization of work: Implications for injury and illness among immigrant Latino poultry-processing workers. *Archives of Environmental & Occupational Health, 62*, 19–26. doi:10.3200/AEOH.62.1.19–26

Hawton, K., & Vislisel, L. (1999). Suicide in nurses. *Suicide and Life-Threatening Behavior, 29*(1), 86–95.

Hay, M. S., & Elig, T. W. (1999). The 1995 Department of Defense Sexual Harassment Survey: Overview and methodology. *Military Psychology, 11*, 233–242. doi:10.1207/s15327876mp1103_2

Heim, E. (1991). Job stressors and coping in health professions. *Psychotherapy and Psychosomatics, 55*, 90–99. doi:10.1159/000288414

Heinrichs, M., Wagner, D., Schoch, W., Soravia, L. M., Hellhammer, D. H., & Ehlert, U. (2005). Predicting posttraumatic stress symptoms from pretraumatic risk factors: A 2-year prospective follow-up study in firefighters. *American Journal of Psychiatry, 162*, 2276–2286. doi:10.1176/appi .ajp.162.12.2276

Hem, E., Berg, A. M., & Ekeberg, Ø. (2001). Suicide in police: A critical review. *Suicide and Life-Threatening Behavior, 31*, 224–233. doi:10.1521/suli.31.2.224.21513

Herloff, B., & Jarvholm, B. (1989). Teachers, stress and mortality. *The Lancet, 1*(8630), 159–160.

Hiott, A. E., Grzywacz, J. G., Davis, S. W., Quandt, S. A., & Arcury, T. A. (2008). Migrant farmworker stress: Mental health implications. *Journal of Rural Health, 24*, 32–39. doi:10.1111/j.1748-0361.2008 .00134.x.

Hoge, C., Castro, C., Messer, S., McGurk, D., Cotting, D., & Koffman, R. (2004). Combat duty in Iraq and Afghanistan, mental health problems, and barriers to care. *New England Journal of Medicine, 351,* 13–22. doi:10.1056/NEJMoa040603

Hoven, C. W., Duarte, C. S., Wu, P., Doan, T., Singh, N., Mandell, D. J., . . . Cohen, P. (2009). Parental exposure to mass violence and child mental health: The First Responder and WTC Evacuee Study. *Clinical Child and Family Psychology Review, 12,* 95–112. doi:0.1007/s10567-009-0047-2

Hovey, J. D., & Magaña, C. G. (2002). Exploring the mental health of Mexican migrant farm workers in the Midwest: Psychosocial predictors of psychological distress and suggestions for prevention and treatment. *Journal of Psychology: Interdisciplinary and Applied, 136,* 493–513. doi:10.1080/00223980209605546

Hu, B. S., Liang, Y. X., Hu, X. Y., Long, Y. F., & Ge, L. N. (2000). Posttraumatic stress disorder in co-workers following exposure to a fatal construction accident in China. *International Journal of Occupational and Environmental Health, 6*(3), 203–207.

Ingersoll, R. M. (2001). Teacher turnover and teacher shortages: An organizational analysis. *American Educational Research Journal, 38,* 499–534. doi:10.3102/00028312038003499

Ingersoll, R. M. (2013, May). *Why schools have difficulty staffing their classrooms with qualified teachers?* New York, NY: United Federation of Teachers Fact Finding Hearing.

Ingersoll, R. M., & May, H. (2012). The magnitude, destinations, and determinants of mathematics and science teacher turnover. *Educational Evaluation and Policy Analysis, 34,* 435–464. doi:10.3102/0162373712454326

Jacobsen, H. B., Caban-Martinez, A., Onyebeke, L. C., Sorensen, G., Dennerlein, J. T., & Reme, S. E. (2013). Construction workers struggle with a high prevalence of mental distress, and this is associated with their pain and injuries. *Journal of Occupational and Environmental Medicine, 55,* 1197–1204. doi:10.1097/JOM.0b013e31829c76b3

Janssen, P. P. M., Bakker, A. B., & de Jong, A. (2001). A test and refinement of the demand-control-support model in the construction industry. *International Journal of Stress Management, 8*(4), 315–332.

Kaplan, M. S., Huguet, N., McFarland, B. H., & Newsom, J. T. (2007). Suicide among male veterans: A prospective population-based study. *Journal of Epidemiology and Community Health, 61,* 619–624. doi:10.1136/jech.2006.054346

Karasek, R. A., Pieper, C., Schwartz, J., Fry, L., & Schier, D. (1985). *Job Content Instrument Questionnaire and user's guide.* New York, NY: Columbia University Job/Heart Project.

Karch, D. L., Logan, J., & Patel, N. (2011). Surveillance for violent deaths: National Violent Death Reporting System, 16 states, 2008. *Centers for Disease Control and Prevention (CDC), Morbidity and Mortality Weekly Report, 60*(10), 1–49.

Kearney, G. D., Rafferty, A. P., Hendricks, L. R., Allen, D. L., & Tutor-Marcom, R. (2014). A cross-sectional study of stressors among farmers in eastern North Carolina. *North Carolina Medical Journal, 75*(6), 384–392.

Kelly, S., Charlton, J., & Jenkins, R. (1995). Suicide deaths in England and Wales, 1982–92: The contribution of occupation and geography. *Population Trends, 80,* 16–25.

Kessler, R. C. (2000). Posttraumatic stress disorder: The burden to the individual and society. *Journal of Clinical Psychiatry, 61*(Suppl. 5), 4–12.

Kolb, L. (1987). A neuropsychological hypothesis explaining posttraumatic stress disorders. *American Journal of Psychiatry, 144*(8), 989–995.

Kubo, T., Fukuda, S., Hirata, K., Shimada, K., Maeda, K., Komukai, K., . . . Yoshikawa, J. (2011). Comparison of coronary microcirculation in female nurses after day-time versus night-time shifts. *American Journal of Cardiology, 108,* 1665–1668. doi:10.1016/j.amjcard.2011.07.028

Kuehn, B. M. (2009). Soldier suicide rates continue to rise. *Journal of the American Medical Association, 301,* 1111–1113. doi:10.1001/jama.2009.342

LaBrash, L. F., Pahwa, P., Pickett, W., Hagel, L. M., Snodgrass, P. R., & Dosman, J. A. (2008). Relationship between sleep loss and economic worry among farmers: A survey of 94 active Saskatchewan noncorporate farms. *Journal of Agromedicine, 13,* 149–154. doi:10.1080/10599240802371862

Landsbergis, P. A. (1988). Occupational stress among health care workers: A test of the job demands-control model. *Journal of Organizational Behavior, 9,* 217–239. doi:10.1002/job.4030090303

Lee, S., Colditz, G. A., Berkman, L. F., & Kawachi, I. (2002). A prospective study of job strain and coronary heart disease in US women. *International Journal of Epidemiology, 31*(6), 1147–1153.

Lee, S., Colditz, G. A., Berkman, L. F., & Kawachi, I. (2004). Prospective study of job insecurity and coronary heart disease in US women. *Annals of Epidemiology, 14*(1), 24–30.

Leung, M.-Y., Chan, I. Y. S., & Yu, J. (2012). Preventing construction worker injury incidents through the management of personal stress and organizational stressors. *Accident Analysis and Prevention, 48,* 156–166. doi:10.1016/j.aap.2011.03.017

Lima, J., Rossini, S., & Reimão, R. (2010). Sleep disorders and quality of life of harvesters rural labourers. *Arquivos de Neuro-Psiquiatria, 68*, 372–376. doi:10.1590/S0004-282X2010000300008

Lingard, H., & Francis, V. (2005). Does work-family conflict mediate the relationship between job schedule demands and burnout in male construction professionals and managers? *Construction Management and Economics, 23*, 733–745. doi:10.1080/01446190500040836

Lingard, H., & Francis, V. (2006). Does a supportive work environment moderate the relationship between work-family conflict and burnout among construction professionals? *Construction Management and Economics, 24*, 185–196. doi:10.1080/14697010500226913

Llorens-Gumbau, M., & Salanova-Soria, M. (2014). Loss and gain cycles? A longitudinal study about burnout, engagement and self-efficacy. *Burnout Research, 1*, 3–11. doi:10.1016/j.burn.2014.02.001

Loo, R. (2003). A meta-analysis of police suicide rates: Findings and issues. *Suicide and Life-Threatening Behavior, 33*, 313–325. doi:10.1521/suli.33.3.313.23209

Magley, V. J., Waldo, C. R., Drasgow, F., & Fitzgerald, L. F. (1999). The impact of sexual harassment on military personnel: Is it the same for men and women? *Military Psychology, 3*, 283–302. doi:10.1207/s15327876mp1103_5

Maguen, S., Metzler, T. J., McCaslin, S. E., Inslicht, S. S., Henn-Haase, C., Neylan, T. C., & Marmar, C. R. (2009). Routine work environment stress and PTSD symptoms in police officers. *Journal of Nervous and Mental Disease, 197*, 754–760. doi:10.1097/NMD.0b013e3181b975f8

Mahon, M., Tobin, J., Cusack, D., Kelleher, C., & Malone, K. (2005). Suicide among regular-duty military personnel: A retrospective case-control study of occupation-specific risk factors for workplace suicide. *The American Journal of Psychiatry, 162*, 1688–1696. doi:10.1176/appi.ajp.162.9.1688

Mandell, W., Eaton, W. W., Anthony, J. C., & Garrison, R. (1992). Alcoholism and occupations: A review and analysis of 104 occupations. *Alcoholism: Clinical and Experimental Research, 16*, 734–746. doi:10.1111/j.1530-0277.1992.tb00670.x

Marzuk, P., Nock, M., Leon, A., Portera, L., & Tardiff, K. (2002). Suicide among New York City police officers, 1977–1996. *American Journal of Psychiatry, 159*, 2069–2071. doi:10.1176/appi.ajp.159.12.2069

Mazzola, J. J., Schonfeld, I., & Spector, P. E. (2011). What qualitative research has taught us about occupational stress. *Stress and Health: Journal of the International Society for the Investigation of Stress, 27*, 93–110. doi:10.1002/smi.1386

McClure, H. H., Martinez, C. R., Jr., Snodgrass, J. J., Eddy, J. M., Jiménez, R. A., Isiordia, L. E., & McDade, T. W. (2010). Discrimination-related stress, blood pressure and Epstein-Barr virus antibodies among Latin American immigrants in Oregon, US. *Journal of Biosocial Science, 42*, 433–461. doi:10.1017/S0021932010000039

McClure, H. H., Snodgrass, J. J., Martinez, C. R., Jr., Squires, E. C., Jiménez, R. A., Isiordia, L. E., . . . Small, J. (2015). Stress, place, and allostatic load among Mexican immigrant farmworkers in Oregon. *Journal of Immigrant Minority Health, 17*(5), 1518–1525. doi:10.1007/s10903-014-0066-z

McFarlane, A. C. (1988). The longitudinal course of posttraumatic morbidity: The range of outcomes and their predictors. *Journal of Nervous and Mental Disease, 176*, 30–39. doi:10.1097/00005053-198801000-00004

Meliá, J. L., & Bercerril, M. (2007). Psychosocial sources of stress and burnout in the construction sector: A structural equation model. *Psicothema, 19*(4), 679–686.

Meliá, J. L., & Bercerril, M. (2009). Health behaviour and safety in the construction sector. *Psicothema, 21*(3), 427–432.

Milliken, C. S., Auchterlonie, J. L., & Hoge, C. W. (2007). Longitudinal assessment of mental health problems among active and reserve component soldiers returning from the Iraq war. *Journal of the American Medical Association, 298*, 2141–2148. doi:10.1001/jama.298.18.2141

Montgomery, C., & Rupp, A. (2005). A meta-analysis for exploring the diverse causes and effects of stress in teachers. *Canadian Education Journal, 28*, 458–486. doi:10.2307/4126479

Mora, D. C., Miles, C. M., Chen, H., Quandt, S. A., Summers, P., & Arcury, T. A. (2016). Prevalence of musculoskeletal disorders among immigrant Latino farmworkers and non-farmworkers in North Carolina. *Archives of Environmental & Occupational Health, 71*, 136–143. doi:10.1080/19338244.2014.988676

Murphy, S. A., Beaton, R. D., Pike, K. C., & Johnson, L. C. (1999). Occupational stressors, stress responses, and alcohol consumption among professional firefighters: A prospective, longitudinal analysis. *International Journal of Stress Management, 6*, 179–196. doi:10.1023/A:1021934725246

National Institute for Occupational Safety and Health. (2015a, March). *Construction safety and health*. Retrieved from www.cdc.gov/niosh/construction

National Institute for Occupational Safety and Health. (2015b, March). *Agricultural safety*. Retrieved from www.cdc.gov/niosh/topics/aginjury/default.html

North, C. S., Tivis, L., McMillen, J., Pfefferbaum, B., Spitznagel, E. L., Cox, J., . . . Smith, E. M. (2002). Psychiatric disorders in rescue workers after the Oklahoma City bombing. *American Journal of Psychiatry, 159*, 857–859. doi:10.1176/appi.ajp.159.5.857

O'Hara, A. F. (2011). The reality of suicide: To the edge and back. In J. M. Violanti, A. F. O'Hara, & T. T. Tate, *On the edge: Recent perspectives on police suicide* (pp. 57–75). Springfield, IL: Charles C. Thomas.

Olson, K. R., & Schellenberg, R. P. (1986). Farm stressors. *American Journal of Community Psychology, 14*, 555–569. doi:10.1007/BF00935358

Parkes, K. R. (1982). Occupational stress among student nurses: A natural experiment. *Journal of Applied Psychology, 67*, 784–796. doi:10.1037/0021-9010.67.6.784

Payne, N. (2001). Occupational stressors and coping as determinants of burnout in female hospice nurses. *Journal of Advanced Nursing, 33*, 3, 396–405. doi:10.1046/j.1365-2648.2001.01677.x

Peck, A. H. (1984). Psychiatric aspects of workmen's compensation problems. *Emotional First Aid, 1*(3), 23–29.

Pegula, S. M. (2004). *An analysis of workplace suicides, 1992–2001.* Washington, DC: Bureau of Labor Statistics.

Pietrzak, R. H., Schechter, C. B., Bromet, E. J., Katz, C. L., Reissman, D. B., Ozbay, F., . . . Southwick, S. M. (2012). The burden of full and subsyndromal posttraumatic stress disorder among police involved in the World Trade Center rescue and recovery effort. *Journal of Psychiatric Research, 46*, 835–842. doi:10.1016/j.jpsychires.2012.03.011

Police Roll of Honour Trust. (2015). Retrieved from www.policememorial.org.uk/index.php?page=roll-2014

Rader, D. (1993, October 10). An actor deals with his dark side. *Parade*, pp. 4–5.

Rathge, R. W., Ekstrom, B. L., & Leistritz, F. L. (1988). The effects of economic strain on stress in farm families. *Farm Research, 45*(4), 19–22.

Reaves, B. A. (2011). *Census of state and local law enforcement agencies, 2008.* Washington, DC: U.S. Department of Justice, Bureau of Justice Statistics.

Reed, D. B., Browning, S. R., Westneat, S. C., & Kidd, P. S. (2006). Personal protective equipment use and safety behaviors among farm adolescents: Gender differences and predictors of work practices. *Journal of Rural Health, 22*, 314–320. doi:10.1111/j.1748-0361.2006.00052.x

Reuters. (1983, February 18). Brush fires in Australia rage on: 69 reported dead and 1,000 hurt. *New York Times.* Retrieved from www.nytimes.com/1983/02/18/world/brush-fires-in-australia-rage-on-69-reported-dead-and-1000-hurt.html

Riese, H., Van Doornen, L. J. P., Houtman, I. L. D., & De Geus, E. J. C. (2004). Job strain in relation to ambulatory blood pressure, heart rate, and heart rate variability among female nurses. *Scandinavian Journal of Work, Environment & Health, 30*, 477–485. doi:10.103TO0278-6133.19.5.429

Roberts, R. E., & Lee, E. S. (1993). Occupation and the prevalence of major depression, alcohol, and drug abuse in the United States. *Environmental Research, 61*(2), 266–278.

Robinson, H. M., Sigman, M. R., & Wilson, J. P. (1997). Duty-related stressors and PTSD symptoms in suburban police officers. *Psychological Reports, 81*, 835–845. doi:10.2466/pr0.1997.81.3.835

Rosenbaum, D. A., Mora, D. C., Arcury, T. A., Chen, H., & Quandt, S. A. (2014). Employer differences in upper-body musculoskeletal disorders and pain among immigrant Latino poultry processing workers. *Journal of Agromedicine, 19*, 384–394. doi:10.1080/1059924X.2014.945710

Schiöler, L., Söderberg, M., Rosengren, A., Järvholm, B., & Torén, K. (2015). Psychosocial work environment and risk of ischemic stroke and coronary heart disease: A prospective longitudinal study of 75 236 construction workers. *Scandinavian Journal of Work, Environment & Health, 41*(3), 280–287. doi:10.5271/sjweh.3491

Schonfeld, I. S. (2000). An updated look at depressive symptoms and job satisfaction in first-year women teachers. *Journal of Occupational and Organizational Psychology, 73*, 363–371. doi:10.1348/096317900167074

Schonfeld, I. S. (2001). Stress in 1st-year women teachers: The context of social support and coping. *Genetic, Social, and General Psychology Monographs, 127*(2), 133–168.

Schonfeld, I. S. (2006). School violence. In E. K. Kelloway, J. Barling, & J. J. Hurrell, Jr. (Eds.), *Handbook of workplace violence* (pp. 169–229). Thousand Oaks, CA: Sage.

Schonfeld, I. S., & Farrell, E. (2010). Qualitative methods can enrich quantitative research on occupational stress: An example from one occupational group. In P. Perrewé & D. C. Ganster (Eds.), *Research in occupational stress and well-being* (pp. 137–197). Bingley, UK: Emerald.

Schonfeld, I. S., & Feinman, S. J. (2012). Difficulties of alternatively certified teachers. *Education and Urban Society, 44*, 215–246. doi:10.1177/0013124510392570

Schulman, M. D., & Armstrong, P. S. (1990). Perceived stress, social support, and survival: North Carolina farm operators and the farm crisis. *Journal of Sociology and Social Welfare, 17*(3), 3–22.

Shirom, A., Oliver, A., & Stein, E. (2009). Teachers' stressors and strains: A longitudinal study of their relationships. *International Journal of Stress Management, 16*, 312–332. doi:10.1037/a0016842

Simmons, L. A., Braun, B., Charnigo, R., Havens, J. R., & Wright, D. W. (2008). Depression and poverty among rural women: A relationship of social causation or social selection? *Journal of Rural Health, 24,* 292–298. doi:10.1111/j.1748-0361.2008.00171.x

Siu, O.-L., Phillips, D. R., & Leung, T.-W. (2004). Safety climate and safety performance among construction workers in Hong Kong: The role of psychological strains as mediators. *Accident Analysis and Prevention, 36,* 359–366. doi:10.1016/S0001-4575(03)00016-2

Smith, J. A., Masuhara, K. L., & Frueh, B. C. (2014). Documented suicides within the British Army during the Crimean War 1854–1856. *Military Medicine, 179,* 721–723. doi:10.7205/MILMED-D-13-00547

Soo, J., Webber, M. P., Gustave, J., Lee, R., Hall, C. B., Cohen, H. W., . . . Prezant, D. J. (2011). Trends in probable PTSD in firefighters exposed to the World Trade Center disaster, 2001–2010. *Disaster Medicine and Public Health Preparedness, 5,* S197–S203. doi:10.1001/dmp.2011.48

Spence Laschinger, H. K., & Finegan, J. (2008). Situational and dispositional predictors of nurse manager burnout: A time-lagged analysis. *Journal of Nursing Management, 16,* 601–607. doi:10.1111/j.1365-2834.2008.00904.x

Spiegel, H. X. (1944). Psychiatric observations in the Tunisian campaign. *American Journal of Orthopsychiatry, 14,* 381–385. doi:10.1111/j.1939-0025.1944.tb04892.x

Stack, S. (2001). Occupation and suicide. *Social Science Quarterly, 82,* 384–396. doi:10.1111/0038-4941.00030

Stellman, J. M., Smith, R. P., Katz, C. L., Sharma, V., Charney, D. S., Herbert, R., . . . Southwick, S. (2008). Enduring mental health morbidity and social function impairment in World Trade Center rescue, recovery, and cleanup workers: The psychological dimension of an environmental health disaster. *Environmental Health Perspectives, 116,* 1248–1253. doi:10.1289/ehp.11164

Stouffer, S. A., Lumsdaine, A. A., Lumsdaine, M. H., Williams, R. M., Jr., Smith, M. B., Janis, I. L., . . . Cottrell, L. S., Jr. (1949). *The American soldier: Combat and its aftermath* (Vol. 2). Princeton, NJ: Princeton University Press.

Stuart, H. (2008). Suicidality among police. *Current Opinion in Psychiatry, 21,* 505–509. doi:10.1097/YCO.0b013e328305e4c1

Swank, R. L. (1949). Combat exhaustion: A descriptive and statistical analysis of causes, symptoms and signs. *Journal of Nervous and Mental Disease, 109,* 475–508. doi:10.1097/00005053-194910960-00001

Swedler, D. I., Simmons, M. M., Dominici, F., & Hemenway, D. (2015). Firearm prevalence and homicides of law enforcement officers in the United States. *American Journal of Public Health, 105,* 2042–2048. doi:10.2105/AJPH.2015.302749

Tanielian, T., & Jaycox, L. H. (2008). *A comprehensive study of the post-deployment health-related needs associated with post-traumatic stress disorder, major depression, and traumatic brain injury among service members returning from Operations Enduring Freedom and Iraqi Freedom.* Santa Monica, CA: Rand.

Tiesman, H. M., Konda, S., Hartley, D., Menéndez, C. C., Ridenour, M., & Hendricks, S. (2015). Suicide in U.S. workplaces, 2003–2010: A comparison with non-workplace suicides. *American Journal of Preventive Medicine, 48,* 674–682. doi:10.1016/j.amepre.2014.12.011

Travers, C. J., & Cooper, C. L. (1993). Mental health, job satisfaction and occupational stress among UK teachers. *Work & Stress, 7,* 137–146. doi:10.1080/02678379308257062

Trinkoff, A. M., Eaton, W. W., & Anthony, J. C. (1991). The prevalence of substance abuse among registered nurses. *Nursing Research, 40,* 172–175. doi:10.1097/00006199-199105000-00011

Ursano, R. J., Kessler, R. C., Stein, M. B., Naifeh, J. A., Aliaga, P. A., Fullerton, C. S., . . . Heeringa, S. G. (2015). Suicide attempts in the US Army during the wars in Afghanistan and Iraq, 2004 to 2009. *Journal of the American Medical Association: Psychiatry, 72*(9), 917–926. doi:10.1001/jamapsychiatry.2015.0987

U.S. Fire Administration. (2014). *Firefighter fatalities in the United States in 2013.* Washington, DC: U.S. Department of Homeland Security, Federal Emergency Management Agency.

U.S. Fire Administration. (2015). *U.S. fire statistics.* Washington, DC: U.S. Department of Homeland Security, Federal Emergency Management Agency. Retrieved from www.usfa.fema.gov/data/statistics

Vasterling, J. J., Proctor, S. P., Friedman, M. J., Hoge, C. W., Heeren, T., King, L. A., & King, D. W. (2010). PTSD symptom increases in Iraq-deployed soldiers: Comparison with nondeployed soldiers and associations with baseline symptoms, deployment experiences, and postdeployment stress. *Journal of Traumatic Stress, 23,* 41–51. doi:10.1002/jts.20487

Violanti, J. M. (2011). Recent national studies on police suicide. In J. M. Violanti, A. F. O'Hara, & T. T. Tate (Eds.), *On the edge: Recent perspectives on police suicide* (pp. 17–31). Springfield, IL: Charles C. Thomas.

Violanti, J. M., Robinson, C. F., & Shen, R. (2013). Law enforcement suicide: A national analysis. *International Journal of Emergency Mental Health and Human Resilience, 15*(4), 289–297.

Violanti, J. M., Vena, J. E., & Petralla, S. (1998). Mortality of a police cohort: 1950–1990. *American Journal of Industrial Medicine, 33*(4), 366–373.

Wagner, D., Heinrichs, M., & Ehlert, U. (1998). Prevalence of symptoms of posttraumatic stress disorder in German professional firefighters. *American Journal of Psychiatry, 155*(12), 1727–1732.

Wang, L., Wheeler, K., Bai, L., Stallones, L., Dong, Y., Ge, J., & Xiang, H. (2010). Alcohol consumption and work-related injuries among farmers in Heilongjiang province, People's Republic of China. *American Journal of Industrial Medicine, 53*, 825–835. doi:10.1002/ajim.20817

The White House. (2003). *Homeland Security Presidential Directive/HSPD-8*. Washington, DC: Author. Retrieved from www.fas.org/irp/offdocs/nspd/hspd-8.html

Wisnivesky, J. P., Teitelbaum, S. L., Todd, A. C., Boffetta, P., Crane, M., Crowley, L., . . . Landrigan, P. J. (2011). Persistence of multiple illnesses in World Trade Center rescue and recovery workers: A cohort study. *The Lancet, 378*(9794), 888–897. doi:10.1016/S0140-6736(11)61180-X

Wulsin, L., Alterman, T., Bushnell, P. T., Li, J., & Shen, R. (2014). Prevalence rates for depression by industry: A claims database analysis. *Social Psychiatry and Psychiatric Epidemiology, 49*, 1805–1821. doi:10.1007/s00127-014-0891-3

Zangaro, G. A., & Soeken, K. L. (2007). A meta-analysis of studies of nurses' job satisfaction. *Research in Nursing & Health, 30*, 445–458. doi:10.1002/nur.20202

EIGHT

Occupational Safety

KEY CONCEPTS AND FINDINGS COVERED IN CHAPTER 8

Risk factors in the physical work environment
Occupational health psychology and occupational safety
>*Individual antecedents of safety performance and workplace accidents and injuries*
>>*Demographics*
>>*Personality*
>>*Ability factors*
>>*Motivation-related differences*
>*Situational antecedents of safety performance and workplace accidents and injuries*
>>*Job characteristics*
>>*Shift work*
>*Implications of considering individual and situational antecedents for safety*
Summary

Occupational safety is an important topic area within occupational health psychology (OHP). Indeed, by any judgment, accidents in the workplace are a major concern for workers and employers alike. Unfortunately, the prevalence of workplace accidents and the resulting fatalities and injuries are disheartening. In each year from 2000 to 2013, between 4,500 and 6,000 U.S. workers suffered fatal injuries at work (Bureau of Labor Statistics [BLS], 2015a), figures that average about 15 workers dying each day. Among the member-countries of the European Union (E.U.), between 3,900 and 5,800 workers suffered fatal injuries at work every year between 2000 and 2012 (Eurostat, 2015), an average of about 13 workers dying each day. Although the numbers of fatal incidents and the fatality rates have declined over recent years (see Table 8.1), the number of fatalities remains a serious concern.

In addition to fatal injuries, the number of nonfatal incidents and the rates of nonfatal occupational injuries and illnesses are also a major concern. Based on the latest statistics, there were about 3 million cases of nonfatal workplace injuries and illnesses reported by private employers in 2013 in the United States, or about 3.3 cases per 100 full-time equivalent workers (BLS, 2015b). In other words, three in every 100 workers were injured or fell sick because of job-related conditions. Of the 3 million injuries and illnesses, over half were serious enough to result in days away from work, job transfers, or job restrictions due to loss of capacity (BLS, 2015b). In 2012, about 3.2 million work-related injuries were reported in the E.U., or about 1.6 cases per 100 full-time equivalent workers (Eurostat, 2015). Taken together, work-related fatalities, injuries, and illnesses represent a severe threat to workers' health and safety.

TABLE 8.1 Work-Related Fatalities in the European Union and United States				
	2000		**2012 or 2013**	
	No. of Fatalities	**1-Year Rate Per 100,000**	**No. of Fatalities**	**1-Year Rate Per 100,000**
E.U.	5,327	2.8	3,918[a]	1.9[a]
U.S.	5,920	4.3	4,585[b]	3.3[b]

[a]Applies to 2012. [b]Applies to 2013.

Although it is difficult to estimate, the financial cost of workplace injuries and illnesses to individual workers and their employers is a major economic burden. The Liberty Mutual Research Institute for Safety (2014) estimated the direct workers' compensation costs associated with the 10 most disabling workplace injuries and illnesses (e.g., overexertion due to lifting, pushing; falls to the same or a different level; having been struck by objects or equipment) that occurred in the United States in 2012. Liberty Mutual found that total direct workers' compensation costs were almost $60 billion. This estimate means that, on average, businesses spent over a billion U.S. dollars per week on injuries.

In addition, Leigh (2011) estimated, using 2007 statistics, the total costs associated with workplace fatal and nonfatal injuries and illnesses. He reported that the costs associated with workplace fatal and nonfatal injures totaled $6 and $186 billion, respectively, a higher estimate than the numbers published by the Liberty Mutual Research Institute for Safety. Moreover, according to Leigh, work-related fatal and nonfatal illnesses were estimated to cost $46 and $12 billion, respectively. These estimates included both direct medical expenses (e.g., hospital stay, doctor's visit, medication; together, these accounted for 27% of the total cost) and indirect costs such as individual workers' lost wages and benefits, employers' cost of hiring and training replacement workers, and workers' compensation administrative costs. These numbers are astonishingly high and do not include other hidden costs for both the remaining workers and their organizations, such as lower employee morale, higher stress, and tarnished organizational reputation (Kaplan & Tetrick, 2011).

Given the seriousness of the issue, it is not surprising that researchers and practitioners from multiple disciplines, including OHP, have been engaged in efforts to identify ways to improve worker safety and reduce risks of injuries and fatalities. In the following sections, we will first briefly review the fields that aim to identify and control risks associated with the physical work environment, and then discuss how the theories and practices associated with OHP complement other disciplinary approaches to improving occupational safety.

RISK FACTORS IN THE PHYSICAL WORK ENVIRONMENT

The approaches that focus on the physical threats to occupational safety include industrial hygiene and ergonomics. According to the U.S. Department of Labor's Occupational Safety and Health Administration (OSHA, 1998), industrial hygiene is "the science of anticipating, recognizing, evaluating, and controlling workplace conditions that may cause workers' injury or illness." These workplace conditions

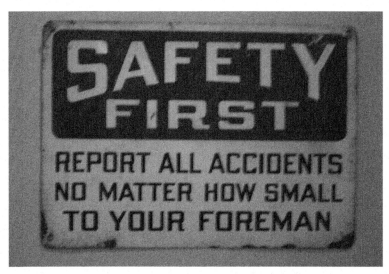

Safety first. (Photographer unknown. Photo courtesy of NIOSH. Public domain.)

include biological, chemical, and physical hazards that may cause or contribute to occupational injuries, illnesses, or discomfort in workers (Herrick & Dement, 2005). Biological hazards refer to "vermin, insects, molds, fungi, viruses, and bacterial contaminants" (Reese, 2008, p. 174). For example, health care workers such as nurses are often exposed to biological hazards, such as blood and viruses, whereas farmers are more likely to be exposed to hazards such as insect bites and animal droppings. Chemical hazards come from "airborne concentration of mists, vapors, gasses, or solids that are in the form of dusts or fumes" (Reese, 2008, pp. 175). Common chemical hazards include pesticides, liquids such as cleaning products and paints, gases such as carbon monoxide and propane, and flammable materials such as gasoline (American Federation of Teachers, 2010). Other hazards include radiation, noise, vibration, and extremes of temperature (Reese, 2008). For example, construction workers who work outdoors may be exposed to extreme weather conditions, and manufacturing workers may be exposed to loud noises on the factory floor.

Industrial hygienists identify workplace hazards by conducting exposure assessments. By taking samples from the workplace (e.g., evaluating air samples to check for chemical hazards), industrial hygienists monitor the extent to which exposures occur (Reese, 2008). Industrial hygienists also help establish the exposure guidelines for various chemical hazards. Because industrial hygiene focuses on the assessment of exposure to hazards, their work is crucial for developing primary intervention programs designed to prevent occupational injuries and illnesses by eliminating those hazards (Herrick & Dement, 2005). However, when the complete removal of hazards is not possible, industrial hygienists may recommend the use of personal protective equipment (e.g., masks or respirators, gloves, earmuffs) to minimize exposure (Reese, 2008).

Ergonomics is concerned with understanding the interaction between humans and their work environments, and focuses on designing jobs, work activities, and work environments to better fit the worker (Reese, 2008). The primary health effect that ergonomics seeks to prevent is musculoskeletal disorders (MSDs). According to the National Institute for Occupational Safety and Health (n.d.), or NIOSH, MSDs

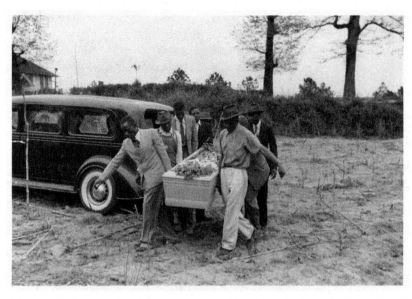

Funeral of a 19-year-old African American sawmill worker, Heard County, Georgia, May 1941. (Photographer is Jack Delano for the U.S. Farm Security Administration. Public domain).

are "injuries or disorders of the muscles, nerves, tendons, joints, cartilage, and disorders of the nerves, tendons, muscles and supporting structures" that result from sudden exertions or "prolonged exposure to physical factors such as repetition, force, vibration, or awkward posture."

Work-related MSDs are one of the leading causes of worker absence and disability (Punnett & Wegman, 2004). In the United States in 2013, MSDs accounted for 33% of all injury and illness cases that required days away from work (BLS, 2014). Workers who reported work-related MSDs took a median of 11 days to recover before returning to work, compared with 8 days for all types of injuries and illnesses (BLS, 2014). Common work-related MSDs include sprains and strains, back pain, and carpal tunnel syndrome (Reese, 2008).

Ergonomists seek to prevent work-related MSDs by conducting ergonomics hazard analyses and redesigning work tasks or modifying workstations to eliminate or minimize hazards (Reese, 2008). Typical ergonomic risk factors that may cause excessive biomechanical load on workers' bodies include force (e.g., lifting heavy objects), repetition, awkward or static postures, and vibration. Once identified, ergonomists may redesign work tasks to limit the duration, frequency, and magnitude of the exposures to hazards (Reese, 2008). In addition, workstations may also be redesigned to better fit the workers and reduce exposure to ergonomic risks. Both approaches can be considered primary interventions as both involve removing exposure risks for workers.

OCCUPATIONAL HEALTH PSYCHOLOGY AND OCCUPATIONAL SAFETY

OHP advances occupational safety and health beyond what the traditional approaches of industrial hygiene and ergonomics contribute. First, OHP applies psychological theory and research to improve workers' overall safety and well-being (Tetrick &

Peiró, 2012). The discipline makes individuals its central concern, and considers how their psychological processes can have implications for health- and safety-related outcomes. OHP considers how individuals perceive, make sense of, and react to the physical and interpersonal environment of the workplace. Psychological interpretations of the work environment may explain variance in employee health and safety beyond what physical, biological, and chemical hazards explain. The strategy known as Total Worker Health™ (TWH), launched by NIOSH in 2011, reflects a perspective that incorporates principles of OHP.[1] TWH integrates the traditional programs of occupational safety and health protection with workplace practices that focus on enhancing physical wellness and psychological well-being (NIOSH, 2015). Central to this strategy is the idea that factors that affect workers' psychological well-being, such as stress and support, also affect physical health and safety. Extant research supports this view by showing that stressors such as job demands, role conflict, and work–family conflict are directly related to workers' injuries and musculoskeletal pain (Bodner, Kraner, Bradford, Hammer, & Truxillo, 2014; Eatough, Way, & Chang, 2012; also see Chapter 4). On the other hand, work characteristics such as organizational support, autonomy, and team cohesion are related to lower risk of injuries and musculoskeletal symptoms (Bodner et al., 2014; Eatough et al., 2012; Sobeih, Salem, Daraiseh, Genaidy, & Shell, 2006). Interventions based on the TWH approach have been shown to lead to changes in workers' health behaviors (e.g., smoking cessation, exercising: Sorensen et al., 2002) and safety-related outcomes (e.g., protection against exposure to hazardous materials: LaMontagne, Stoddard, Youngstrom, Lewiton, & Sorensen, 2005).

A second contribution is that a line of OHP research has demonstrated the efficacy of integrating psychological processes with the traditional approaches to occupational safety. For example, Sauter and Swanson (1996) proposed an ecological model to understand the joint effects of physical task demands (and the resulting biomechanical strain) combined with workplace psychosocial characteristics (and the resulting psychological strain) on workers' musculoskeletal injuries. This model not only explicitly recognizes that psychological strain may exacerbate the effects of biomechanical strain on musculoskeletal injuries, but also involves decision-making processes to highlight how individuals, given the same task with similar biomechanical load, may report different levels of symptoms depending on the psychosocial work environment. Although some of the earlier research did not consistently support the implications of psychosocial characteristics of the workplace and work stress on musculoskeletal injuries (e.g., Swanson & Sauter, 2006), more recent research (e.g., Chang, Bernard, Bloswick, & Johnson, 2015; Eatough et al., 2012; Golubovich, Chang, & Eatough, 2014) has underlined the importance of stress-related mechanisms in employees' reports and reactions to musculoskeletal injuries. For example, Golubovich et al. (2014) showed that poor safety climate, which was conceptualized as a stressor, was related to higher employee frustration, which, in turn, was related to higher levels of musculoskeletal pains in the neck, shoulders, upper back, and lower back regions, controlling for physical job demands. This tendency was attenuated when employees reported high levels of psychological hardiness, suggesting that people vary in resilience in the context of stress and frustration.

---

[1] TWH is reprised in Chapter 11.

Similarly, controlling for physical job demands, Eatough et al. (2012) found that the effects of stressors (e.g., role conflict) on musculoskeletal symptoms was mediated by emotional strain. Chang et al. (2015) found that perceived supervisor support lessened the connection between musculoskeletal injuries and employee absenteeism, suggesting that employees may use different coping strategies to deal with discomfort, depending on the psychosocial context of their workplace.

A third contribution of OHP to occupational safety is its focus on contextual factors that can influence safety-related outcomes (Tetrick & Peiró, 2012). OHP researchers regard occupational safety as embedded within a psychosocial and interpersonal context. Hazards in the workplace cannot be addressed in isolation. Rather, characteristics of the psychosocial environment, such as group cohesion, workplace support, leadership, and workplace climate, can have important implications for occupational safety (Tetrick & Peiró, 2012). Chapter 6 provides more comprehensive coverage of issues related to climate and leadership and their effects on occupational health and safety.

A fourth contribution of OHP is its refinement of the criteria for evaluating workplace safety. Building on the performance management literature within industrial and organizational psychology, OHP highlights the distinction between two types of safety-related criteria: safety performance versus safety outcomes (Kaplan & Tetrick, 2011). The former refers to workers' behaviors that contribute to the maintenance and enhancement of workplace safety, and can be further differentiated along two dimensions: safety compliance and safety participation. Compliance reflects the core, required behaviors to maintain workplace safety, such as following safety protocols and wearing protective gear (Neal & Griffin, 2006). Participation refers to behaviors, although not prescribed by management, that enhance workplace safety by supporting a safety-conscious psychosocial environment. Safety participation includes behaviors such as serving on safety committees and assisting coworkers with safety-related problems (Neal & Griffin, 2006). Safety outcomes, on the other hand, reflect accidents, near misses, and occupational injuries (Kaplan & Tetrick, 2011). The key distinction between safety performance and safety outcomes is that although safety performance is largely under the control of individual workers, external factors, such as nature of the tasks and industries (along with safety performance) may influence safety outcomes. Differentiating between safety performance and safety outcomes allows researchers and practitioners to identify safety-related criteria at either the safety-performance or safety-outcome level, and then design interventions to target outcome criteria relevant to either or both levels.

Finally, OHP not only differentiates between safety behaviors and safety outcomes, but also builds the conceptual clarity of the safety performance construct. For example, Neal and Griffin (2006) distinguished between safety compliance and participation, with the former being more in-role and compulsory, and the latter, more extrarole and voluntary. Hofmann, Morgeson, and Gerras (2003) also differentiated between in- and extrarole safety performance. Their conceptualization focused on extrarole safety performance. They also identified six extrarole safety performance dimensions: helping, voice, stewardship, whistle-blowing, civic virtue, and initiating safety-related change. Burke, Sarpy, Tesluk, and Smith-Crowe (2002), after reviewing the research literature and safety training materials from the hazardous waste industry, proposed a four-dimensional structure for safety performance constructs. These dimensions include using personal protective equipment, engaging in practices that reduce risks of accidents, communicating information related to health and safety, and exercising employee rights and responsibilities. The efforts of Neal and Griffin (2006), Hofman et al. (2003), and Burke et al. (2002) have refined the construct clarity of safety performance and delineated the criterion space needed to better understand factors contributing to various safety-related outcomes. In the next section, we discuss key antecedents for safety performance and accidents and injuries in the workplace.

Individual Antecedents of Safety Performance and Workplace Accidents and Injuries

Historically, most OHP research on antecedents of safety-related outcomes concerned individual differences and characteristics of the work environment. In this section, we will discuss the major findings pertaining to individual characteristics as antecedents for safety-related outcomes.

Demographics

Research on occupational health disparities has consistently identified differences in the risk of accidents and injuries across demographic groups, including genders and racial, ethnic, and age groups. In general, male workers are more likely to be employed by high-injury/illness occupations, and tend to have higher rates of occupational fatalities (Steege, Baron, Marsh, Menédez, & Myers, 2014). Racial and ethnic minorities such as Blacks and Hispanics also tend to be employed in high-risk occupations, and they tend to suffer higher rates of injuries, illnesses, and fatalities (Stanbury & Rosenman, 2014; Steege et al., 2014). For example, work-related homicide rates were higher for Blacks and foreign-born workers (Steege et al., 2014). Moreover, compared with Whites, Blacks were more likely to suffer from work-related illnesses such as silicosis and asthma; in addition, Hispanics had higher rates of pesticide-related injuries and illnesses than non-Hispanics (Stanbury & Rosenman, 2014). Finally, older workers are more likely to suffer from workplace fatalities compared with younger workers (Steege et al., 2014).

Although these research findings suggest that demographic factors may predict safety-related outcomes, much of the literature also indicates some of the sources of the observed differences between genders and racial/ethnic and age groups may be attributable to other factors. First, males, racial/ethnic minority group members, and older workers are more likely to be employed in lower paid and higher risk occupations (e.g., Krieger, 2009; Murray, 2003; Stanbury & Rosenman, 2014). As such, they are likely exposed to more occupational hazards, and thus exhibit higher rates of illnesses, injuries, and fatalities.

Moving beyond specific occupational types to demographic characteristics, Landsbergis, Grzywacz, and LaMontagne (2014) found that racial and ethnic minorities and individuals in lower socioeconomic positions are more exposed to troublesome organizational conditions. These conditions include job insecurity, less autonomy, less support, fewer opportunities to learn new skills, and reduced employer concern for worker safety. Such conditions are linked to higher risk for occupational injuries and illnesses. Okechukwu, Souza, Davis, and de Castro (2014) synthesized research on workplace experiences of racial/ethnic minority workers. Okechukwu et al. (2014) showed that minority workers are likely to experience more workplace injustice, such as discrimination, harassment, abuse, and bullying. Unfair treatment may contribute not only directly to adverse health and safety outcomes, but also indirectly by leading to "differential assignment to hazardous duties" (Okechukwu et al., 2014). Similarly, Meyer (2014) found that among Black workers, race-based discrimination in hiring and promotion was related to lower levels of perceived job control, which, in turn, predicted poorer self-rated health (see Chapter 4) 10 years later, controlling for self-rated health at baseline. For White workers, perceived job control did not mediate the relationship between discrimination (discrimination was rarely reported by Whites) and self-rated health. Research results suggest that the poor treatment that minority group members receive may contribute to the incidents of occupational illnesses and injuries.

Personality

Personality refers to individuals' predispositions to behave in a particular way across different situations. The most widely accepted model of personality is the Big Five model (Levy, 2013). The Big Five model characterizes individuals' traits along five broad dimensions: openness to experience, conscientiousness, extraversion, agreeableness, and neuroticism. Openness reflects individuals' general appreciation for a variety of experiences and willingness to try new and different things. Conscientiousness refers to an orientation for achievement and the tendency to demonstrate self-discipline. Extroverted individuals enjoy interacting with other people, and derive energy from engaging in interpersonal interactions. Agreeableness reflects individuals' general concern for social harmony and getting along with others. Finally, individuals who are high on neuroticism tend to experience more negative emotions such as anger, anxiety, and depression, and are more reactive to challenging or demanding situations (Costa & McCrae, 1992).

Conscientiousness, compared with the other dimensions of personality, has been a consistent predictor of safety performance. Multiple meta-analyses have shown that a high level of conscientiousness is related to increased safety behaviors at work (e.g., Christian, Bradley, Wallace, & Burke, 2009; Beus, Dhanani, & McCord, 2015). In addition, empirical studies have shown that conscientiousness predicted greater self- and other-rated safety compliance and safety participation above and beyond situational variables such as leadership (e.g., Inness, Turner, Barling, & Stride, 2010) and safety climate (e.g., Wallace & Chen, 2006). Meta-analytic results also suggest that agreeableness is associated with higher levels of safety behaviors at work, whereas extraversion is related to lower levels (Beus et al., 2015). Interestingly, neuroticism exhibited a complex pattern of relationship with safety behaviors. Although some facets of neuroticism, such as anger and impulsiveness, were related to lower levels of safety behaviors, anxiety, another facet of neuroticism, was related to increased safety behaviors (Beus et al., 2015). This pattern of findings suggests that a finer-grained approach may be helpful for understanding the relationships between personality traits and safety performance.

In addition to safety performance, personality traits have also been linked to safety outcomes. Conscientiousness has been shown to be consistently, and negatively, related to workplace accidents and injuries (e.g., Beus et al., 2015; Christian et al., 2009; Clarke & Robertson, 2008). Meta-analytic findings have also shown that agreeableness is negatively related to workplace accidents (Beus et al., 2015; Clarke & Robertson, 2005, 2008). On the other hand, neuroticism has appeared to have a consistent, positive association with accidents (Clarke & Robertson, 2005, 2008) and injuries (Christian et al., 2009). Finally, some meta-analytic studies have found a positive relationship between openness to experiences and accidents (e.g., Beus et al.,

2015; Clarke & Robertson, 2005), whereas other studies (e.g., Christian et al., 2009; Clarke & Robertson, 2008) have found only limited support for this relationship.

Importantly, researchers tend to agree that personality traits are related to safety-related outcomes through an individual's values and motivations. For example, Christian et al. (2009) found that high conscientiousness is associated with increased motivation for safety, which, in turn, leads to higher safety performance. Beus et al. (2015) showed that agreeableness and conscientiousness were related to fewer accidents through increased safety performance. On the other hand, the investigators found that the relationship of extraversion and neuroticism to increased accident risk was mediated by lower safety performance. Taken together, it is possible to argue that personality traits may drive individuals' values and priorities at work, which, in turn, influence attention and effort regarding safety-related behaviors.

In addition to the Big Five personality traits, other researchers have examined additional stable traits and the traits' relationships with safety-related outcomes. Some of these traits are similar to the Big Five traits and have demonstrated similar patterns of relationships with safety-related outcomes. For example, negative affectivity (NA) refers to individuals' tendency to experience more negative emotions and has been linked to neuroticism. Research on NA has shown that it is associated with lower safety compliance and participation (Inness et al., 2010). Similarly, compliance, which can be viewed as a facet of conscientiousness, was positively related to safety performance (Hogan & Foster, 2013). Other researchers have focused on relationships of self-evaluations and attributes to safety-related outcomes. Meta-analytic findings suggest that a high internal locus of control, or the belief that one controls the events in one's own life, is positively related to safety compliance and participation (Christian et al., 2009). On the other hand, having a positive general evaluation of oneself may be both a benefit and a liability. Whereas some studies (e.g., Yuan, Li, & Lin, 2014) have shown that a high self-evaluation is associated with high safety performance, other research suggests that a high level of confidence in one's own ability is negatively related to construction workers' safety performance (Salanova, Lorente, & Martínez, 2012). It is also possible that self-evaluation may have a curvilinear relationship with safety-related outcomes. Although a moderate level of positive self-evaluation is beneficial for safety performance, extremely high levels of efficacy beliefs may result in workers ignoring safety rules because they believe that they can perform tasks without taking the necessary precautions.

Ability Factors

Research on ability factors and safety-related outcomes has focused mostly on cognitively related abilities and attention regulation. Interestingly, results concerning workers' cognitive ability or general intelligence and safety-related outcomes have been equivocal. Some studies found that cognitive ability was positively related to safety performance (Postlethwaite, Robbins, Rickerson, & McKinniss, 2009). By contrast, other studies found that after controlling for traits such as Big Five personality factors, cognitive ability was unrelated to accident involvement (Hansen, 1989; Kotzé & Steyn, 2013). Still other research has examined the interactive effects of cognitive ability and personality traits. For example, Postlethwaite et al. (2009) found that cognitive ability interacted with conscientiousness in predicting workers' safety behavior. In particular, cognitive ability was positively related to safety performance when conscientiousness was low, and unrelated to safety performance when conscientiousness was high. In this case, cognitive ability appears to buffer the negative effects of low conscientiousness on safety-related outcomes.

In addition to general cognitive ability, research has also underlined the importance of cognitive and emotional safety engagement. "Cognitive safety engagement" refers to "attention to, and concentration on the safe execution of work tasks" (Wachter & Yorio, 2014, p. 125); "emotional safety engagement" refers to enthusiasm for and pride in workplace safety programs. Both cognitive and emotional safety engagement were found to be negatively related to workplace injuries (Wachter & Yorio). Moreover, positive safety management practices were related to higher levels of workers' cognitive and emotional safety engagement (Wachter & Yorio).

Interestingly, considerably more research has examined the implications of workers' ineffective regulation of cognitive attention and memory, or "cognitive failure," on safety-related outcomes. According to Wallace and Vodanovich (2003), cognitive failure refers to "a breakdown in cognitive functioning that results in a cognitively based mistake [in the execution of a task] that a person should normally be capable of completing" (p. 316). It also shows some trait-like stability over time. Cognitive failure has been linked to lower safety performance rated by self and supervisors (Wallace & Chen, 2005; Wallace & Vodanovich, 2003). In addition, cognitive failure was found to have positive association with self-reported micro-accidents, serious accidents, and injuries (Wallace & Chen, 2005; Wallace & Vodanovich, 2003). Cognitive failure also mediated the effects of work interruptions on near misses in a nursing sample, such that nurses who were interrupted during a task were more likely to report failures in their attention and memory, which in turn were associated with higher incidents of near misses. Day, Brasher, and Bridger (2012), employing a case-control design, compared cognitive failure in sailors in the Royal Navy who were involved in an accident and sailors who were not. Day et al. (2012) found that after controlling for gender, age, and job level, those who were involved in accidents reported higher levels of cognitive failure. Overall, failure to regulate one's memory and attention at work appeared to have detrimental effects on occupational safety.

In addition to its main effect, cognitive failure at work may have spillover effects on workers' safety in nonwork settings. For example, Elfering, Grebner, and Haller (2012) found that cognitive failure at work was positively related to risky driving behaviors during workers' commute from work to home. Cognitive failure at work was also positively related to traffic accidents and near misses during commutes to and from work (Elfering, Grebner, & de Tribolet-Hardy, 2013). Finally, work-related cognitive failure was positively related to domestic falls (Elfering, Grebner, & Boillat, 2013).

Much like cognitive ability, cognitive failure also interacted with conscientiousness in predicting safety behaviors and accidents. Cognitive failure had a weaker, positive relationship with unsafe behavior and accidents when employees reported high levels of conscientiousness (Elfering et al., 2013; Wallace & Vodanovich, 2003). This finding suggests that high cognitive failure accentuates the negative association between conscientiousness and unsafe behaviors and accidents. Taken together, these results underscore the importance of effective cognitive attention and memory regulation on workers' safety.

Motivation-Related Differences

A number of motivation-related individual differences have been thought to be antecedents of safety-related outcomes. A meta-analysis (Christian et al., 2009) showed that employees' safety motivation is positively related to safety compliance. Safety motivation was negatively related to OSHA recordable injuries and injuries that resulted in days away from work (Wachter & Yorio, 2014). Importantly, safety motivation appeared to mediate the effects of other distal individual traits and situational characteristics on safety-related outcomes. For example, safety motivation mediated the positive relation of conscientiousness to safety behaviors (Christian et al., 2009). The effect of safety management practice on OSHA recordable injuries and injuries that resulted in days away from work was mediated by safety motivation (Wachter & Yorio, 2014).

Relatedly, research has examined organizational practices that may promote employees' motivation to work in a safe manner. In particular, goal-setting practices (e.g., being "accident free" for 30 consecutive days) and associated compensation or rewards (e.g., giving everyone a $100 bonus if the goal of being accident free for 30 days is met) have been implemented to promote safety. Empirical evidence suggests that lack of goal setting at the workplace is associated with an increased likelihood for injuries (Leung, Chan, & Yu, 2012). Moreover, case studies have suggested that both outcome- (i.e., accident free) and behavior-based (i.e., safety performance) incentive programs can reduce accidents (Yeow & Goomas, 2014). Finally, a behavior-based safety program that incorporates goal setting, feedback, and praise for workers' safe behaviors has been shown to lead to increases in safety performance (Choudhry, 2014).

In addition to examining the effects associated with the general safety motivation, researchers have also applied a self-regulation framework to better understand the mechanisms underlying employees' safety behaviors. Among the different theories associated with self-regulation, "regulatory focus" theory (Higgins, 1997, 1998) has received a good deal of attention. Regulatory focus theory describes how individuals regulate their behaviors through two coexisting motivational systems that satisfy different needs during goal-related pursuits (Higgins & Spiegel, 2004; Scholer & Higgins, 2008). "Promotion focus" is activated when individuals self-regulate around nurturance needs and involves striving for ideals through advancement and accomplishment. This focus encourages behaviors intended to move people closer to desired end-states. On the other hand, a "prevention focus" regulates the pursuit of security needs and involves fulfilling duties and obligations through vigilant and responsible behaviors. This focus orients individuals to avoid conditions that pull them away from desired end-states.

Empirical research findings have emphasized the implications of promotion and prevention foci on employees' safety-related outcomes. Because its orientation is toward security and emphasis on vigilant behaviors, a high prevention focus is expected to be beneficial for safety-related outcomes. However, having a promotion focus may be detrimental to safety-related outcomes because individuals may focus on the pursuit of advancement at the expense of safety. Indeed, Lanaj, Chang, and Johnson (2012) summarized relationships between regulatory focus and safety performance, and found that although prevention focus has a positive relationship to safety performance, promotion focus is associated with lower safety performance. Wallace and Chen (2006) demonstrated that work-based regulatory focus mediated the effects of conscientiousness on safety performance. In particular, conscientiousness had a positive effect on supervisor-rated safety compliance via a dampened promotion focus and an increased prevention focus. Taken together, these findings underline the importance of considering characteristics associated with individual motivation and self-regulation in the context of occupational safety.

Situational Antecedents of Safety Performance and Workplace Accidents and Injuries

Beyond the individual characteristics just discussed, OHP has also identified a number of situational variables that predict safety-related outcomes. We focus on two contextual variables concerning job and work design—job characteristics and shift work. For more discussion of other psychosocial characteristics that are antecedents of occupational safety (e.g., safety climate, transformational leadership), please see Chapter 6.

Job Characteristics

Hackman and Oldham (1980) postulated five core job dimensions that characterize the structure of jobs: skill variety, task identity, task significance, autonomy, and feedback. "Skill variety" refers to the extent to which the job requires employees to develop and apply a range of skills and abilities. "Task identity" captures the degree to which the job requires workers to complete a sequence of tasks to achieve a visible outcome, such as producing a component of a product or serving a customer. "Task significance" refers to how important the job is to other stakeholders (e.g., coworkers, customers, or even the general public). Together, having jobs high on these three dimensions can lead employees to experience greater meaningfulness with regard to their work.

"Autonomy" refers to the extent to which a job provides employees with independence and decision-making latitude to determine how to carry out work-related tasks. Jobs high on autonomy allow employees to experience a greater sense of responsibility for outcomes of their work. Finally, "feedback" concerning performance provides workers with knowledge of results. Positive outcomes, such as increased motivation and performance and higher satisfaction, are associated with each of the five job characteristics (e.g., Humphrey, Nahrgang, & Morgeson, 2007).

In terms of safety-related outcomes, job characteristics have been linked to safety performance and accidents and injuries. In terms of safety performance in a nursing sample, knowledge-based job characteristics, including skill variety and job complexity, are positively related to safety compliance and participation (Lievens & Vlerick, 2014). Interestingly, a meta-analysis (Nahrgang, Morgeson, & Hofmann, 2011) revealed a negative relationship between job complexity and safety behavior. These results suggest that jobs that are overly complicated may be detrimental to employee safety. Autonomy has consistently been linked to better safety performance (Nahrgang et al., 2011). Feedback concerning safety-related performance and incidents (e.g., Choudhry, 2014; Lee, Shon, & Oah, 2014) has been linked to increases in employees' safety performance. In addition, research has found that feedback to supervisors about their communications regarding the integration of production and safety-related concerns during daily exchanges with employees resulted in improvement in safety climate and employees' safety behavior (Zohar & Polachek, 2014). Moreover, such feedback to supervisors enhanced employees' performance during a safety audit conducted by independent observers. Finally, employees in jobs high on skill variety were less likely to report musculoskeletal injuries (Grzywacz et al., 2007).

Shift Work

"Shift work" refers to "a job schedule in which employees work hours other than the standard hours of 8 a.m. to 5 p.m. or a schedule other than the standard workweek"

(Grosswald, 2004, p. 414). A review of the relevant research literature concluded that safety may be compromised by shift work (Folkard & Tucker, 2003). In particular, relative risks for accidents and injuries are higher for night shifts compared with day or afternoon shifts, and the risks increase with successive night shifts (i.e., working during successive nights) and with more hours on duty (Baker, Olson, & Morisseau, 1994; Folkard & Tucker, 2003). These increases in risks are likely associated with disruptions of workers' sleep schedules and circadian rhythms (Folkard, Lombardi, & Tucker, 2005).

Indeed, multiple studies have demonstrated linkages between sleep quality and safety-related outcomes. In terms of safety performance, insomnia symptoms have been shown to be negatively associated with construction workers' safety performance (Kao, Spitzmueller, Cigularov, & Wu, 2016). In addition, workers with sleep disorders (e.g., obstructive sleep apnea syndrome) had a higher likelihood of involvement in occupational accidents (Ulfberg, Carter, & Edling, 2000). Sleep disturbances such as insomnia, difficulties falling asleep, and poor sleep quality were also found to predict higher rates of occupational injuries among workers of different occupations, such as construction workers (Kao et al., in press), nurses (Shao, Chou, Yeh, & Tzeng, 2010), and public sector employees (Salminen et al., 2010). Finally, Barnes and Wagner (2009) demonstrated that sleep loss due to daylight saving time change (i.e., spring forward) was associated with increases in occupational injuries. Taken together, research supports the view that shift work and associated sleep disruptions have negative effects on occupational safety, including reductions in safety performance and increased risk for accidents and injuries.

Implications of Considering Individual and Situational Antecedents for Safety

Before reflecting on the implications of research on individual and situational antecedents for safety, a caveat is suggested. With a few exceptions (e.g., Neal & Griffin, 2006), the majority of the studies cited in this chapter were cross-sectional in design. Research on the impact of individual and situational variables on safety could benefit from an increased focus on longitudinal designs with their greater prospects for assessing causal models.

We underline the importance of safety by stressing the implications of the cited research. Understanding individual differences and situational characteristics as antecedents of safety-related outcomes has important implications for the human resource functions within organizations. First, organizations interested in promoting safety performance may include measures of some individual difference factors (e.g., conscientiousness and cognitive failure) as part of a selection test battery used during recruitment. Selecting potential candidates on the basis of these characteristics may help ensure the recruitment of a workforce that is predisposed to value workplace safety and follow proper procedures and practices to protect themselves.

Tetrick and Peiró (2012) suggested that OHP can improve the practice of safety training, which is often considered to be one of the most important activities for improving workplace safety and preventing occupational accidents and injuries (Huang, Leamon, Courtney, Chen, & DeArmond, 2007). For example, applications of learning principles that require active participation (e.g., behavioral modeling; hands-on activities) aimed at engaging trainees have been shown to lead to better safety training (e.g., Burke et al., 2006). In addition, incorporating a dialogic learning perspective that includes structured interpersonal discussion and guided intrapersonal reflection can promote greater understanding during safety training, thereby achieving better safety-related outcomes (Burke, Holman, & Birdi, 2006). Moreover, understanding individual difference factors that predict safety-related outcomes may inform potential aptitude-by-treatment interactions, and identify individual employees who will benefit from more frequent safety refresher training sessions, an alternative training delivery method, or a differently paced training program.

Third, research on safety motivation and its effects points to the potential for organizations to incorporate safety performance as part of their performance management system. Doing so may not only highlight the importance of workplace safety, but also encourage employee motivation for safety. Specifically, safety performance should be regularly reviewed and included as part of employees' performance portfolio. During the performance feedback session, employees and their managers may include discussions concerning setting performance goals to promote workplace safety and prevent accidents and injuries. Rewards and recognition should be given to those who demonstrate good safety-related performance.

Finally, given the positive implications of job characteristics for safety-related outcomes, interventions designed to broaden the job scope may contribute to enhanced safety performance and reduced risk of accidents and injuries. For example, skill variety can be improved by rotating employees through different positions that require different abilities. Participative decision-making and employee involvement can help increase autonomy. Providing employees with timely and actionable feedback may also contribute to improving safety (Choudhry, 2014; Lee et al., 2014).

SUMMARY

Despite decades of academic research, industrial effort, and public policy changes, occupational safety continues to be a serious concern for worker health and well-being. Data collected in the E.U. and the U.S. indicate that substantial numbers of workers are killed or seriously injured on the job every year, and the trend seems to be steady, rather than gradually decreasing. In this chapter, we introduced the OHP approach to occupational safety and discussed the key research findings. With its emphasis on psychological processes, OHP research on safety complements work based on other approaches (e.g., industrial hygiene and ergonomics). OHP research on occupational safety has focused on identifying individual characteristics (e.g., demographics, personality) and contextual factors (e.g., job characteristics and shift work) that are antecedents to workplace accidents and injuries. Demographic risk factors include membership in racial or ethnic minority groups and the male sex. An example of a personality trait that is related to high levels of safety performance is conscientiousness. Other evidence suggests that conscientiousness and agreeableness are related to safety motivation, which in turn is related to lower accident risk. The experience of cognitive failure is related to lower safety performance and micro-accidents as well as less safe driving on the commute home from work. Individuals high on prevention regulatory focus, who are motivated to follow rules and fulfill obligations, tend to show better safety performance. By contrast, those high on promotion focus, who are motivated by pursuing ideals and desirable outcomes, tend to show lower safety performance. Some organizational goal-setting practices may improve safety outcomes by influencing employees' safety motivation (e.g., providing a financial reward for being accident free for 30 days).

Situational job characteristics such as job complexity and skill variety have been linked to safety compliance and participation. High levels of job complexity, however, have been implicated in reduced safety behavior. Job-related autonomy has been linked to better safety performance. Safety-related feedback from supervisors has been found to be related to better safety climate and safe behaviors. Injuries and accidents are more likely to occur during night shifts than during day shifts. Poor sleep quality is related to impaired safety performance. These findings have implications for implementing appropriate human resources practices (e. g., selection and training) and work designs (e.g., reward systems and work tasks) to promote safety.

REFERENCES

American Federation of Teachers. (2010). *Health and safety for workers in schools and colleges.* Retrieved from https://www.osha.gov/dte/grant_materials/fy10/sh-20839-10/circle_chart.pdf

Baker, K., Olson, J., & Morisseau, D. (1994). Work practices, fatigue, and nuclear power plant safety performance. *Human Factors, 36,* 244–257. doi:10.1177/001872089403600206

Barnes, C. M., & Wagner, D. T. (2009). Changing to daylight saving time cuts into sleep and increases workplace injuries. *Journal of Applied Psychology, 94,* 1305–1317. doi:10.1037/a0015320

Beus, J. M., Dhanani, L. Y., & McCord, M. A. (2015). A meta-analysis of personality and workplace safety: Addressing unanswered questions. *Journal of Applied Psychology, 100,* 481–498. doi:10.1037/a0037916

Bodner, T., Kraner, M., Bradford, B., Hammer, L., & Truxillo, D. (2014). Safety, health, and well-being of municipal utility and construction workers. *Journal of Occupational and Environmental Medicine, 56,* 771–778. doi:10.1097/JOM.0000000000000178

Bureau of Labor Statistics. (2014, December). *Nonfatal occupational injuries and illnesses requiring days away from work, 2013.* Retrieved from www.bls.gov/news.release/pdf/osh2.pdf

Bureau of Labor Statistics. (2015a, June). *Census of fatal occupational injuries (CFOI): Current and revised data.* Retrieved from www.bls.gov/iif/oshcfoi1.htm

Bureau of Labor Statistics. (2015b, June). *Industry injury and illness data.* Retrieved from www.bls.gov/iif/oshsum.htm

Burke, M. J., Holman, D., & Birdi, K. (2006). A walk on the safe side: The implications of learning theory for developing effective safety and health training. In G. P. Hodgkinson & J. K. Ford (Eds.), *International review of industrial and organizational psychology* (pp. 1–44). London, UK: Wiley.

Burke, M. J., Sarpy, S. A., Smith-Crowe, K., Chan-Serafin, S., Islam, G., & Salvador, R. (2006). Relative effectiveness of worker safety and health training methods. *American Journal of Public Health, 96,* 315–324. doi:10.2105/AJPH.2004.059840

Burke, M. J., Sarpy, S. A., Tesluk, P. E., & Smith-Crowe, K. (2002). General safety performance: A test of a grounded theoretical model. *Personnel Psychology, 55,* 429–457. doi:10.1111/j.1744-6570.2002.tb00116.x

Chang, C.-H., Bernard, T. E., Bloswick, D. S., & Johnson, R. E. (2015, May). Employee behavioral reactions to musculoskeletal symptoms: Supervisor support as a moderator. In K. S. Jennings & T. W. Britt (Chairs), *Supporting employees in high stress jobs: Benefits of social support for physical and psychological health.* Symposium presented at the 11th International Conference on Occupational Stress and Health: Work, Stress, and Health 2015, Atlanta, GA.

Choudhry, R. M. (2014). Behavior-based safety on construction sites: A case study. *Accident Analysis and Prevention, 70,* 14–23. doi:10.1016/j.aap.2014.03.007

Christian, M. S., Bradley, J. C., Wallace, J. C., & Burke, M. J. (2009). Workplace safety: A meta-analysis of the roles of person and situation factors. *Journal of Applied Psychology, 94,* 1103–1127. doi:10.1037/a0016172

Clarke, S., & Robertson, I. T. (2005). A meta-analytic review of the big five personality factors and accident involvement in occupational and non-occupational settings. *Journal of Occupational and Organizational Psychology, 78,* 355–376. doi:10.1348/096317905X26183

Clarke, S., & Robertson, I. (2008). An examination of the role of personality in work accidents using meta-analysis. *Applied Psychology: An International Review, 57,* 94–108. doi:10.1111/j.1464-0597.2007.00267.x

Costa, P. T., Jr., & McCrae, R. R. (1992). *Revised NEO Personality Inventory (NEO-PI-R) and NEO Five-Factor Inventory (NEO-FFI) manual*. Odessa, FL: Psychological Assessment Resources.

Day, A. J., Brasher, K., & Bridger, R. S. (2012). Accident proneness revisited: The role of psychological stress and cognitive failure. *Accident Analysis and Prevention, 49*, 532–535. doi:10.1016/j.aap.2012.03.028

Eatough, E. M., Way, J. D., & Chang, C.-H. (2012). Understanding the link between psychosocial work stressors and work-related musculoskeletal complaints. *Applied Ergonomics, 43*, 554–563. doi:10.1016/j.apergo.2011.08.009

Elfering, A., Grebner, S., & Boillat, C. (2013). Busy at work and absent-minded at home: Mental workload, cognitive failure, and domestic falls. *Swiss Journal of Psychology, 72*, 219–228. doi:10.1024/1421-0185/a000114

Elfering, A., Grebner, S., & de Tribolet-Hardy, F. (2013). The long arm of time pressure at work: Cognitive failure and commuting near-accidents. *European Journal of Work and Organizational Psychology, 22*, 737–749. doi:10.1080/1359432X.2012.704155

Elfering, A., Grebner, S., & Haller, M. (2012). Railway-controller-perceived mental work load, cognitive failure and risky commuting. *Ergonomics, 55*, 1463–1475. doi:10.1080/00140139.2012.718802

Eurostat. (2015, June). *Accident at work statistics*. Retrieved from http://ec.europa.eu/eurostat/statistics-explained/index.php/Accidents_at_work_statistics

Folkard, S., Lombardi, D. A., & Tucker, P. T. (2005). Shiftwork: Safety, sleepiness, and sleep. *Industrial Health, 43*, 20–23. doi:10.2486/indhealth.43.20

Folkard, S., & Tucker, P. (2003). Shift work, safety and productivity. *Occupational Medicine, 53*, 95–101. doi:10.1093/occmed/kqg047

Golubovich, J., Chang, C.-H., & Eatough, E. M. (2014). Safety climate, hardiness, and musculoskeletal complaints: A mediated moderation model. *Applied Ergonomics, 45*, 757–766. doi:10.1016/j.apergo.2013.10.008

Grosswald, B. (2004). The effects of shift work on family satisfaction. *Families in Society: The Journal of Contemporary Social Services, 85*, 413–423. doi:10.1606/1044-3894.1503

Grzywacz, J. G., Arcury, T. A., Marín, A., Carrillo, L., Coates, M. L., Burke, B., & Quandt, S. A. (2007). The organization of work: Implications for injury and illness among immigrant Latino poultry-processing workers. *Archives of Environmental & Occupational Health, 62*, 19–26. doi:10.3200/AEOH.62.1.19-26

Hackman, J. R., & Oldham, G. R. (1980). *Work redesign*. Upper Saddle River, NJ: Pearson.

Hansen, C. P. (1989). A causal model of the relationship among accidents, biodata, personality, and cognitive factors. *Journal of Applied Psychology, 74*, 81–90. doi:10.1037//0021-9010.74.1.81

Herrick, R., & Dement, J. (2005). Industrial hygiene. In L. Rosenstock, M. R. Cullen, C. A. Brodkin, & C.A. Redlich (Eds.), *Textbook of clinical occupational and environmental medicine* (2nd ed., pp. 45–75). Philadelphia, PA: Elsevier Saunders.

Higgins, E. T. (1997). Beyond pleasure and pain. *American Psychologist, 52*, 1280–1300. doi:10.1037/0003-066X.52.12.1280

Higgins, E. T. (1998). Promotion and prevention: Regulatory focus as a motivational principle. *Advances in Experimental Social Psychology, 30*, 1–46. doi:10.1016/S0065-2601(08)60381-0

Higgins, E. T., & Spiegel, S. (2004). Promotion and prevention strategies for self-regulation: A motivated cognition perspective. In R. F. Baumeister & K. D. Vohs (Eds.), *Handbook of self-regulation: Research, theory, and applications* (pp. 171–187). New York, NY: Guilford Press.

Hofmann, D. A., Morgeson, F. P., & Gerras, S. J. (2003). Climate as a moderator of the relationship between leader-member exchange and content specific citizenship: Safety climate as an exemplar. *Journal of Applied Psychology, 88*, 170–178. doi:10.1037/0021-9010.88.1.170

Hogan, J., & Foster, J. (2013). Multifaceted personality predictors of workplace safety performance: More than conscientiousness. *Human Performance, 26*, 20–43. doi:10.1080/08959285.2012.736899

Huang, Y. H., Leamon, T. G., Courtney, T. K., Chen, P. Y., & DeArmond, S. (2007). Corporate financial decision-makers' perceptions of workplace safety. *Accident Analysis and Prevention, 39*, 767–775. doi:10.1016/j.aap.2006.11.007

Humphrey, S. E., Nahrgang, J. D., & Morgeson, F. P. (2007). Integrating motivational, social, and contextual work design features: A meta-analytic summary and theoretical extension of the work design literature. *Journal of Applied Psychology, 92*, 1332–1356. doi:10.1037/0021-9010.92.5.1332

Inness, M., Turner, N., Barling, J., & Stride, C. B. (2010). Transformational leadership and employee safety performance: A within-person, between jobs design. *Journal of Occupational Health Psychology, 15*, 279–290. doi:10.1037/a0019380

Kao, K.-Y., Spitzmueller, C., Cigularov, K., & Wu, H. (2016). Linking insomnia to workplace injuries: A moderated mediation model of supervisor safety priority and safety behavior. *Journal of Occupational Health Psychology, 21,* 91–104. doi:10.1037/a0039144

Kaplan, S., & Tetrick, L. E. (2011). Workplace safety and accidents: An industrial and organizational psychology perspective. In S. Zedeck (Ed.), *APA Handbook of industrial and organizational psychology* (Vol. 1, pp. 455–472). Washington, DC: American Psychological Association.

Kotzé, M., & Steyn, L. (2013). The role of psychological factors in workplace safety. *Ergonomics, 56,* 1928–1939. doi:10.1080/00140139.2013.851282

Krieger, N. (2009). Workers are people too: Societal aspects of occupational health disparities: An ecosocial perspective. *American Journal of Industrial Medicine, 53,* 104–115. doi:10.1002/ajim.20759

LaMontagne, A. D., Stoddard, A. M., Youngstrom, R. A., Lewiton, M., & Sorensen, G. (2005). Improving the prevention and control of hazardous substance exposures: A randomized controlled trial in manufacturing worksites. *American Journal of Industrial Medicine, 48,* 282–292. doi:10.1002/ajim.20218

Lanaj, K., Chang, C.-H., & Johnson, R. E. (2012). Regulatory focus and work-related outcomes: A meta-analysis. *Psychological Bulletin, 138,* 998–1034. doi:10.1037/a0027723

Landsbergis, P. A., Grzywacz, J. G., & LaMontagne, A. D. (2014). Work organization, job insecurity, and occupational health disparities. *American Journal of Industrial Medicine, 57,* 495–515. doi:10.1002/ajim.22126

Lee, K., Shon, D., & Oah, S. (2014). The relative effects of global and specific feedback on safety behaviors. *Journal of Organizational Behavior Management, 34,* 16–28. doi:10.1080/01608061.2013.878264

Leigh, J. P. (2011). Economic burden of occupational injury and illness in the United States. *The Milbank Quarterly, 89,* 728–772. doi:10.1111/j.1468-0009.2011.00648.x

Leung, M.-Y., Chan, I. Y. S., & Yu, J. (2012). Preventing construction worker injury incidents through the management of personal stress and organizational stressors. *Accident Analysis and Prevention, 48,* 156–166. doi:10.1016/j.aap.2011.03.017

Levy, P. E. (2013). *Industrial/organizational psychology: Understanding the workplace* (4th ed.). New York, NY: Palgrave Macmillan.

Liberty Mutual Research Institute for Safety. (2014). *2014 Liberty Mutual workplace safety index.* Retrieved from www.libertymutual.com/researchinstitute

Lievens, I., & Vlerick, P. (2014). Transformational leadership and safety performance among nurses: The mediating role of knowledge-related job characteristics. *Journal of Advanced Nursing, 70,* 651–661. doi:10.1111/jan.12229

Meyer, J. D. (2014). Race-based job discrimination, disparities in job control, and their joint effects on health. *American Journal of Industrial Medicine, 57,* 587–595. doi:10.1002/ajim.22255

Murray, L. R. (2003). Sick and tired of being sick and tired: Scientific evidence, methods, and research implications for racial and ethnic disparities in occupational health. *American Journal of Public Health, 93,* 221–226. doi:10.2105/AJPH.93.2.221

Nahrgang, J. D., Morgeson, F. P., & Hofmann, D. A. (2011). Safety at work: A meta-analytic investigation of the link between job demands, job resources, burnout, engagement, and safety outcomes. *Journal of Applied Psychology, 96,* 71–94. doi:10.1037/a0021484

National Institute for Occupational Safety and Health. (n.d.). *Musculoskeletal disorders.* Retrieved from https://www.cdc.gov/niosh/programs/msd

National Institute for Occupational Safety and Health. (2015). *Total Worker Health™.* Retrieved from www.cdc.gov/niosh/twh/totalhealth.html

Neal, A., & Griffin, M. A. (2006). A study of the lagged relationships among safety climate, safety motivation, safety behavior, and accidents at the individual and group levels. *Journal of Applied Psychology, 91,* 946–953. doi:10.1037/0021-9010.91.4.946

Occupational Safety and Health Administration. (1998). *Industrial hygiene* (OSHA No. 3143). Retrieved from https://www.osha.gov/Publications/OSHA3143/OSHA3143.htm#Industrial

Okechukwu, C. A., Souza, K., Davis, K. D., & de Castro, A. B. (2014). Discrimination, harassment, abuse, and bulling in the workplace: Contribution of workplace injustice to occupational health disparities. *American Journal of Industrial Medicine, 57,* 573–586. doi:10.1002/ajim.22221

Postlethwaite, B., Robbins, S., Rickerson, J., & McKinniss, T. (2009). The moderation of conscientiousness by cognitive ability when predicting workplace safety behavior. *Personality and Individual Differences, 47,* 711–716. doi:10.1016/j.paid.2009.06.008

Punnett, L., & Wegman, D. H. (2004). Work-related musculoskeletal disorders: The epidemiologic evidence and the debate. *Journal of Electromyography Kinesiology, 14,* 13–23. doi:10.1016/j.jelekin.2003.09.015

Reese, C. D. (2008). *Occupational health and safety management: A practical approach* (2nd ed.). Boca Raton, FL: CRC Press and Taylor & Francis Group.

Salanova, M., Lorente, L., & Martínez, I. M. (2012). The dark and bright sides of self-efficacy in predicting learning, innovative and risky performances. *The Spanish Journal of Psychology, 15,* 1123–1132. doi:10.5209/rev_SJOP.2012.v15.n3.39402

Salminen, S., Oksanen, T., Vahtera, J., Sallinen, M., Härmä, M., Salo, P., . . . Kivimäki, M. (2010). Sleep disturbances as a predictor of occupational injuries among public sector workers. *Journal of Sleep Research, 19,* 207–213. doi:10.1111/j.1365-2869.2009.00780.x

Sauter, S. L., & Swanson, N. G. (1996). An ecological model of musculoskeletal disorders in office work. In S. L. Sauter & S. D. Moon (Eds.), *Beyond biomechanics: Psychosocial aspects of musculoskeletal disorders in office work* (pp. 3–20). Bristol, PA: Taylor & Francis.

Scholer, A. A., & Higgins, E. T. (2008). Distinguishing levels of approach and avoidance: An analysis using regulatory focus theory. In A. J. Elliot (Ed.), *Handbook of approach and avoidance motivation* (pp. 489–504). New York, NY: Psychology Press.

Shao, M. F., Chou, Y. C., Yeh, M. Y., & Tzeng, W. C. (2010). Sleep quality and quality of life in female shift-working nurses. *Journal of Advanced Nursing, 66,* 1565–1572. doi:10.1111/j.1365-2648.2010.05300.x

Sobeih, T. M., Salem, O., Daraiseh, N., Genaidy, A., & Shell, R. (2006). Psychosocial factors and musculoskeletal disorders in the construction industry: A systematic review. *Theoretical Issues in Ergonomics Science, 7,* 329–344. doi:10.1080/14639220500090760

Sorensen, G., Stoddard, A. M., LaMontagne, A. D., Emmons, K., Hunt, M. K., Youngstrom, R., . . . Christiani, D. C. (2002). A comprehensive worksite cancer prevention intervention: Behavior change results from a randomized controlled trial (United States). *Cancer Causes & Control, 13,* 493–502. doi:10.1023/A:1016385001695

Stanbury, M., & Rosenman, K. D. (2014). Occupational health disparities: A state public health-based approach. *American Journal of Industrial Medicine, 57,* 596–604. doi:10.1002/ajim.22292

Steege, A. L., Baron, S. L., Marsh, S. M., Menédez, C. C., & Myers, J. R. (2014). Examining occupational health and safety disparities using national data: A cause for continuing concern. *American Journal of Industrial Medicine, 57,* 527–538. doi:10.1002/ajim.22297

Swanson, N. G., & Sauter, S. L. (2006). A multivariate evaluation of an office ergonomic intervention using longitudinal data. *Theoretical Issues in Ergonomics Science, 7,* 3–17. doi:10.1080/1463922051 2331335124

Tetrick, L. E., & Peiró, J. M. (2012). Occupational safety and health. In S. W. J. Kozlowski (Ed.), *The Oxford handbook of organizational psychology* (Vol. 2, pp. 1228–1244). New York, NY: Oxford University Press.

Ulfberg, J., Carter, N., & Edling, C. (2000). Sleep-disordered breathing and occupational accidents. *Scandinavian Journal of Work, Environment, & Health, 26,* 237–242. doi:10.5271/sjweh.537

Wachter, J. K., & Yorio, P. L. (2014). A system of safety management practices and worker engagement for reducing and preventing accidents: An empirical and theoretical investigation. *Accident Analysis and Prevention, 68,* 117–130. doi:10.1016/j.aap.2013.07.029

Wallace, J. C., & Chen, G. (2005). Development and validation of work-specific measure of cognitive failure: Implications for occupational safety. *Journal of Occupational and Organizational Psychology, 78,* 615–632. doi:10.1348-096317905X37442

Wallace, J. C., & Chen, G. (2006). A multilevel integration of personality, climate, self-regulation, and performance. *Personnel Psychology, 59,* 529–557. doi:10.1111/j.1744-6570.2006.00046.x

Wallace, J. C., & Vodanovich, S. J. (2003). Workplace safety performance: Conscientiousness, cognitive failure, and their integration. *Journal of Occupational Health Psychology, 8,* 316–327. doi:10.1037/1076-8998.8.4.316

Yeow, P. H. P., & Goomas, D. T. (2014). Outcome-and-behavior-based safety inventive program to reduce accidents: A case study of a fluid manufacturing plant. *Safety Science, 70,* 429–437. doi:10.1016/j.ssci.2014.07.016

Yuan, Z., Li, Y., & Lin, J. (2014). Linking challenge and hindrance stress to safety performance: The moderating effect of core self-evaluation. *Personality and Individual Differences, 68,* 154–159. doi:10.1016/j.paid.2014.04.025

Zohar, D., & Polachek, T. (2014). Discourse-based intervention for modifying supervisory communication as leverage for safety climate and performance improvement: A randomized field study. *Journal of Applied Psychology, 99,* 113–124. doi:10.1037/a0034096

NINE

Work–Family Balance

KEY CONCEPTS AND FINDINGS COVERED IN CHAPTER 9

In the past few decades, there have been dramatic changes in work and family structure, including increases in women's participation in paid employment, greater numbers of dual-earner households and single-parent families, and a growing trend among working adults to bear responsibilities for caring for their children *and* their elderly relatives (Neal & Hammer, 2007). These changes challenge the traditional assumption that the workplace must be designed to separate work and family demands in order to maximize employees' productivity (Kanter, 1977). Indeed, as workplaces become more diverse and family structures more complex, employees must juggle competing role expectations from both work and family domains. This experience can be stressful, especially when individuals face a culture of competitiveness, driving them to consider work as their uppermost priority and sacrifice their personal lives to be successful.

According to a 2012 survey of a representative sample of U.S. adults, 56% of working mothers and 50% of working fathers found it difficult to balance the responsibilities of their job and their family (Parker & Wang, 2013). Although working fathers spent an average of 10 hours per week on housework and 7 hours on childcare-related activities, up from 4 and 2.5 hours based on a 1965 survey, working mothers remain the primary care providers in the family realm. Moreover, whereas working fathers tend to consider having a high-paying job more important than balancing work and family responsibilities, working mothers are more generally concerned with flexible work arrangements (Parker & Wang, 2013). Unfortunately, although workers place higher importance on concerns for balancing work and personal lives, they also experience less support from their employers. For example, only about one-third (36%) of the workers in the United States were satisfied with the support provided by their employers to help balance demands from work and personal domains (Clay, 2011). A survey by Society for Human Resource Management (2010) found that many firms were reducing or eliminating family-friendly benefits, such as flexible work arrangements and eldercare referral. Similarly, employer provision of full-time pay during maternity leave has also seen a decline (Shellenbarger, 2008).

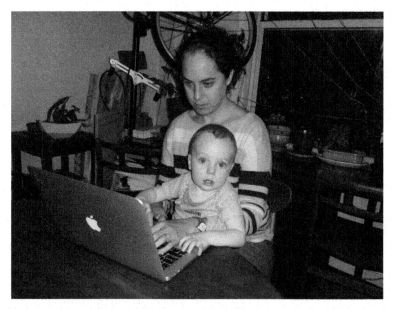

Mother working while her child sits on her lap. (Photo by Irvin Sam Schonfeld.)

Given the rising challenges faced by workers to meet demands from work and domains outside of work, work–family research—the study of "positive and negative processes, antecedents, and outcomes related to work and family roles" (Kossek, Baltes, & Matthews, 2011, p. 352)—is vital to informing organizational practices and helping individual employees manage their responsibilities. In what follows, the negative and positive aspects of the work–family interface are discussed. These negative and positive aspects of the work–family interface have implications for employees' general health and well-being (e.g., stress symptoms, satisfaction with their experiences) and functioning in either domain. Those implications will be explored. Relevant research using different methodologies, including longitudinal and cross-national designs, will be discussed. The research findings will then be integrated, and the concept of work–family balance will be introduced. Alternative conceptualizations of work–family balance will also be discussed. Finally, broader contextual factors and policy implications of work–family research will be presented.

NEGATIVE WORK–FAMILY INTERFACE: WORK–FAMILY CONFLICT (WFC)

Work–family conflict (WFC) is one of the most studied aspects of the interface of work and the family. The research captures the negative side of the work–family interface (Greenhaus & Allen, 2011). WFC occurs when role demands from work and family are mutually incompatible, such that meeting role expectations in one domain makes it difficult to meet role expectations in the other domain (Greenhaus & Beutell, 1985). WFC is a bidirectional phenomenon; fulfilling responsibilities from either domain can hamper an individual's ability to fulfill responsibilities in the other domain (Gutek, Searle, & Klepa, 1991). Specifically, work interference with family (WIF) occurs when participation in the work role hinders participation in the family role (Mesmar-Magnus & Viswesvaran, 2005). For example, an employee may miss his or her child's soccer match because the employee has to work overtime to complete a job assignment. On the other hand, family interference with work (FIW) reflects the fulfillment of family responsibilities impeding an individual's meeting a work-related responsibility. An example of FIW is missing an important work meeting because the employee has to stay at home to care for a sick child.

In addition to bidirectionality, research has also identified different forms of WFC. According to Greenhaus and Beutell (1985), three types of WFC may occur: time-based conflict, strain-based conflict, and behavior-based conflict. Time-based WFC occurs when time spent fulfilling one role interferes with participation in the other role (Carlson, Kacmar, & Williams, 2000). The two examples of WIF and FIW described in the previous paragraph reflect time-based conflict. Strain-based WFC occurs when strain (e.g., negative emotions; fatigue) experienced in one role interferes with the participation in the other role (Carlson et al., 2000). For example, employees may experience high levels of anxiety at work owing to low job security, which, in turn, makes them more irritable when interacting with family members. Alternatively, worry about a family member's illness may preoccupy an employee, preventing the employee from paying full attention at work. Finally, behavior-based WFC occurs when behaviors necessary in one domain are incompatible with what is required to fulfill the demands of the other domain (Carlson et al., 2000). For example, nurturing behaviors that are needed in the family domain may not be effective on the job if employees work in a highly competitive environment. Similarly, directive behaviors that exemplify effective leadership at work can create problems when employees interact with spouses at home.

Situational Antecedents of WFC

Because the concept of WFC is rooted in role theory, studies that examined the antecedents of WFC have typically focused on factors that can shape employees' role expectations in the work or family realms. Some factors have been thought to contribute to different forms of WIF and FIW. In particular, researchers tend to adopt, explicitly or implicitly, the demand–control–support framework (Johnson & Hall, 1988; Karasek, 1979) of stress (see Chapter 3) when examining the antecedents of WFC. In particular, variables in the work and family domains that reflect high demands, low control, and/or low support are considered candidate factors that are likely linked with WFC.

High psychological and physical workload, number of working hours, shift work (including working Sundays), and a higher number of dependents have been found to be associated with WFC (e.g., Barnes-Farrell et al., 2008). High work demands are typically reflected by structural characteristics of the job (e.g., working hours), individual employees' devotion to work (e.g., job involvement), and work stressors that may be perceived as threatening or challenging to the employees (e.g., work role ambiguity or workplace aggression). High family demands, on the other hand, can also be defined by the structural characteristics of the family (e.g., number of dependent children), family role devotion (e.g., family centrality), and stressors derived from family (e.g., family role overload that comes with having a sick or disabled child; Michel, Kotrba, Mitchelson, Clark, & Baltes, 2011). Research has consistently found associations between heavy work demands and FIW and WIF. Byron's (2005) meta-analysis showed that long work hours, job involvement, and role overload at work were related to WIF. In addition, family demands such as hours spent on family tasks and number of dependent children living at home were positively related to FIW. Beyond the evidence assembled by Byron (2005), Michel, Kotrba, et al.'s (2011) more recent meta-analysis also found that both work stressors (e.g., role ambiguity) and family stressors (e.g., family role ambiguity) contributed to FIW and WIF.

In addition to meta-analytic evidence, empirical studies have assessed specific stressors at work and home that predict WFC. For example, Demsky, Ellis, and Fritz (2014) found that workplace mistreatment was related to WIF as rated by both the focal employees *and* their significant others. In addition, Lambert, Minor, Wells, and Hogan (2015) found that the extent of danger staff members at correctional facilities perceived at work was related to WIF. Similarly, Hepburn and Barling (1996) found that the number of hours spent caring for elderly relatives is related to FIW. Taken together, research supports the idea that the extensiveness of demands from either the work or the family domain is associated with increased WFC.

The second category of situational antecedents includes factors that reflect control in the work or family domain. For example, Michel, Kotrba, et al.'s (2011) meta-analysis found that job autonomy is related to lower levels of WIF, and that the relationship is stronger among males than females. In addition to assessing the effect of perceived control or autonomy on WFC directly, research on control has also focused on the effects of flexible work arrangements, which refer to organizational policies and practices that afford employees flexibility and control over how, when, and where work is completed (Lambert, Marler, & Gueutal, 2008). Indeed, Byron (2005) found that schedule flexibility is related to both reduced WIF and FIW. In addition, Michel, Kotrba, et al.'s (2011) quantitative review also showed that schedule flexibility was negatively related to WIF, particularly for married employees and those with dependent children.

Allen, Johnson, Kiburz, and Shockley (2013), in their quantitative review, further compared the effects of different types of flexibility on WFC. They found that in terms of flexible work locations (flexplace), only the amount of use, but not the availability, of flexplace, was negatively related to WIF. On the other hand, flexible schedule availability, or flextime, was negatively related to WIF, whereas the extensiveness of use of a flexible schedule was unrelated to WIF. Finally, FIW was negatively related to flexplace availability but unrelated to the other flexible work arrangements, regardless of availability or actual use.

Primary studies focused on establishing the boundary conditions of the effectiveness of control and flexible work arrangements on WFC. In a study of a nationally representative U.S. sample, DiRenzo, Greenhaus, and Weer (2011) found that job level moderated the effects of job autonomy on WIF in employed adults living with a spouse or partner and having at least one child at home. Specifically, the inverse relationship between job autonomy and WIF was stronger when participants' job level was at a higher rather than a lower organizational rank. The finding further suggests that autonomy may not protect against WIF when employees are lower in the organizational hierarchy. Kossek, Lautsch, and Eaton (2006) found that perceived control was negatively related to FIW. However, employees who attempted to integrate the work and family domains by simultaneously fulfilling role expectations from the two domains tended to experience higher levels of FIW. Shockley and Allen (2007) found that both flextime and flexplace were negatively related to WIF when family responsibility was high, and unrelated to WIF when family responsibility was low. The results were a little different for FIW. As with WIF, both types of flexible work arrangements were negatively related to FIW when family responsibility was high. Both, however, were *positively* related to FIW when family responsibility was low. In other words, flexible work arrangements tended to be beneficial in terms of FIW when family responsibility was high, but detrimental when family responsibility was low.

Finally, research on the effects of telecommuting also offers insights on the effects of flexibility on WFC. Gajendran and Harrison's (2007) meta-analysis revealed an overall negative relationship between telecommuting and WFC. Interestingly, Golden, Viega, and Simsek (2006) found that telecommuting was negatively related to WIF, especially for employees who reported high, in contrast to low, scheduling flexibility. However, telecommuting was positively related to FIW, particularly for those with a larger family. Taken together, these findings suggest that although perceived control and flexibility are generally associated with lower WIF, their effects on FIW are more equivocal and may depend on contextual factors.

In terms of support, meta-analytic results have been consistent with the view that support from supervisors and coworkers at work, and support from spouses or other family members, are negatively associated with both WIF and FIW (Byron, 2005; Michel, Kotrba, et al., 2011). In another meta-analysis, Kossek, Pichler, Bodner, and Hammer (2011) further compared the effects of general support and support specifically targeted at assisting employees with family-related concerns (e.g., expressed empathy toward an employee wanting to maintain a balance between work and family). The investigators also compared the effects of support from different sources (i.e., organization versus supervisor). The researchers found that both general and family-specific support from supervisors were positively related to family-specific support from the organization, which, in turn, was related to lower WIF. On the other hand, general support from the organization had limited effect on employees' WIF. These results suggest that perceived support, especially a type of support oriented toward assisting employees with work–family matters, is associated with lower WFC.

Some studies have found that gender may be an important boundary condition for the effect of support. In a Dutch sample, van Daalen, Williemsen, and Sanders (2006) found that in addition to the main effect, gender moderated the effect of support from different sources on time- and strain-based WIF and FIW. For example, supervisor support was related to lower time-based WIF in male employees but to increased WIF in female employees. Similarly, coworker support was negatively related to strain-based FIW in men but not in women. Interestingly, gender did not moderate the negative relationships between support from the spouse and coworkers with time-based FIW. Taken together, these studies suggest that female employees may be particularly vulnerable when it comes to WFC, regardless of the level of support that they may receive.

Finally, scholars have identified some broader contextual factors that may contribute to WFC beyond the focal employees' immediate organizational and familial characteristics. For example, Young and Wheaton (2013) examined the effect of neighborhood similarity in terms of socioeconomic status, family composition, and ethnicity on workers' WFC. They found that neighborhood similarity was related to lower WFC for female residents only, and explained this effect by suggesting that such similarity may not only foster the development of shared normative expectations about how to manage work and family responsibilities, but also generate assumptions about the support availability. Dierdorff and Ellington (2008) examined how occupational characteristics of interdependence, responsibility for others, and interpersonal conflict could predict WIF beyond individual-based work and family characteristics (e.g., time pressure, role overload, schedule flexibility). They found that after controlling for these individual characteristics, interdependence and responsibility for others at the occupational level predicted higher levels of WIF. These studies point to the importance of considering the broader contextual factors that may have implications for workers' WFC.

Taken together, these findings suggest that situational characteristics in the work and family domains that reflect high demands (e.g., long work hours; more dependent children), low control (e.g., inflexible work arrangement), and/or low support (e.g., family-specific support from supervisors or organizations; spousal support) tend to be associated with high WFC. Moreover, characteristics beyond the work and family domains, such as features of the community, may also have implications for employees' WFC.

Dispositional Antecedents of WFC

In terms of dispositional antecedents, multiple meta-analyses have revealed significant relationships between workers' personality traits and WFC. Michel, Clark, and Jaramillo (2011) found that in employees, high levels of extraversion, agreeableness, and conscientiousness were related to lower levels of WFC, whereas high levels of neuroticism were related to higher levels of WFC. Allen et al. (2012) conducted a finer-grained analysis and summarized the relationships between various individual traits with different types of WIF and FIW. Overall, in terms of the Big Five[1] personality characteristics, Allen et al.'s (2012) results were consistent with Michel, Clark, et al.'s (2011) findings. However, Allen et al.'s (2012) additional analysis showed that positive affectivity (PA)[2] and self-efficacy were negatively related to WIF and FIW, whereas negative affectivity (NA) was related to higher levels of WIF and FIW. Moreover, Allen et al.'s (2012) finer-grained analyses indicated that when compared across different types of WIF and FIW, neuroticism tended to have the weakest relationship with time-based conflict compared with other types of conflict. Their findings also suggest that time-based WFC may be more affected by structural characteristics of work and family (e.g., working hours) than by stable individual differences.

In addition to meta-analytic summaries, empirical studies have examined the extent to which different types of dispositional and situational antecedents were predictive of WFC. Carlson (1999) found that NA was a unique predictor of time- and

---

[1] The Big Five personality traits refer to conscientiousness, extraversion (or its opposite, introversion), agreeableness, neuroticism (which approximately corresponds to negative affectivity), and openness to experience.

[2] PA refers to the propensity to experience positive emotions.

strain-based WFC, whereas both NA and Type A personality predicted behavior-based WFC. Hargis, Kotrba, Zhdanova, and Baltes (2011), on the other hand, compared both situational characteristics (job and family stress; supervisor and family support; job and family involvement; work hours; number of children; age of the youngest child) and dispositional traits (locus of control, positive and NA) as possible antecedents of different types of WIF and FIW. They found that job stress emerged as a dominant predictor consistently across different types of WIF. Age of the youngest child was a dominant predictor of time- and strain-based WIF, and NA was a dominant predictor of strain- and behavior-based WIF. Finally, job stress and NA were the most dominant predictors of all three types of FIW.

Taken together, these findings support the view that employees with certain characteristics (e.g., high neuroticism or NA; low agreeableness, conscientiousness, extraversion, and PA) tend to report higher levels of WFC. Moreover, research findings suggest that when considered together, both situational characteristics and dispositional traits emerge as significant antecedents of WFC. Thus, although certain individuals are predisposed to experience more conflict between domains, these tendencies may be exacerbated by situational factors.

Outcomes of WFC

Two theoretical perspectives provide explanations of the relationships between WFC and its outcomes. First, the "cross-domain hypothesis" (Frone, Russell, & Cooper, 1992) suggests that WFC should have stronger implications for outcomes within the domain that is being affected. For example, in the case of WIF, stronger effects on outcomes in the family domain are expected (e.g., effects on family satisfaction; interaction among family members) because work responsibilities prevent the focal employees from meeting family role expectations. On the other hand, FIW should have stronger effects on outcomes in the work domain, such as job attitudes and work behaviors. Consistent with this perspective, research has found significant relationships between WIF and family domain outcomes, including reduced marital satisfaction, family satisfaction, and family-related performance (Amstad, Meier, Fasel, Elfering, & Semmer, 2011). On the other hand, FIW has significant implications for outcomes in the work domain, including lower work satisfaction and organizational commitment, higher levels of turnover intentions, and lower work performance and helping behaviors (Amstad et al., 2011).

The second theoretical perspective is the "matching hypothesis," or the "source attribution framework" (Amstad et al., 2011; Shockley & Singla, 2011). According to this perspective, individuals appraise and attribute the negative spillover to the source of the conflict, and therefore, outcomes in the source domain should suffer more. Based on this perspective, workers experiencing WIF (FIW) likely attribute blame to the work (family) domain, and as a result, their well-being and effectiveness in the source domain should suffer more.

Although both perspectives make intuitive sense and have received empirical support, recent meta-analyses tend to provide stronger support for the matching hypothesis than for the cross-domain hypothesis. For example, Kossek and Ozeki's (1998) meta-analysis showed that compared with FIW, WIF had a stronger negative relationship with job satisfaction, consistent with the matching hypothesis. In another meta-analysis, Shockley and Singla (2011) compared the extent to which FIW and WIF predicted job and family satisfaction. They found that when both were included in a path model,[3] WIF had a stronger, negative relationship with job satisfaction, compared with WIF's relationship with family satisfaction. In addition, FIW had a stronger, negative relationship with family satisfaction compared with FIW's relationship with job satisfaction. Shockley and Singla's results thus support the matching hypothesis.

Moving beyond satisfaction, Amstad et al.'s (2011) meta-analysis compared the relationships of WIF and FIW with a number of outcomes in the work and family domains. Overall, their results were consistent with the matching hypothesis, with a few exceptions. For example, compared with FIW, WIF had stronger negative relationships with outcomes in the work domain, including work satisfaction, organizational commitment, and organizational citizenship[4] behavior. Moreover, the positive relationships between WIF and turnover intention, burnout, and job stress were also stronger than FIW's relationships with these outcomes. Finally, consistent with the matching hypothesis, compared with WIF, FIW had stronger negative relationships with marital satisfaction and family satisfaction. However, Amstad et al. (2011) also found some support for the cross-domain hypothesis. In particular, FIW had a stronger negative relationship with employees' work performance; WIF, compared with FIW, had a stronger negative relationship with workers' family-related performance (how well one manages one's family-related responsibilities).

In the area of diagnosable mental health problems, Grzywacz and Bass (2003) found that work-to-family and family-to-work conflicts were related to elevated risk of depressive and anxiety disorders and drinking problems in a nationally representative U.S. sample. Nohe, Meier, Sonntag, and Michel (2015), taking a rigorous approach to meta-analyses, limited their analyses to longitudinal studies of WFC. They examined relationships involving WIF, FIW, general strain (e.g., psychological distress, depression), and work-related strain (e.g., burnout). The investigators found that both WIF and FIW predict strain, and strain predicts both WIF and FIW. Consistent with the matching hypothesis, WIF, compared with FIW, was more strongly associated with work-related strain (burnout; there were insufficient data to examine family-related strain, e.g., parental stress).

Overall, research findings appear to provide stronger support for the matching hypothesis, such that individuals attribute the WFC to the source of the spillover, and their well-being and effectiveness in the source domain tend to suffer more compared with the domain that is being influenced. In particular, WIF tends to have stronger negative relationships with well-being and effectiveness outcomes in the work domain, whereas negative relationships between FIW and outcomes in the family domain tend to be stronger.

Experience Sampling and Longitudinal Research

In order to better capture the natural fluctuations in WFC over time, more recent research has adopted experience sampling methodology (see the section on diary

---

[3] Without being overly technical, suffice it to say that a path model is a variety of statistical model.

[4] Organizational citizenship behaviors refer to voluntary behaviors on the part of an employee that are helpful to an organization (e.g., attending a meeting although not required to; helping another worker learn to complete a task).

methods in Chapter 2) or longer, more standard longitudinal designs to investigate dynamic relationships involving WFC and its various antecedents and outcomes. In a daily diary study, U.S. workers reported their daily job demands, daily control, and WIF at the end of each day for 14 consecutive days (Butler, Grzywacz, Bass, & Linney, 2005). Results showed significant within-person variance in these variables, suggesting that participants experienced different levels of demands, control, and WIF each day. In addition, similar to findings from more common between-person studies, in the diary study daily demands were found to be related to daily WIF; this relationship, however, was weaker on days where participants had higher control. In another study with a similar design, Singaporean university workers reported their daily workload, daily support from supervisors, and daily WIF experiences for 5 days (Goh, Ilies, & Wilson, 2015). Results showed that daily workload was related to daily WIF, and this relationship was stronger on days where supervisor support was low. Finally, in an experience sampling study with U.S. service workers, engaging in emotional labor (i.e., regulating one's emotional display at work to comply with organizational requirements) was positively associated with workers' anxiety level in the afternoon, which, in turn, predicted evening strain-based WIF (Wagner, Barnes, & Scott, 2014). These findings suggest that WFC may not be a stable construct, and examining its changes over time can be informative.

In addition to research on the relationship between antecedents and WFC, experience-sampling methodology has been applied to research that examines the effects of WFC on various outcomes. For example, in a study that followed U.S. workers for 14 days, Ilies et al. (2007) found that daily WIF was negatively related to workers' social interactions with their children and spouse, as rated by spouses. In a daily diary study conducted in China, Wang, Liu, Zhan, and Shi (2010) found that daily WIF, but not daily FIW, was predictive, over a period of 5 weeks, of employees' daily alcohol use after work. Moreover, the relationship between daily WIF and alcohol consumption was greater when participants perceived strong peer drinking norms, and when family support was low. Finally, Judge, Ilies, and Scott (2006) examined U.S. workers' daily WFC experience and their affective reactions at work and at home. The investigators found that over a period of 2 weeks, daily FIW was positively related to participants' guilt and hostility at work. On the other hand, daily WIF was positively related to participants' guilt and hostility at home. Moreover, hostility partially mediated the effect of WIF on marital satisfaction. Overall, these studies employing experience-sampling methods provide support for the cross-domain hypothesis (Frone et al., 1992). It is possible that evidence is more supportive of the cross-domain hypothesis when examining within-person effects of WFC, whereas evidence is more supportive of the matching domain hypothesis when examining between-person effects.

Beyond outcomes specific to the work or family domain, studies have also examined the effects of WFC on non–domain-specific outcomes. For example, in a U.S. study, Shockley and Allen (2013) examined the effects of WIF and FIW on physical health indicators, including heart rate, systolic blood pressure, and diastolic blood pressure, using an experience-sampling design. They found that over a 10-day study period, WIF incidents, but not FIW incidents, were related to increases in participants' heart rate. In addition, daily FIW incidents were related to higher daily systolic and diastolic blood pressure when participants reported low supervisor support for family. In a study conducted in China, Liu et al. (2015), using a daily diary design, explored the effects of WIF and FIW on employees' displaced aggression against various targets. The investigators found that the indirect effect of daily WIF on displaced aggression against workers' supervisors, coworkers, and family members was mediated by emotional exhaustion. The effect was also moderated by workplace interpersonal conflict. More specifically, daily WIF had a significant, indirect effect on displaced aggression only when daily conflict was high. Daily FIW also had significant indirect effects on workers' displaced aggression via emotional exhaustion, but this tendency was attenuated if employees perceived high levels of family-related support from supervisors.

Finally, research employing longitudinal designs examined the relationships between WFC and its antecedents or outcomes using different time lags. Results have been somewhat different across studies. For example, some studies with a 6-month lag (e.g., Kelloway, Gottlieb, & Barham, 1999) found that WFC was an outcome of stress symptoms, whereas others with similar or longer time lags (e.g., Frone, Russell, & Cooper, 1997; Grant-Vallone & Donaldson, 2001) found that WFC was predictive of subsequent adverse mental (e.g., increased depressive symptoms, excessive alcohol consumption) and physical health (e.g., increased blood pressure) effects. Still others (e.g., Rantanen, Kinnunen, Feldt, & Pulkkinen, 2008) found that WIF was unrelated to psychological well-being (e.g., emotional exhaustion, GHQ[5]) across 1- and 6-year time lags. Although these results seemed equivocal, the findings from Nohe et al.'s (2015) meta-analysis of longitudinal studies were consistent with the view that WFC and strain are reciprocally related. More specifically, Nohe et al. (2015) found that prior WFC is predictive of subsequent increases in strain, and prior strain is predictive of subsequent increases in WFC.

Other longitudinal studies have identified different patterns of relationships involving WFC for men and women. For example, in a study conducted in Finland, Kinnunen, Geurts, and Mauno (2004) found that time 1 WIF was unrelated to well-being outcomes assessed 1 year later for male participants. However, WIF at time 1 was related to female participants' lower job satisfaction and higher parental stress and psychological distress 1 year later. Interestingly, the different relationship patterns for male and female participants are not always replicated across studies. For example, Hammer, Cullen, Neal, Sinclair, and Shafiro (2005), in a U.S. study, found no difference between men and women for relationships between WFC and depressive symptoms assessed 1 year later.

Taken together, it appears that the temporal dynamics for WFC and its antecedents and outcomes need to be better understood, and studies using different time frames and multiple measurement points will be useful to help capture these changes over time. In particular, studies with an experience-sampling design may identify more transitory, within-individual variations in WFC and the relationship of those variations with antecedents and outcomes over short periods of time. More standard longitudinal studies, with their lengthier time frames, will be helpful in tracking the long-term implications of WFC.

Cross-National Research

Although the majority of the research on WFC has been conducted in the Western countries, there has been an increase in the past decade in WFC studies taking a

---

[5] See Chapter 3 regarding the psychological symptom measure known as the GHQ.

perspective that is even more international in scope. Interestingly, studies conducted in non-Western countries do not consistently replicate findings obtained in Western countries. For example, although work demands have been shown to predict WFC based on studies conducted in the Western settings, demands were also found to predict WFC in India (Aryee, Srinivas, & Tan, 2005) and Hong Kong (Aryee, Luk, Leung, & Lo, 1999), but not in Japan (Matsui, Ohsawa, & Onglatco, 1995). Similarly, although some studies found that scheduling flexibility was related to reduced WIF in Eastern countries (Hill, Erickson, Homes, & Ferris, 2010), others found that compared with workers in English-speaking countries, flexible work arrangements such as flextime and telecommuting had limited effects in reducing workers' time- or strain-based WIF in Asian and Latin American countries (Masuda et al., 2012). Finally, whereas studies in India (Aryee et al., 2005) and Singapore (Aryee, 1992) found a negative association between WFC and job satisfaction, other research conducted in Asia failed to find this relationship (e.g., Yang, 2005).

Cross-national studies, in which data were collected in multiple countries, have provided some support for the view that WFC and its relationship with antecedents or outcomes may be stronger in nations with individualistic cultures (Chang & Spector, 2011). Individualistic cultural values emphasize personal achievement and the maximization of individual gains. On the other hand, collectivistic cultural values emphasize the welfare of the social group, and members are motivated to fulfill their assigned group roles and obligations (Hofstede, 2001; Triandis, 2001). Yang, Chen, Choi, and Zou (2000) argued that these cultural values may affect how individuals evaluate the work–family interface. In particular, employees from individualistic cultures may view work as time spent away from their family; whereas those from collectivistic cultures may view work as time spent to fulfill the responsibility of providing for a family. Indeed, large-scale cross-national studies have suggested that work demands are positively related to WFC for workers in English-speaking countries (e.g., the U.S., Canada, Australia, and U.K.), but unrelated to WFC for workers in Asian (e.g., China) and Latin American countries (Spector, Sanchez, Siu, Salgado, & Ma, 2004; Spector et al., 2007). Overall, it appears that meaningful between-country variance exists in how employees experience WFC.

POSITIVE WORK–FAMILY INTERFACE: WORK–FAMILY ENHANCEMENT (WFE)

In addition to negative interference, a positive interface between work and family domains can also occur. In the past few decades, the positive interface has been approached from different perspectives, and several distinct, yet highly related, constructs have been developed to reflect this positive experience (Greenhaus & Allen, 2011). Positive spillover refers to the transfer of positively valenced experiences (e.g., affective reactions, behaviors) from one domain to the other, and is expected to benefit the receiving domain (Hanson, Hammer, & Colton, 2006). Enrichment occurs when experiences in one domain improve the quality and the effectiveness of individuals' functioning in the other domain (Greenhaus & Powell, 2006). Finally, facilitation refers to the extent to which experiences in one domain provide developmental, affective, and efficacious gains that contribute to the improved functioning of another domain (Wayne, Grzywacz, Carlson, & Kacmar, 2007). Although the role enhancement perspective of improved functioning in one role due to experiences in the other role is embedded in both enrichment and facilitation concepts, facilitation is intended to be a broader concept as it emphasizes system-level functioning (Grzywacz, Carlson, Kacmar, & Wayne, 2007). For the remainder of the chapter, we use the term "enhancement" as a generic term intended to capture the positive interface between work and family domains. This terminology is consistent with the underlying mechanism of role enhancement process, and has been adopted by the most recent comprehensive review of the work–family literature (Allen, 2012).

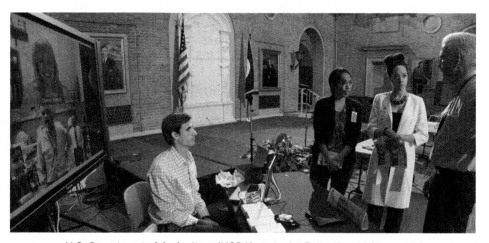

U.S. Department of Agriculture (USDA) strategist Debra Arnold (on screen)
uses a teleconferencing system to demonstrate telework systems and abilities, during
National Work and Family Month Open House and Expo, October 2014, Washington, DC.
(Photographer is Lance Cheung. Public Domain.)

Much like WFC, work–family enhancement (WFE) is presumed to be a bidirectional construct. Work enhancement of family (WEF) occurs when work experiences benefit participation in the family domain, whereas family enhancement of work (FEW) captures the positive spillover effect in the opposite direction (Allen, 2012). Different scholars have proposed different ways to characterize and operationalize WFE experiences. For example, van Steenbergen, Ellemers, and Mooijaart (2007) suggested that WFE can be understood within the framework of four dimensions. "Time-based enhancement" suggests that time spent in one domain allows individuals to better function or enjoy their role in the other domain. "Energy-based enhancement" refers to individuals gaining energy from their participation in one role and then using the energy gained to perform their role in the other domain. "Behavioral enhancement" occurs when behavior or skills learned in one domain facilitate one's performance in the other domain. Finally, "psychological facilitation" occurs when positive experiences in one domain allow individuals to better concentrate and perform in the other domain. Carlson, Kacmar, Wayne, and Grzywacz (2006) proposed an alternative conceptualization. Their taxonomy focuses on the types of gains or resources individuals develop that transfer to the other domain. In particular, gains can be differentiated into three types: development or acquisition of skills; affect; and capital or security. Finally, Wiese, Seiger, Schmid, and Freund (2010) proposed another approach to examine WFE. In particular, their conceptualization focuses on the transfer of competencies, transfer of positive mood, and cross-domain compensation, with the last dimension capturing individuals' experiences of engagement in one domain facilitating their ability to address failure in the other domain.

Although different researchers have different ways to characterize the WFE experience, the majority of the studies in this area examine the antecedents and outcomes of the overall WEF or FEW, rather than the specific dimensions of WFE. Moreover, with a few exceptions, results involving different dimensions of WFE tend to be similar. Thus, unless specifically noted, the research findings in the following sections are based on studies examining aggregated WEF and FEW experiences.

Situational Antecedents of WFE

Wayne et al. (2007) proposed a conceptual model of WFE that highlighted three categories of environmental predictors for WFE. The first category is energy resources. Specifically, work-based energy resources such as enriched jobs and developmental opportunities are expected to positively predict WEF, whereas family-based energy resources such as family developmental opportunities (e.g., family helps the focal individual acquire new knowledge relevant to being a good worker) are expected to positively predict FEW. Consistent with this perspective, Carlson et al. (2006) found that work-based energy resources, including job autonomy and developmental experiences at work, were related to WEF. Family mutuality, or the extent to which family members cooperate and share responsibilities, was positively related to FEW. Similarly, Skinner and Ichii (2015) found that Australians working in jobs that provided high levels of autonomy and skill utilization reported higher levels of WFE[6] after controlling for the effects of job and family demands. Skinner and Ichii also found that cohesive neighborhoods and social support from neighbors were positively related to WFE.

The second category of situational antecedents comprises support resources. Matthews, Mills, Trout, and English (2014) showed that family-supportive supervisor behaviors are distinguishable from more generally supportive supervisor behaviors. Wayne et al. (2007) argued that support from coworkers and supervisors should predict WEF, whereas support from family members is expected to predict FEW. In a U.S. study, Wadsworth and Owens (2007) compared how well support from different sources predicted WEF and FEW. They found that supervisor, coworker, and organizational support predicted WEF, whereas support from family sources (e.g., spouse) was not a significant predictor. On the other hand, spousal support and support from children predicted FEW, and none of the support from work-based sources predicted FEW. In a study conducted in China, Ho, Chen, Cheung, Liu, and Worthington (2013) examined the spillover and the cross-over effects of work and family support on WEF and FEW for husband–wife dyads. Ho et al. found that for husbands, family support was predictive of their own FEW, which reflects a positive spillover effect. Their partners' work support was positively related to their own WEF and FEW, consistent with the cross-over effect of support on WFE experiences. For wives, family support was related to FEW and WEF, and work support, to FEW. However, no cross-over effect of husbands' perceived support was found for wives' WFE experience.

---

[6] In this study, WFE reflects neither WEF nor FEW, but assesses the value of having both work and family responsibilities. See Marshall and Barnett (1993) for the WFE measure used by Skinner and Ichii.

Finally, Wayne et al. (2007) identified condition resources as another category of situational predictors for WFE. Condition resources, such as job prestige, may provide individuals with greater social, economic, emotional, and intellectual gains that can lead to positive enhancement experiences. Unfortunately, existing research has not focused enough on this particular set of situational predictors. As such, the extent to which condition resources may be linked to WFE is unclear.

Taken together, having enriched, energizing experiences in one domain appears to encourage the positive spillover to the other domain. Additionally, research has consistently found that support from work and family domain is an important predictor for positive work–family interface.

Dispositional Antecedents of WFE

Wayne and colleagues (Wayne, Randel, & Stevens, 2006; Wayne et al., 2007) enumerated three personal characteristics that are likely to predict WFE. In particular, Wayne et al. (2006, 2007) proposed that individuals who experience positive affective states and self-efficacy are likely to report high levels of WFE. In other words, individuals who tend to experience positive emotions and mood or who have positive beliefs about their ability are likely to experience a positive interface between work and family domains. In addition, Wayne and colleagues advanced the view that those who are high on work and family identity (the importance an individual places on work or family in terms of self-definition) should experience more WEF/FEW respectively, because strong domain identity orients individuals to be more engaged in that domain, and as such, they may be more likely to generate positive gains to be transferred to the other domain.

Research on personality predictors of WFE tends to support Wayne et al.'s (2007) proposition regarding the association between PA and WFE. For example, in a nationally representative U.S. sample, Wayne, Musisca, and Fleeson (2004) found that extraversion, a personality trait that is similar to PA, is associated with WEF and FEW. In addition, neuroticism, which reflects individuals' tendency to experience negative emotions, was inversely related to WEF. In an Indian study, Aryee et al. (2005) found a negative association between neuroticism and FEW. Finally, there is also meta-analytic (Michel, Clark, et al., 2011) support for the view that extraversion and PA are directly related to WFE, and that neuroticism and NA are inversely related to WFE.

In terms of efficacy as a predictor, Wayne et al. (2007) argued that individuals who are high on self-efficacy are more likely to view role expectations as challenges, and more effectively utilize resources in one domain to facilitate their functioning in the other domain. Empirical research, however, has provided mixed support for this view. In a study that directly examined the effect of participants' generalized self-efficacy on their WFE, Boyar and Mosley (2007) found that efficacy predicted neither WEF nor FEW. By contrast, Tement (2014) found that self-efficacy mediated the effect of family support on participants' work engagement. This result implicates efficacy in the family-to-work facilitation process.

Unlike findings related to efficacy, research has provided consistent support for the association between domain identity and WFE. For example, in their U.S. study, Wayne et al. (2006) found that work identity predicted WEF but not FEW, and family identity predicted FEW but not WEF. Similarly, Ho et al. (2013), in their Chinese sample, found that participants' family orientation predicted FEW but not WEF. Taken together, these results are consistent with Wayne et al.'s (2006, 2007) view that domain identity allows individuals to gain more positive resources from that domain, which can then be transferred to the other domain.

Finally, there appeared to be consistent demographic differences in WFE. For example, women appeared to experience more WFE than men (Aryee et al., 2005; van Steenbergen et al., 2007). Wiese et al. (2010) found that in addition to gender, parents and nonparents also experienced different levels of WFE. In general, female participants and those who were parents tended to use work experiences to compensate for frustration experienced in the family domain, whereas male and nonparent participants were more likely to use family experiences to compensate for their experiences in the work domain.

Taken together, research findings suggest that stable individual characteristics such as demographic and personality traits may predict different WFE experiences. In addition, having a strong identity or orientation toward a particular domain may also promote WFE.

Outcomes of WFE

Research on outcomes of WFE has typically focused on employees' well-being, attitudes, and behaviors at work and at home. In terms of well-being outcomes, a meta-analysis (McNall, Nicklin, & Masuda, 2010) has shown that WEF and FEW are related to better employee mental and physical health. In an Israeli study, Dishon-Berkovits (2014) found that WFE is related to lower levels of burnout symptoms. Finally, in their nationally representative U.S. sample, Grzywacz and Bass (2003) found different relationships between WEF and FEW with depression, anxiety disorder, and problem drinking in employees. Specifically, FEW was related to lower risk of depression and problem drinking, but unrelated to anxiety disorder; WEF was not a significant predictor of any of these outcomes.

Research on attitudinal outcomes of WFE tends to focus on satisfaction and commitment in the work and family domains. For example, meta-analytic findings have shown that WEF and FEW are related to job satisfaction, family satisfaction, and affective organizational commitment (McNall et al., 2010). In a study conducted in India, Srivastava and Srivastava (2014) found that both WEF and FEW predicted workers' marital satisfaction. Using employees of a U.S. insurance company, Wayne et al. (2006) found that in addition to affective organizational commitment (i.e., emotional attachment to the job), WEF was also associated with a construct called "continuance organizational commitment," a type of commitment that is based on lack of better alternatives and fear of losing existing investments (e.g., retirement package).

In their meta-analysis, Shockley and Singla (2011) compared the cross-domain and matching hypotheses with regard to relationships between WEF and FEW, on the one hand, and job and family satisfaction, on the other. They found that when both WEF and FEW were included in a path model, WEF had a stronger relationship with job satisfaction compared with WEF's relationship with family satisfaction. By contrast, FEW had a stronger relationship with family satisfaction than with job satisfaction. This pattern is consistent with the matching hypothesis.

Interestingly, research regarding the effects of WFE on employees' turnover intentions is somewhat inconsistent. Although a meta-analysis (McNall et al., 2010) reported near-zero relationships between WEF and FEW, on the one hand, and turnover intentions, on the other, other studies have shown a significant negative relationship between WFE and turnover intentions (e.g., Odle-Dusseau, Britt,

& Greene-Shortridge, 2012). McNall et al.'s (2010) meta-analysis, however, showed large, between-study variance in the WFE-turnover intentions relationship, variance that could not be explained by sampling error or measurement unreliability. These results suggest that moderators may exist that alter the nature of the relationship between WFE and employee turnover intentions.

Finally, studies from Albania (Karatepe & Bektechi, 2008), India (Srivastava & Srivastava, 2014), the United States (Odle-Dusseau et al., 2012), and The Netherlands (van Steenbergen et al., 2007) bear on the relationship of WFE to job performance. More specifically, Karatepe and Bektechi (2008) and Srivastava and Srivastava (2014) found that WFE is directly related to employees' job performance. However, Odle-Dusseau et al. (2012) found that only WEF, but not FEW, was predictive of job performance. Other research (van Steenbergen et al., 2007) indicated that gender moderated the association of WEF and FEW with job performance. Specifically, energy-based FEW and psychological facilitation of WEF (e.g., work experience that helps put home-related matters in perspective) were positively related to job performance in men but not in women. However, behavior-based and psychological FEW were positively related to job performance in women but unrelated to performance in men.

Taken together, research has provided consistent support for positive relationships between WFE and outcomes reflecting employees' health and well-being (e.g., burnout, job satisfaction, marital satisfaction). However, the association between WFE and effectiveness outcomes (e.g., withdrawal intentions, performance) may depend on the type of effectiveness outcome assessed and the individual characteristics of the focal employees.

Experience Sampling and Longitudinal Research

Experience sampling (see the Diary Studies section in Chapter 2) has not been as commonly employed in WFE research as in research on WFC, although we underline its use in studies conducted in the United States (Butler et al., 2005; Lawson, Davis, McHale, Hammer, & Buxton, 2014) and Spain (Sanz-Vergel, Demerouti, Moreno-Jiménez, & Mayo, 2010). Existing research is consistent with the view that WFE varies significantly within persons over time, and its relationship with antecedents and outcomes may also change over time. Butler et al. (2005) found that within-person variation accounted for 69% of the variance in WFE. In addition, they showed that daily job demands were inversely related to employees' daily WFE. By contrast, daily control and skill utilization were directly related to daily WFE. Sanz-Vergel et al. (2010) found that employees' recovery after work breaks and the expression of positive emotions at work predicted WFE at night. In addition, recovery after work breaks and the expression of positive emotions at home were positively predictive of employee vigor at home.

In addition to predictors of WFE, daily diary designs have also been used to examine within-person relationships between WFE and outcomes. Lawson et al. (2014) examined the effects of mothers' WEF on children's health indicators. Specifically, they found that mothers' positive work experiences were related to lower negative mood after work, which, in turn, was predictive of lower negative mood and fewer physical symptoms in their children. On the other hand, mothers' negative work experience was related to their lower positive mood after work, which, in turn, was associated with their children's lower positive mood, poorer sleep quality, and shorter sleep duration. These findings suggest that not only will work-to-home spillover affect the focal employees, but the effect will carry over to employees' children.

There have not been many empirical studies examining the effects associated with WFE longitudinally, and findings from two U.S. studies (Carlson et al., 2011; Hammer et al., 2005) have been inconsistent. On one hand, Hammer et al. (2005) found no significant relationship between WFE and employees' depressive symptoms assessed 1 year later. On the other hand, Carlson et al. (2011) found that WEF was positively related to participants' physical health assessed 4 months later, which, in turn, was negatively related to their actual turnover assessed 8 months later. In their Netherlands sample, van Steenbergen and Ellemers (2009) found that WEF at baseline was associated with lower cholesterol, body mass index, and rates of sickness absence, and increased performance 1 year later, controlling for the outcome measures as assessed at time 1. More longitudinal research is needed to better examine the effects of WFE over time.

Taken together, less research on WFE has utilized either an experience-sampling methodology or longitudinal designs compared with research on WFC. The extant research using a daily diary design appears to show that WFE experiences can have meaningful micro-level, within-person fluctuations over a short period of time, and can cross over to children. However, research involving WFE with longer time lapses is less consistent.

WORK–FAMILY BALANCE

According to Kossek (2008), work–family balance refers to the extent to which individuals perceive their work and family roles to be compatible and at equilibrium with each other. Unlike the clear conceptualization of positive and negative interfaces between work and family, work–family balance has been defined and discussed in a variety of ways, with some scholars strongly endorsing the term and others rejecting it (see Greenhaus & Allen, 2011 for a review). In what follows, we discuss three common ways that work–family balance has been defined, and introduce Greenhaus and Allen's framework for integrating these different perspectives.

The first common way to define work–family balance is to consider balance as the absence of WFC and/or the presence of WFE. Duxbury and Higgins (2001) underlined the condition in which employees are unable to balance work and family responsibilities such that the time and energy required to participate in one role is incompatible with participation in the other role. In other words, participation in one role hinders participation in the other role. Frone (2003) proposed that work–family balance represents low WFC in combination with high WFE. This approach to work–family balance tends to overlap with an examination of positive versus negative interfaces of the work and family domains.

A second approach to understanding work–family balance is to consider balance as high involvement in both work and family roles. For example, focusing on the personal resources such as time and energy, Kirchmeyer (2000) defined work–family balance as how well employees can distribute their limited personal resources across different domains. Similarly, Marks and MacDermid (1996) suggested that balance is achieved when employees fully engage themselves in all the roles and responsibilities across the different domains. This approach focuses on the extent to which employees can meet their role expectations from different domains, and consider that balance is accomplished when employees fully engage in their different roles and responsibilities.

Finally, a third approach considers work–family balance as high performance and satisfaction across different roles (e.g., Caligiuri & Lazarova, 2005; Grzywacz & Carlson, 2007). Based on this approach, high involvement in different roles across domains is not quite enough. Rather, individuals must be effective (e.g., successful at work, effective as a spouse and/or a parent) and derive enjoyment (e.g., experience satisfaction) from their different roles across domains in order to be considered balanced (Greenhaus & Allen, 2011).

In their review, Greenhaus and Allen (2011) regarded the first approach to work–family balance as running "counter to everyday conceptions," as balance cannot always be equated to low WFC. For example, individuals may create WFC by more fully participating in work and family roles. Greenhaus and Allen advanced the idea that WFC and WFE may be mechanisms through which individuals achieve work–family balance.

Combining this argument and the second and the last approaches to work–family balance, Greenhaus and Allen (2011) proposed a more elaborate, integrated model where WFC and WFE are considered antecedents to work–family balance. In accordance with the third approach to balance, the effects of WFC and WFE on balance are mediated by effectiveness[7] in and satisfaction with the work and family domains (see Figure 9.1). Finally, this integrated model includes individuals' life values. At this juncture, one particular life value, the individual's "life role priority," comes into play. A person's life role priority can be family focused, career focused, or career and family focused. Greenhaus and Allen (2011) argued that, at any point in a person's life, the individual's life role priority moderates the relationship of effectiveness and satisfaction (within the context of each domain) to work–family balance.

In particular, for individuals who place high priorities on both work and family roles, they can achieve work–family balance only if they judge themselves to be effective and experience satisfaction within both domains. However, for those who place priority on either the work or the family role, they feel balanced when they are effective and satisfied with their experiences in the domain they prioritize, irrespective of the effectiveness or satisfaction they experience in the other domain. Based on this approach, balance is defined differently for different people, and is achieved when

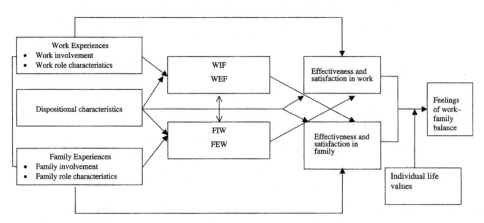

Figure 9.1 Greenhaus and Allen's model of work–family balance.
FEW, family enrichment of work; FIW, family interference with work; WEF, work enrichment of family; WIF, work interference with family. Figure republished with the permission of the authors and the American Psychological Association. From Greenhaus and Allen (2011).

---

[7] Effectiveness is gauged by standards internal to the individual.

individuals experience high levels of effectiveness and satisfaction in the domain(s) onto which they place high priority (Greenhaus & Allen, 2011).

CONSIDERATION OF THE BROADER CONTEXT

In the current chapter, we discussed the positive and negative aspects of work–family interface, and also the new perspective of work–family balance. Our discussion of situational antecedents for WFC and WFE has focused mainly on factors within the boundary of the organization. However, broader contextual factors, particularly those related to social policies relevant to facilitating individuals' meeting work and family responsibilities, can have significant implications for employees' experiences (Heymann, Earle, & Hayes, 2007). We now discuss the implications of social policies bearing on work–family issues.

Esping-Anderson's (1990) welfare regime typology has often been applied to organize differences in social policy across countries. On the basis of this typology, countries can be categorized as having liberal, conservative, or social democratic regimes, depending on the roles played by the state, the market, and the family in managing the interface between work and family domains. Liberal[8] regimes are characterized by market-domination, with minimum state-provided welfare (Eikemo & Bambra, 2008). Individuals in this regime need to rely on their own resources to meet role expectations from the work and family domains, and organizations will implement "family-friendly policies" if such policies contribute positively to the bottom line (den Dulk, 2005). Conservative[9] regimes are characterized by state-domination, and welfare is typically administered to employers (Eikemo & Bambra, 2008). Individuals in this regime can rely on collaboration between the state and employers to provide workers with support and services to help manage demands from both work and family domains. Finally, social democratic regimes are also state-dominated, and welfare is provided by a state with egalitarian goals (Eikemo & Bambra, 2008). In this case, individuals can rely on state-provided services and benefits, such as childcare and parental leave, to help meet their role expectations from different domains.

As a country of liberal regime, the United States is often criticized for lagging behind other industrialized countries in terms of its social policies to assist employees to better manage work and family responsibilities (Allen, 2012). For example, in a recent comprehensive study of 185 countries and territories around the world, Addati, Cassirer, and Gilchrist (2014) found that all but two countries provide women with paid maternity leave. The two exceptions are Papua New Guinea and the United States. Among the developed economies, 95% of the countries offer paid maternity leave of 14 weeks or longer; these countries also have the highest leave benefits (at least two thirds of previous earnings; Ghosheh, 2013), with the United States lagging behind at 12 weeks of unpaid maternity leave at the federal level. It is worth noting that several U.S. states have passed legislation to guarantee employees paid maternity leave, including California, New Jersey, and Washington (Ray, Gornick, & Schmitt, 2009). In addition, several large U.S. companies, including Google, Facebook, and KPMG, also offer paid maternity or parental leave for their employees.

---

[8] The term "liberal" here is rooted in 19th-century classical liberalism, and not the more familiar social liberalism of Franklin Roosevelt's New Deal.

[9] The conservative model is aligned with the ideas of the Prussian statesman Otto von Bismarck.

Unfortunately, limited research is available linking the social policy at the country level with individual outcomes, such as WFC or WFE. However, existing research supports the view that general health outcomes tend to be better for individuals in countries with social democratic regimes (e.g., Chung & Muntaner, 2007). Moreover, research on family-friendly policies enacted by organizations (e.g., flexible work arrangement policies) tends to support their efficacy in eliminating WFC for employees. More research is necessary to better establish the connection between national policy and individual employees' work–family interface.

SUMMARY

In this chapter, we reviewed key concepts and processes associated with understanding how workers manage their work and family roles. WIF and FIW reflect the two possible directions of the general negative work–family intersections, or WFC, and capture the incompatible demands on workers' time, energy, and behaviors from the two domains. The situational antecedents of WFC have been understood from the theoretical approach of the demand–control–support framework, and research has generally supported the view that WFC is predicted by high work or family demands (e.g., high workload or number of dependent children living at home) and low control or flexibility at work or home. Moreover, family-specific support at work appears to be negatively related to WFC. In addition to situational antecedents, individuals who are high on negative affectivity and low on conscientiousness, agreeableness, and positive affectivity tend to experience higher levels of WFC. In terms of outcomes of WFC, research tends to support the matching hypothesis, or source attribution framework, such that workers' WFC has stronger negative implications for their well-being and effectiveness in the source domain (i.e., work domain for WIF and family domain for FIW). Finally, research has examined the temporal dynamics of WFC and its relationships with antecedents and consequences. Daily experience sampling studies have shown that individuals' WFC experiences can fluctuate from day to day. On the other hand, longitudinal studies with longer time frames have yielded more equivocal results regarding the outcomes of WFC.

Positive work–family interface, or WFE, can also occur bi-directionally. Research on WEF and FEW has typically supported the view that engaged, energizing experiences in one domain tend to promote the positive spillover for workers. Moreover, support from work and family is associated with higher levels of WFE. Individuals high on positive affectivity and low on negative affectivity tend to experience higher levels of WFE. In terms of outcomes, WFE has been found to have positive implications for workers' health and well-being. Finally, compared to WFC, fewer empirical studies have been conducted to examine the temporal dynamics of WFE. However, available findings indicate that important variance in WFE changes over time. More research, however, is needed to understand the temporal dynamics of WFE.

REFERENCES

Addati, L., Cassirer, N., & Gilchrist, K. (2014). *Maternity and paternity at work: Law and practice across the world*. Geneva, Switzerland: International Labour Organization.

Allen, T. D. (2012). The work and family interface. In S. W. J. Kozlowski (Ed.), *The Oxford handbook of organizational psychology* (Vol. 2, pp. 1163–1198). New York, NY: Oxford University Press.

Allen, T. D., Johnson, R. C., Kiburz, K. M., & Shockley, K. M. (2013). Work-family conflict and flexible work arrangements: Deconstructing flexibility. *Personnel Psychology, 66,* 345–376. doi:10.1111/peps.12012

Allen, T. D., Johnson, R. C., Saboe, K. N., Cho, E., Dumani, S., & Evans, S. (2012). Dispositional variables and work-family conflict: A meta-analysis. *Journal of Vocational Behavior, 80,* 17–26. doi:10.1016/j.jvb.2011.04.004

Amstad, F. T., Meier, L. L., Fasel, U., Elfering, A., & Semmer, N. K. (2011). A meta-analysis of work-family conflict and various outcomes with a special emphasis on cross-domain versus matching-domain relations. *Journal of Occupational Health Psychology, 16,* 151–169. doi:10.1037/a0022170.

Aryee, S. (1992). Antecedents and outcomes of work-family conflict among married professional women: Evidence from Singapore. *Human Relations, 45,* 813–837. doi:10.1177/001872679204500804

Aryee, S., Luk, V., Leung, A., & Lo, S. (1999). Role stressors, interrole conflict, and well-being: The moderating influence of spousal support and coping behaviors among employed parents in Hong Kong. *Journal of Vocational Behavior, 54,* 259–278. doi:10.1006/jvbe.1998.1667

Aryee, S., Srinivas, E. S., & Tan, H. H. (2005). Rhythms of life: Antecedents and outcomes of work-family balance in employed parents. *Journal of Applied Psychology, 90,* 132–146. doi:10.1037/0021-9010.90.1.132

Barnes-Farrell, J. L., Davies-Schrils, K., McGonagle, A., Walsh, B., Di Milia, L., Fischer, F. M., . . . Tepas, D. (2008). What aspects of shiftwork influence off-shift well-being of healthcare workers? *Applied Ergonomics, 39,* 589–596. doi:10.1016/j.apergo.2008.02.019

Boyar, S. L., & Mosley, D. C., Jr. (2007). The relationship between core self-evaluations and work and family satisfaction: The mediating role of work-family conflict and facilitation. *Journal of Vocational Behavior, 71,* 265–281. doi:10.1016/j.jvb.2007.06.001

Butler, A. B., Grzywacz, J. G., Bass, B. L., & Linney, K. D. (2005). A daily diary study of job characteristics, work-family conflict and work-family facilitation. *Journal of Occupational and Organizational Psychology, 78,* 155–169. doi:10.1348/096317905X40097

Byron, K. (2005). A meta-analytic review of work-family conflict and its antecedents. *Journal of Vocational Behavior, 67,* 169–198. doi:10.1016/j.jvb.2004.08.009

Caligiuri, P., & Lazarova, M. (2005). Work-life balance and the effective management of global assignees. In S. A. Y. Poelmans (Ed.), *Work and family: An international research perspective* (pp. 121–145). Mahwah, NJ: Erlbaum.

Carlson, D. S. (1999). Personality and role variables as predictors of three forms of work-family conflict. *Journal of Vocational Behavior, 55,* 236–253. doi:10.1006/jvbe.1999.1680

Carlson, D. S., Grzywacz, J. G., Ferguson, M., Hunter, E. M., Clinch, C. R., & Arcury, T. A. (2011). Health and turnover of working mothers after childbirth via the work–family interface: An analysis across time. *Journal of Applied Psychology, 96,* 1045–1054. doi:10.1037/a0023964

Carlson, D. S., Kacmar, K. M., Wayne, J. H., & Grzywacz, J. G. (2006). Measuring the positive side of the work-family interface: Development and validation of work-family enrichment scale. *Journal of Vocational Behavior, 68,* 131–164. doi:10.1016/j.jvb.2005.02.002

Carlson, D. S., Kacmar, K. M., & Williams, L. L. (2000). Construction and initial validation of a multidimensional measure of work-family conflict. *Journal of Vocational Behavior, 56,* 249–276. doi:10.1006/jvbe.1999.1713

Chang, C.-H., & Spector, P. E. (2011). Cross-cultural occupational health psychology. In J. Quick & L. Tetrick (Eds.), *Handbook of occupational psychology* (2nd ed., pp. 119–137). Washington, DC: American Psychological Association.

Chung, H., & Muntaner, C. (2007). Welfare state matters: A typological multilevel analysis of wealthy countries. *Health Policy, 80,* 328–339.

Clay, R. (2011). Is stress getting to you? *Monitor on Psychology, 42,* 58. Washington, DC: American Psychological Association.

Demsky, C. A., Ellis, A. M., & Fritz, C. (2014). Shrugging it off: Does psychological detachment from work mediate the relationship between workplace aggression and work-family conflict? *Journal of Occupational Health Psychology, 19,* 195–205. doi:10.1037/a0035448

den Dulk, L. (2005). Workplace work-family arrangements: A study and explanatory framework of differences between organizational provisions in different welfare states. In S. A. Y. Poelmans (Ed.), *Work and family: An international research perspective* (pp. 211–238). Mahwah, NJ: Erlbaum.

Dierdorff, E., & Ellington, J. K. (2008). It's the nature of the work: Examining behavior-based sources of work-family conflict across occupations. *Journal of Applied Psychology, 93,* 883–892. doi:10.1037/0021-9010.93.4.883

DiRenzo, M. S., Greenhaus, J. H., & Weer, C. H. (2011). Job level, demands, and resources as antecedents of work-family conflict. *Journal of Vocational Behavior, 78,* 305–314. doi:10.1016/j.jvb.2010.10.002

Dishon-Berkovits, M. (2014). Burnout: Contributing and protecting factors within the work-family interface. *Journal of Career Development, 41,* 467–486. doi:10.1177/0894845313512181

Duxbury, L., & Higgins, C. (2001). *Work–life balance in the new millennium: Where are we? Where do we need to go?* (CPRN discussion paper No. W/12). Ottawa, Ontario, Canada: Canadian Policy Research Networks.

Eikemo, T. A., & Bambra, C. (2008). The welfare state: A glossary for public health. *Journal of Epidemiology and Community Health, 62,* 3–6. doi:10.1136/jech.2007.066787

Esping-Anderson, G. (1990). *The three worlds of welfare capitalism.* London, UK: Polity.

Frone, M. R. (2003). Work-family balance. In J. C. Quick & L. E. Tetrick (Eds.), *Handbook of occupational health psychology* (pp. 143–162). Washington, DC: American Psychological Association.

Frone, M. R., Russell, M., & Cooper, M. L. (1992). Antecedents and outcomes of work-family conflict: Testing a model of the work-family interface. *Journal of Applied Psychology, 77,* 65–78. doi:10.1037/0021-9010.77.1.65

Frone, M., R., Russell, M., & Cooper, M. L. (1997). Relation of work-family conflict to health outcomes: A four-year longitudinal study of employed parents. *Journal of Occupational and Organizational Psychology, 70,* 325–335. doi:10.1111/j.2044-8325.1997.tb00652.x

Gajendran, R. S., & Harrison, D. A. (2007). The good, the bad, and the unknown about telecommuting: Meta-analysis of psychological mediators and individual consequences. *Journal of Applied Psychology, 92,* 1524–1541. doi:10.1037/0021-9010.92.6.1524

Ghosheh, N. (2013). *Working conditions laws report 2012: A global review.* Geneva, Switzerland: International Labour Organization.

Goh, Z., Ilies, R., & Wilson, K. S. (2015). Supportive supervisors improve employees' daily lives: The role supervisors play in the impact of daily workload on life satisfaction via work-family conflict. *Journal of Vocational Behavior, 89,* 65–73. doi:10.1016/j.jvb.2015.04.009

Golden, T. D., Viega, J. F., & Simsek, Z. (2006). Telecommuting's differential impact on work-family conflict: Is there no place like home? *Journal of Applied Psychology, 91,* 1340–1350. doi:10.1037/0021-9010.91.6.1340

Grant-Vallone, E. J., & Donaldson, S. I. (2001). Consequences of work-family conflict on employee well-being over time. *Work & Stress, 15,* 214–226. doi:10.1080/02678370110066544

Greenhaus, J. H., & Allen, T. D. (2011). Work-family balance: A review and extension of the literature. In J. C. Quick & L. E. Tetrick (Eds.), *Handbook of occupational health psychology* (2nd ed., pp. 165–183). Washington, DC: American Psychological Association.

Greenhaus, J. H., & Beutell, J. N. (1985). Sources of conflict between work and family roles. *Academy of Management Review, 10,* 76–88. Retrieved from www.jstor.org/stable/258214

Greenhaus, J. H., & Powell, G. N. (2006). When work and family are allies: A theory of work-family enrichment. *Academy of Management Review, 31,* 72–92. doi:10.5465/AMR.2006.19379625

Grzywacz, J. G., & Bass, B. L. (2003). Work, family, and mental health: Testing different models of work-family fit. *Journal of Marriage and Family, 65,* 248–262. doi:10.1111/j.1741-3737.2003.00248.x

Grzywacz, J. G., & Carlson, D. S. (2007). Conceptualizing work-family balance: Implications practice and research. *Advances in Development Human Resources, 9,* 455–471. doi:10.1177/1523422307305487

Grzywacz, J. G., Carlson, D. S., Kacmar, K. M., & Wayne, J. H. (2007). A multi-level perspective on the synergies between work and family. *Journal of Occupational and Organizational Psychology, 80,* 559–574. doi:10.1348/096317906X163081

Gutek, B. A., Searle, S., & Klepa, L. (1991). Rational versus gender role explanations for work-family conflict. *Journal of Applied Psychology, 76,* 560–568. doi:10.1037/0021-9010.76.4.560

Hammer, L. B., Cullen, J. C., Neal, M. B., Sinclair, R., R., & Shafiro, M. V. (2005). The longitudinal effects of work-family conflict and positive spillover on depressive symptoms among dual-earner couples. *Journal of Occupational Health Psychology, 10,* 138–154. doi:10.1037/1076-8998.10.2.138

Hanson, G. C., Hammer, L. B., & Colton, C. L. (2006). Development and validation of a multidimensional scale of perceived work-family positive spillover. *Journal of Occupational Health Psychology, 11,* 249–265. doi:10.1037/1076-8998.11.3.249

Hargis, M. B., Kotrba, L. M., Zhdanova, L., & Baltes, B. B. (2011). What's really important? Examining the relative importance of antecedents to work-family conflict. *Journal of Managerial Issues, 23,* 386–408. doi:10.1037/t06070-000

Hepburn, C. G., & Barling, J. (1996). Eldercare responsibilities, interrole conflict and employee absence: A daily study. *Journal of Occupational Health Psychology, 1,* 311–318. doi:10.1037/1076-8998.1.3.311

Heymann, J., Earle, A., & Hayes, J. (2007). *The work, family, and equity index: How does the United States measure up?* Boston, MA: Project on Global Working Families. Retrieved from http://www.hreonline.com/pdfs/08012009Extra_McGillSurvey.pdf

Hill, E. J., Erickson, J. J., Homes, E. K., & Ferris, M. (2010). Workplace flexibility, work hours, and work-life conflict: Finding an extra day or two. *Journal of Family Psychology, 24,* 349–358. doi:10.1037/a0019282

Ho, M. Y., Chen, X., Cheung, F. M., Liu, H., & Worthington, E. L., Jr. (2013). A dyadic model of the work-family interface: A study of dual-earner couples in China. *Journal of Occupational Health Psychology, 18,* 53–63. doi:10.1037/a0030885

Hofstede, G. (2001). *Cultural consequences: Comparing values, behaviors, institutions and organizations across nations* (2nd ed.). Thousand Oaks, CA: Sage.

Ilies, R., Schwind, K. M., Wagner, D. T., Johnson, M. D., DeRue, D. S., & Ilgen, D. R. (2007). When can employees have a family life? The effects of daily workload and affect on work-family conflict and social behaviors at home. *Journal of Applied Psychology, 92,* 1368–1379. doi:10.1037/0021-9010.92.5.1368

Johnson, J. V., & Hall, E. M. (1988). Job strain, work place social support, and cardiovascular disease: A cross-sectional study of a random sample of the Swedish working population. *American Journal of Public Health, 78,* 1336-1342. doi:10.2105/AJPH.78.10.1336

Judge, T. A., Ilies, R., & Scott, B. A. (2006). Work-family conflict and emotions: Effects at work and at home. *Personnel Psychology, 59,* 779–814. doi:10.1111/j.1744-6570.2006.00054.x

Kanter, R. M. (1977). *Work and family in the United States: A critical review for research and policy.* New York, NY: Russell Sage Foundation.

Karasek, R. A. (1979). Job demands, job decision latitude and mental strain: Implications for job redesign. *Administrative Science Quarterly, 24,* 285–308.

Karatepe, O. M., & Bektechi, L. (2008). Antecedents and outcomes of work-family facilitation and family-work facilitation among frontline hotel employees. *International Journal of Hospitality Management, 27,* 517–528. doi:10.1016/j.ijhm.2007.09.004

Kelloway, E. K., Gottlieb, B. H., & Barham, L. (1999). The source, nature, and direction of work and family conflict: A longitudinal investigation. *Journal of Occupational Health Psychology, 4,* 337–346. doi:10.1037/1076-8998.4.4.337

Kinnunen, U., Geurts, S., & Mauno, S. (2004). Work-to-family conflict and its relationship with satisfaction and well-being: A one-year longitudinal study on gender differences. *Work & Stress, 18,* 1–22. doi:10.1080/02678370410001682005

Kirchmeyer, C. (2000). Work-life initiatives: Greed or benevolence regarding workers' time? In C. L. Cooper & D. M. Rousseau (Eds.), *Trends in organizational behavior* (Vol. 7, pp. 79–93). West Sussex, UK: Wiley.

Kossek, E. E. (2008). Work-family balance. In S. J. Clegg & J. R. Bailey (Eds.), *International encyclopedia of organization studies* (pp. 1630–1635). Thousand Oaks, CA: Sage.

Kossek, E. E., Baltes, B. B., & Matthews, R. A. (2011). How work-family research can finally have an impact in organizations. *Industrial and Organizational Psychology, 4,* 352–369.

Kossek, E. E., Lautsch, B. A., & Eaton, S. C. (2006). Telecommuting, control, and boundary management: Correlates of policy use and practice, job control, and work-family effectiveness. *Journal of Vocational Behavior, 68,* 347–367. doi:10.1016/j.jvb.2005.07.002

Kossek, E. E., & Ozeki, C. (1998). Work-family conflict, policies, and the job-life satisfaction relationship: A review and directions for organizational behavior–human resources research. *Journal of Applied Psychology, 83,* 139–149. doi:10.1037/0021-9010.83.2.139

Kossek, E. E., Pichler, S., Bodner, T., & Hammer, L. B. (2011). Workplace social support and work-family conflict: A meta-analysis clarifying the influence of general and work-family-specific supervisor and organizational support. *Personnel Psychology, 64,* 289–313. doi:10.1111/j.1744-6570.2011.01211.x

Lambert, A. D., Marler, J. H., & Gueutal, H. G. (2008). Individual differences: Factors affecting employee utilization of flexible work arrangements. *Journal of Vocational Behavior, 73,* 107–117. doi:10.1016/j.jvb.2008.02.004

Lambert, E. G., Minor, K. I., Wells, J. B., & Hogan, N. L. (2015). Leave your job at work: The possible antecedents of work-family conflict among correctional staff. *The Prison Journal, 95,* 114–134. doi:10.1177/0032885514563284

Lawson, K. M., Davis, K. D., McHale, S. M., Hammer, L. B., & Buxton, O. M. (2014). Daily positive spillover and crossover from mothers' work to youth health. *Journal of Family Psychology, 28,* 807–907. doi:10.1037/fam0000028

Liu, Y., Wang, M., Chang, C.-H., Shi, J., Zhou, L., & Shao, R. (2015). Work-family conflict, emotional exhaustion, and displaced aggression toward others: The moderating roles of workplace interpersonal conflict and perceived managerial family support. *Journal of Applied Psychology, 100,* 793–808. doi:10.1037/a0038387

Marks, S. R., & MacDermid, S. M. (1996). Multiple roles and the self: A theory of role balance. *Journal of Marriage and the Family, 58,* 417–432. doi:10.2307/353506

Marshall, N. L., & Barnett, R. C. (1993). Work-family strains and gains among two-earner couples. *Journal of Community Psychology, 21*, 64–78. doi:10.1002/1520-6629(199301)21:13.0.CO;2-P

Masuda, A. D., Poelmans, S. A. Y., Allen, T. D., Spector, P. E., Lapierre, L. M., Cooper, C. L., . . . Moreno-Velazquez, I. (2012). Flexible work arrangements availability and their relationship with work-to-family conflict, job satisfaction, and turnover intentions: A comparison of three country clusters. *Applied Psychology: An International Review, 61*, 1–29. doi:10.1111/j.1464-0597.2011.00453.x

Matsui, T., Ohsawa, T., & Onglatco, M.-L. (1995). Work-family conflict and the stress-buffering effects of husband support and coping behavior among Japanese married working women. *Journal of Vocational Behavior, 47*, 178–192. doi:10.1006/jvbe.1995.1034

Matthews, R. A., Mills, M. J., Trout, R. C., & English, L. (2014). Family-supportive supervisor behaviors, work engagement, and subjective well-being: A contextually dependent mediated process. *Journal of Occupational Health Psychology, 19*, 168–181. doi:10.1037/a0036012

McNall, L. A., Nicklin, J. M., & Masuda, A. D. (2010). A meta-analytic review of the consequences associated with work-family enrichment. *Journal of Business & Psychology, 25*, 381–396. doi:10.1007/s10869-009-9141-1

Mesmar-Magnus, J., & Viswesvaran, C. (2005). Convergence between measures of work-to-family and family-to-work conflict: A meta-analytic examination. *Journal of Vocational Behavior, 67*, 215–232. doi:10.1016/j.jvb.2004.05.004

Michel, J. S., Clark, M. A., & Jaramillo, D. (2011). The role of the five factor model of personality in the perceptions of negative and positive forms of work-nonwork spillover: A meta-analytic review. *Journal of Vocational Behavior, 79*, 191–203. doi:10.1016/j.jvb.2010.12.010

Michel, J. S., Kotrba, L. M., Mitchelson, J. K., Clark, M. A., & Baltes, B. B. (2011). Antecedents of work-family conflict: A meta-analytic review. *Journal of Organizational Behavior, 32*, 689–725. doi:10.1002/job.695

Neal, M. B., & Hammer, L. B. (2007). *Working couples caring for children and aging parents: Effects on work and well-being.* Mahwah, NJ: Lawrence Erlbaum.

Nohe, C., Meier, L., Sonntag, K., & Michel, A. (2015). The chicken or the egg? A meta-analysis of panel studies of the relationship between work-family conflict and strain. *Journal of Applied Psychology, 100*, 522–536. doi:10.1037/a0038012

Odle-Dusseau, H. N., Britt, T. W., & Greene-Shortridge, T. M. (2012). Organizational work-family resources as predictors of job performance and attitudes: The process of work-family conflict and enrichment. *Journal of Occupational Health Psychology, 17*, 28 40. doi:10.1037/a0026428

Parker, K., & Wang, W. (2013). *Modern parenthood: Roles of moms and dads converge as they balance work and family.* Washington, DC: Pew Research Center. Retrieved from www.pewsocialtrends.org/2013/03/14/modern-parenthood-roles-of-moms-and-dads-converge-as-they-balance-work-and-family

Rantanen, J., Kinnunen, U., Feldt, T., & Pulkkinen, L. (2008). Work-family conflict and psychological well-being: Stability and cross-lagged relations within one- and six-year follow-ups. *Journal of Vocational Behavior, 73*, 37–51. doi:10.1016/j.jvb.2008.01.001

Ray, R., Gornick, J. C., & Schmitt, J. (2009). *Parental leave policies in 21 countries: Assessing generosity and gender equality.* Washington, DC: Center for Economic and Policy Research.

Sanz-Vergel, A. I., Demerouti, E., Moreno-Jiménez, B., & Mayo, M. (2010). Work–family balance and energy: A day-level study on recovery conditions. *Journal of Vocational Behavior, 76*, 118–130. doi:10.1016/j.jvb.2009.07.001

Shellenbarger, S. (2008, June 11). Downsizing maternity leave: Employers cut pay, time off. *The Wall Street Journal*, p. D1.

Shockley, K. M., & Allen, T. D. (2007). When flexibility helps: Another look at the availability of flexible work arrangements and work-family conflict. *Journal of Vocational Behavior, 71*, 479–493. doi:10.1016/j.jvb.2007.08.006

Shockley, K. M., & Allen, T. D. (2013). Episodic work-family conflict, cardiovascular indicators, and social support: An experience-sampling approach. *Journal of Occupational Health Psychology, 18*, 262–275. doi:10.1037/a0033137

Shockley, K. M., & Singla, N. (2011). Reconsidering work-family interactions and satisfaction: A meta-analysis. *Journal of Management, 37*, 861–886. doi:10.1177/0149206310394864

Skinner, N., & Ichii, R. (2015). Exploring a family, work, and community model of work-family gains and strains. *Community, Work, & Family, 18*, 79–99. doi:10.1080/13668803.2014.981507

Society for Human Resource Management. (2010). *2010 employee benefits: Examining employee benefits in the midst of a recovering economy.* Alexandria, VA: Society for Human Resource Management.

Spector, P. E., Allen, T. D., Poelmans, S. A. Y., Lapierre, L. M., Cooper, C. L., O'Driscoll, M., . . . Widerszal-Bazyl, M. (2007). Cross-national differences in relationships of work demands, job satisfaction, and turnover intentions with work-family conflict. *Personnel Psychology, 60*, 805–835. doi:10.1111/j.1744-6570.2007.00092.x

Spector, P. E., Sanchez, J. I., Siu, O. L., Salgado, J., & Ma, J. (2004). Eastern versus Western control beliefs at work: An investigation of secondary control, socioinstrumental control, and work locus of control in China and the US. *Applied Psychology: An International Review, 53*, 38–60. doi:10.1111/j.1464-0597.2004.00160.x

Srivastava, S., & Srivastava, U. R. (2014). Work and non-work related outcomes of work-family facilitation. *Social Science International, 30*, 353–372.

Tement, S. (2014). The role of personal and key resources in the family-to-work enrichment process. *Scandinavian Journal of Psychology, 55*, 489–496. doi:10.1111/sjop.12146

Triandis, H. C. (2001). Individualism-collectivism and personality. *Journal of Personality, 69*, 907–924. doi:10.1111/1467-6494.696169

van Daalen, G., Williemsen, T. M., & Sanders, K. (2006). Reducing work-family conflict through different sources of social support. *Journal of Vocational Behavior, 69*, 462–476. doi:10.1016/j.jvb.2006.07.005

van Steenbergen, E. F. & Ellemers, N. (2009). Is managing the work-family interface worthwhile? Benefits for employee health and performance. *Journal of Organizational Behavior, 30*, 617–642. doi:10.1002/job.5

van Steenbergen, F., Ellemers, N., & Mooijaart, A. (2007). How work and family can facilitate each other: Distinct types of work-family facilitation and outcomes for women and men. *Journal of Occupational Health Psychology, 12*, 279–300. doi:10.1037/1076-8998.12.3.279

Wadsworth, L. L., & Owens, B. P. (2007). The effects of social support on work-family enhancement and work-family conflict in the public sector. *Public Administration Review, 67*, 75–86. doi:10.1111/j.1540-6210.2006.00698.x

Wagner, D. T., Barnes, C. M., & Scott, B. A. (2014). Driving it home: How workplace emotional labor harms employee home life. *Personnel Psychology, 67*, 487–516. doi:10.1111/peps.12044

Wang, M., Liu, S., Zhan, Y., & Shi, J. (2010). Daily work-family conflict and alcohol use: Testing the cross-level moderation effects of peer drinking norms and social support. *Journal of Applied Psychology, 95*, 377–386. doi:10.1037/a0018138

Wayne, J. H., Grzywacz, J. G., Carlson, D. S., & Kacmar, K. M. (2007). Work-family facilitation: A theoretical explanation and model of primary antecedents and consequences. *Human Resource Management Review, 17*, 63–76. doi:10.1016/j.hrmr.2007.01.002

Wayne, J. H., Musisca, N., & Fleeson, W. (2004). Considering the role of personality in the work-family experience: Relationships of the Big Five to work-family conflict and facilitation. *Journal of Vocational Behavior, 64*, 108–130. doi:10.1016/S0001-8791(03)00035-6

Wayne, J. H., Randel, A. E., & Stevens, J. (2006). The role of identity and work-family support in work-family enrichment and its work-related consequences. *Journal of Vocational Behavior, 69*, 445–461. doi:10.1016/j.jvb.2006.07.002

Wiese, B. S., Seiger, C. P., Schmid, C. M., & Freund, A. M. (2010). Beyond conflict: Functional facets of the work-family interplay. *Journal of Vocational Behavior, 77*, 104–117. doi:10.1016/j.jvb.2010.02.011

Yang, N. (2005). *Individualism-collectivism and work-family interfaces: A Sino-U.S. comparison.* Mahwah, NJ: Erlbaum.

Yang, N., Chen, C. C., Choi, J., & Zou, Y. (2000). Sources of work-family conflict: A Sino-U.S. comparison of the effects of work and family demands. *Academy of Management Journal, 43*, 113–123. doi:10.2307/1556390

Young, M., & Wheaton, B. (2013). The impact of neighborhood composition on work-family conflict and distress. *Journal of Health and Social Behavior, 54*, 481–497. doi:10.1177/0022146513504761

TEN

Interventions in Occupational Health Psychology

KEY CONCEPTS AND FINDINGS COVERED IN CHAPTER 10

Integrated model for intervention in OHP
    Primary interventions to improve work–life balance
    Secondary interventions to improve work–life balance
    Tertiary interventions to improve work–life balance
    Primary interventions to improve physical health and safety
    Secondary interventions to improve physical health and safety
    Tertiary interventions to improve physical health and safety
    Primary interventions to improve psychological health and well-being
    Secondary and tertiary interventions to improve psychological health and well-being
Summary

Occupational health psychology (OHP) involves the application of psychological theories and principles for the purpose of understanding and enhancing the safety, health, and well-being of workers. To these ends, the primary purpose of OHP is to prevent physical illness, mental health problems, and injuries and to promote workers' health and well-being through the creation of work environments that are supportive of employee health, safety, and well-being (Sauter, Hurrell, Fox, Tetrick, & Barling, 1999; Tetrick & Quick, 2011). In this chapter, we review OHP-related interventions that promote worker health, safety, and well-being. Specifically, we first discuss a general framework for understanding different approaches to interventions within OHP. Common interventions designed to promote worker safety, health, and well-being will be introduced and their efficacy and effectiveness will be reviewed. We use the term "efficacy" to represent the extent to which an intervention implemented in the context of experimental and quasi-experimental research benefits participants in the experimental group; we use the term "effectiveness" to represent the extent to which an intervention implemented under the usual conditions of work benefits workers.

INTEGRATED MODEL FOR INTERVENTION IN OHP

Before discussing specific interventions and their efficacy and effectiveness, it is helpful to introduce an integrated model for intervening in the workplace. The model proposed by Tetrick and Quick (2011) is based on a combination of two approaches, the Practices for Achieving Total Health, or PATH, model (Grawitch, Gottschalk, & Munz, 2006) and the public health prevention model (Schmidt, 1994).

The PATH model (Grawitch et al., 2006) identifies five areas through which workplace practices can be enhanced in order to promote occupational health: work–life balance, employee growth and development, health and safety, recognition, and employee involvement. When organizations invest resources to advance these five areas, the investment is not only likely to enhance employee well-being, but also improve the organization as a whole. Grawitch et al. (2006) regarded employee well-being as comprising both physical and psychological facets of health. Markers of well-being are reflected in physical health indicators, mental health indicators, stress and resilience, and morale at work. Organizational improvement refers to individual performance outcomes that have advantages at the organizational level (Grawitch et al., 2006) such as reduced absenteeism and turnover, reduced accident and injury rates (which are also reflective of employee physical health), and improved productivity and customer service. All translate into overall betterment of the organization.

The second approach is the public health prevention model (Schmidt, 1994). In this model, interventions are classified according to three categories: primary interventions (primary prevention), secondary interventions (secondary prevention), and tertiary interventions (tertiary prevention). Targets of primary interventions are individuals who are not at risk.

The goal of primary interventions is prevention. Primary interventions are often population based, such that interventions are applicable to all the employees within an organization (or all workers within a particular unit of an organization). Examples of primary interventions include health education or promotion campaigns in which a message about the benefits of regular exercise or the harm associated with smoking is broadcast to reach to all members of an organization (Tetrick & Quick, 2003, 2011). Another type of primary intervention would involve changing task structures such that workers would have more latitude in making task-related decisions, presuming increased latitude would have a beneficial effect on health and morale.

Secondary interventions target individuals who are at risk for illness, injury, or ill-being. Rather than reaching out to all the workers in the organization or an organizational unit, secondary interventions tend to target specific groups or individuals who are exposed to various risk factors. For example, safety tips and personal protective equipment may be provided to workers who are exposed to physical, biological, or chemical hazards on the job (Tetrick & Quick, 2011).

Finally, tertiary interventions are directed toward individuals who have experienced health decrements and are intended to restore their health and well-being. Tertiary interventions are typically individual-based, but group-based tertiary interventions designed to alleviate the symptoms of individuals who suffer from a similar illness or injury are also possible. For example, individual counseling or group therapy to treat those with work-related burnout symptoms can be considered a tertiary intervention (Tetrick & Quick, 2011).

In integrating the PATH model with the public health model, Tetrick and Quick (2011) proposed a taxonomy of interventions that are designed to protect and promote workers' health, safety, and well-being. Specifically, they argued that primary, secondary, and tertiary interventions could be implemented by an organization to enhance the five areas highlighted by the PATH model. For example, in the area of employee growth and involvement, organizations may offer all employees training in both job-related skills and general interpersonal skills. Such training can be considered a primary intervention because it may facilitate communication among workers and reduce the likelihood of interpersonal conflict, a major stressor. The intervention may also improve job performance. As a secondary intervention, organizations may design specific training aimed at meeting the needs of a subset of employees. For example, technology training for older workers may be helpful (Levy, 2013). Finally, tertiary intervention may involve remedial training for employees who have experienced occupational illnesses or injuries. For example, organizations may provide training for individuals who need special accommodation (e.g., utilization of additional equipment, alternative work arrangements) due to their occupational injuries.

In the following sections, we will introduce primary, secondary, and tertiary interventions designed to address OHP topic areas discussed elsewhere in the book and summarize the evidence for their efficacy and effectiveness where possible. In doing so, we will focus on two of the five areas discussed in the PATH model, namely, work–life balance and health and safety (including psychological health and well-being), as these areas are the focal concerns of this book.

Primary Interventions to Improve Work–Life Balance

Primary interventions designed to improve work–life balance typically provide employees with benefits such as flexible work arrangements or personal days off (Tetrick & Quick, 2011). These benefits are available to all employees and are designed to prevent work duties interfering with family responsibilities and vice versa. Flexible work arrangements include practices such as flextime, a compressed workweek, part-time options, job-sharing, and telecommuting (Levy, 2013). Flextime refers to flexibility in work schedule, where organizations may designate a "core period" during which all employees must be available (e.g., 11 a.m. to 3 p.m.), and beyond that, individual employees have the flexibility to structure their workday (e.g., when to start and finish work) or workweek provided that they complete a predetermined number of working hours (Baltes, Briggs, Huff, Wright, & Neuman, 1999). A compressed workweek also offers flexibility in terms of schedule, such that the workweek is compressed into fewer than 5 days by increasing the number of hours employees work each day. The most common compressed workweek in the United States is a 4-day, 40-hour workweek, such that employees work 4 days a week for 10 hours a day (Latack & Foster, 1985). Organizations have adopted other configurations of the compressed workweek, such as 3-day, 36-hour workweek or the 3-day, 40-hour workweek.

Both part-time options and job-sharing are practices designed to reduce individual employees' workload in order to provide them with flexibility (Kelly et al., 2008). Finally, telecommuting offers individuals flexibility regarding work location (Levy, 2013). Garrett and Danziger (2007) identified three forms of telework for organizational employees on the basis of their primary work location. The first type is the fixed-site teleworkers; these workers perform some of their job tasks at home or in a satellite office. A second type is the mobile teleworkers, who work predominantly in the field. Finally, the last category is the flexiworkers, who mix office work with work in the home and the field. In a cross-sectional survey, Garrett and Danziger compared these three types of teleworkers in the United States. The researchers found that, although the three types of teleworkers reported similarly high levels of job satisfaction, (a) flexiworkers tended to report higher influence over their job and (b) mobile workers appeared to be better able to keep up with the workload.

Research on the effectiveness of the flexible work arrangements often distinguishes between the availability of such policies in the workplace and the actual use of these policies (Kelly et al., 2008). In terms of availability, a nationally representative sample of medium and large employers (i.e., those with 50 or more employees) in the United States revealed that various flexible work arrangement practices have been widely adopted. For example, 68% of the companies make flextime available, 46% provide a compressed workweek, and 35% provide a teleworking arrangement (Bond, Galinsky, Kim, & Brownfield, 2005). However, the availability of flexible work arrangements alone may not be enough for achieving work–life balance and preventing work interference with family responsibilities and vice versa. Kelly et al. (2008) concluded from their qualitative review that studies of the availability of flexible work arrangements tend to yield mixed results. Consistent with Kelly et al.'s conclusion, Allen, Johnson, Kiburz, and Shockley's (2013) meta-analysis of mainly cross-sectional surveys showed that flextime availability was associated with lower work interference with family; however, the availability of flexible work location (e.g., telecommuting) was unrelated to work interference with family. The meta-analysis also found that flexplace availability was associated with lower family interference with work and that flextime availability, however, was unrelated to family interference with work. To sum up, Allen et al.'s results suggest that availability of different types of flexible work arrangement may have different effects on different aspects of work–life balance.

Beyond availability, results tend to show that the actual use of flexible work arrangements helps individuals achieve work–life balance. For example, in their meta-analysis of experimental-control group, pre–post, and experimental-normative group studies, Baltes, Briggs, Huff, Wright, and Neuman (1999) found that compared with employees working under traditional work arrangements, those who utilized flextime practices reported higher job satisfaction and satisfaction with their work schedule. Similarly, those working under a compressed workweek schedule reported higher job satisfaction and satisfaction with their work schedule compared with those working under traditional work arrangements. Gajendran and Harrison's (2007) meta-analysis of predominantly cross-sectional studies revealed an overall negative relationship between telecommuting and work–family conflict, thus linking flexible work location and better work–life balance. Consistent with Gajendran and Harrison (2007), Allen et al.'s (2013) meta-analysis also suggested that the use of flexible work location arrangements was negatively related to work interference with family. However, their results indicated that flextime use was not significantly related to work interference with family. Interestingly, Baltes et al. found that the positive effects associated with the use of flextime weaken the longer individuals work under a flexible schedule. This finding suggests that the long-term effect of such interventions may gradually wear off as individuals become more accustomed to a flexible work schedule.

A rigorous examination of primary interventions is needed. Although it is unlikely that we will see the introduction of experiments and quasi-experiments to assess primary interventions oriented toward evaluating the impact of flexible time arrangements on work–life balance, it is possible for researchers to capitalize on natural experiments and time series designs (see Chapter 2) to better document the effects of such time arrangements. Overall, existing research evidence is consistent with the view that flexible work arrangements have been widely adopted by organizations as a way to enhance employees' work–life balance. However, making these policies available may not be sufficient to prevent conflict between work and nonwork domains. Actual use of these flexible work arrangements appears to be more important to the goal of improving work–life balance.

Secondary Interventions to Improve Work–Life Balance

Secondary interventions designed to improve work–life balance tend to focus on providing family-friendly benefits that apply to employees with family responsibilities (Tetrick & Quick, 2011). These benefits do not apply to all employees, but are designed to assist those who are at risk for experiencing work–family conflict and to help those individuals better meet their work *and* family responsibilities. For example, providing childcare and eldercare benefits and offering paid leaves to help workers meet their responsibilities outside of work constitute organizational programs and policies that are viewed as secondary interventions to improve work–life balance (Levy, 2013). In terms of benefits associated with childcare/eldercare, the most common practice is to provide employees pre–tax spending accounts for dependent care; almost half (45%) of medium to large U.S. companies reported the availability of such benefits for their employees (Bond et al., 2005). The provision of information and referral services to help employees obtain high-quality dependent care is also a common practice. One-third of medium to large U.S. companies report that they provide such information (Bond et al., 2005). A much smaller percentage of the U.S. companies (7%) offer on-site childcare (Bond et al., 2005). In much of Europe, the provision of childcare is considered a public responsibility (i.e., supported by the government) rather than a benefit associated with one's particular employment (European Union, 2016). As such, it is not common for organizations to provide childcare as a secondary intervention for workers because provision is governed and supported by national policy.

Organizations can also offer paid leaves to help their employees achieve work–life balance. Although the United States is one of the two countries that do not have a national policy regarding paid maternity leave (Addati, Cassirer, & Gilchrist, 2014), almost half (46%) of medium to large U.S. employers offer employees at least partially paid family leaves (Bond et al., 2005). Other companies offer full- or partially paid sabbaticals or paid time-off to engage in activities for personal growth and development. For example, Google, a company that has routinely been ranked number 1 on the list of "100 Best Companies to Work For" published by *Fortune* magazine, offers employees 20 paid days off a year to engage in voluntary work. Kimpton Hotels and Restaurants, which also ranked highly on *Fortune* magazine's list, offers employees 4 weeks of paid sabbatical after employees have been working for the company for 7 years. The paid time-off is intended to help employees achieve better work–life balance.

Beyond organizational policies concerning family-specific benefits, researchers have also focused on developing other types of secondary interventions to improve the work–family balance of at-risk employees. One example is the intervention designed to enhance organizational support for employees to better handle work–family conflict. Specifically, Hammer, Kossek, Anger, Bodner, and Zimmerman (2011) described a study designed to evaluate the efficacy of a supervisor training and self-monitoring intervention that built on ideas underlined in an earlier cross-sectional study. In that earlier study, Hammer, Kossek, Yragui, Bodner, and Hanson (2009) identified family-supportive behaviors that include supervisors' actions that provide emotional support (e.g., showing care for employees' work–family demands) and instrumental support (e.g., changing an employee's shift so that he or she can meet family responsibilities), role-modeling behaviors (e.g., demonstrating how to balance work–family demands), and creative work–family management (e.g., restructuring work to facilitate employee effectiveness at work and at home). Hammer et al. (2009) found that these family-supportive behaviors were negatively related to employees' work interference with family and positively related to their family-to-work enhancement. Employees whose supervisors engaged in these family-supportive behaviors also tended to report higher job satisfaction and lower turnover intentions.

Building on the idea that supervisors' family-supportive behaviors benefit employees, Hammer et al. (2011) developed an intervention that included two features. One was a training program to teach supervisors family-supportive behaviors. The other was a behavioral self-monitoring component to ensure that supervisors transfer what they learned during training to practice in the workplace.

In this study, Hammer et al. (2011) randomly assigned six grocery stores in a midwestern U.S. grocery chain to receive the intervention, while another six stores served as control sites. The researchers trained mid- and high-level managers in the intervention sites and asked the subordinates in the experimental and control sites to report work–family conflict, job satisfaction, and physical health on a pre–post intervention basis. Results showed that compared with employees at the control sites, employees at the intervention sites reported better physical health after controlling for baseline health. The intervention interacted with subordinates' baseline family interference with work in predicting their physical health and job satisfaction postintervention. Specifically, family interference with work was negatively associated with employees' physical health only for those whose supervisors did not receive the intervention; interference was unrelated to health for employees whose supervisors received the intervention. Surprisingly, family interference with work had a weak relationship with employees' job satisfaction only among those whose supervisors did not receive the intervention; interference was *positively* related to job satisfaction for those whose supervisors were in the treatment group. Finally, employees' perceptions of supervisor family-supportive behaviors mediated these main and interaction effects.

Hammer et al.'s (2011) research was a prelude to another study, namely, the Work, Family, and Health Study (WFHS), a large intervention study designed by an interdisciplinary team. The aim of this newer, larger intervention, referred to as "STAR" (Support Transform Achieve Results; Hammer et al., 2016), was to help employees achieve work–life balance by enhancing supervisor family-supportive behaviors. A second component, which was applicable to all employees regardless of family status, was designed to provide employees with greater control over when and where they work. This multiyear, multisite study was a group-randomized field experiment that took place at two firms representing different industries: the information technology (IT) division of a large, *Fortune 500* company and an extended-care/nursing home company with multiple worksites. Different worksites of these two companies were randomly assigned to intervention and practice-as-usual (i.e., control) conditions. Employees and their managers were assessed at baseline, and at 6, 12, and 18 months postintervention. More information about the overall study can be found at www.WorkFamilyHealthNetwork.org.

To date, the research has demonstrated the efficacy of the STAR intervention. Kelly et al. (2014) found that, at the 6-month follow-up, IT employees in the intervention condition, compared with IT employees in the control group, perceived higher levels of supervisor family-supportive behaviors and reduced work–family conflict. Davis et al. (2015) showed that IT employees in the STAR intervention group reported spending more time with their children at the 12-month follow-up postintervention. Given carryover to home life, children of parents in the STAR group, compared with control children, took less time to fall asleep at night (McHale et al., 2015). Olson et al. (2015) found that the STAR intervention resulted in improved sleep quality and quantity among IT employees at the 12-month follow-up. Finally, Hammer et al. (2016) found that the STAR intervention protected low-wage health care employees against a decline in safety compliance behaviors and organizational citizenship behaviors at the 6- and 12-month follow-ups, respectively. Taken together, these results demonstrate that this intervention not only benefits professionals, but also can help those in lower-wage occupations. The latter group is particularly vulnerable as some organizational benefits seen in other workplaces (e.g., paid time-off to achieve work–life balance) may not be readily available to them. The STAR intervention represents a potential avenue for organizations to improve work–life balance for lower-wage workers.

Tertiary Interventions to Improve Work–Life Balance

In terms of tertiary interventions designed to support employees with health decrements due to work–life imbalance, Tetrick and Quick (2011) underlined the importance of employee assistance programs (EAPs) and the role such programs play in supporting employees who experience difficulties with responsibilities outside of work. According to Berridge, Cooper, and Highley (1997), EAPs provide a set of services such as counseling, advice, and assistance. EAPs are funded by organizations in order to help employees with personal difficulties and performance problems. In some cases, EAPs provide services such as individual and family counseling to help employees (a) cope with harmful symptoms (e.g., high levels of burnout symptoms) induced by work–family conflict and (b) develop strategies to better meet both work and family responsibilities. Because EAPs usually involve a broad set of services designed to help employees cope with symptoms resulting from a wide range of problems beyond work–family conflict (Arthur, 2000; Berridge & Cooper, 1994), there is no clear evidence that speaks directly to the effectiveness of EAPs as a tertiary intervention for improving work–life balance. However, evaluation results tend to show high user satisfaction with EAPs and that EAP participation is associated with overall improvement in quality of life (e.g., Macdonald, Lothian, & Wells, 1997; Macdonald, Wells, Lothian, & Shain, 2000). Evidence for EAP participation and improvement based on objective criteria is more mixed. For example, only about half of the employees reported improvement in productivity or lower absenteeism after EAP use (e.g., Attridge, 2003; Harlow, 2006).

Unfortunately, research on EAPs as a tertiary intervention tends to employ weak study designs, which limit our ability to speak directly about the outcomes of EAP participation. Given the wide range of services available through EAPs, more research is needed to further determine which types of EAP services are most beneficial in reducing work–life conflict.

Primary Interventions to Improve Physical Health and Safety

Primary interventions to improve workers' physical health and safety may involve general health- and safety-promotion programs and training efforts that are applicable to an entire organization (Tetrick & Quick, 2011). To illustrate, primary interventions have been conducted with the aim of reducing sitting or sedentary work, which is a risk for cardiovascular disease, obesity, and overall mortality (Shrestha et al., 2016). These interventions include changes in the physical work space (e.g., use of sit-stand desks, treadmill desks, cycling work stations), policy changes (e.g., walking meetings), the provision of tools and feedback (e.g., use of pedometers), and education and counseling to promote more physical activity at work. In a recent review of studies utilizing controlled pre- and postdesigns, Shrestha et al. (2016) concluded that adopting sit-stand desks helped reduce participants' sitting time at work at the 3- and 6-month follow-up. The positive effect of desks, however, weakened over time. Other studies using experimental or quasi-experimental designs revealed similar benefits associated with sit-stand desks; however, the effects of active work stations (e.g., treadmill and cycling desks) were less consistent. Having a policy of walking meetings did not much alter participants' sitting time. Interventions that provided participants with pedometers as a way to encourage more physical activities during the day also had inconsistent effects (Freak-Poli, Cumpston, Peeters, & Clemes, 2013). Finally, Shrestha et al. (2016) found that while counseling reduced participants' sitting time at work, other types of training or computer prompts to move around did not have a consistent effect.

Other primary interventions are designed to improve the general psychosocial environment of the organization in order to improve workers' physical health and safety. In a randomized controlled study, Zohar and Polachek (2014) designed a discourse-based intervention to improve workplace safety by enhancing the safety climate in a manufacturing company. As discussed in Chapters 6 and 8, safety climate refers to how much priority employees perceive that their work organization places on safety. Safety climate has been linked to important safety-related outcomes, such as safety performance, occupational accidents, and worker injuries (Beus, Payne, Bergman, & Arthur, 2010; Christian, Bradley, Wallace, & Burke, 2009). Zohar and Polachek's (2014) intervention used feedback to train supervisors to communicate messages to their subordinates in a way that integrated both safety- and productivity-related topics. Supervisors in the control group received no feedback. Data on safety climate perceptions, safety behaviors, and safety audits were collected 8 weeks before the intervention, and again after the 12-week intervention ended. Results showed that subordinates in the experimental group reported significant pre- to postimprovement in safety climate perceptions and safety behaviors after the intervention; by contrast, climate perceptions and safety performance remained unchanged for those in the control group. In addition to the self-reported data, safety audits were conducted before and after the intervention by two external, independent safety experts to evaluate the adequacy of risk protection for employees on the basis of walk-around tours of the company. Zohar and Polachek (2014) found a significant improvement in safety audit results in the experimental group but not in the control group.

In a study in which 51 organizational units from 11 businesses were randomly assigned to experimental and control conditions, Naveh and Katz-Navon (2015) examined the impact of an intervention that was designed to develop and maintain a road safety management system. The system had (a) a training component to teach participants safe driving behaviors; (b) a participatory decision-making component to involve both managers and subordinates in planning and executing strategies to monitor road safety behaviors; and (c) a reward component to motivate and sustain safe driving behaviors. Road safety climate was reported by participants 3 months before the intervention and 1 year after the beginning of the intervention. The number of traffic violation tickets received by employees was recorded 1 year before the intervention and 1 year after the beginning of the intervention. Naveh and

Katz-Navon (2015) found that drivers in units assigned to the experimental group reported higher levels of safety climate after the intervention, whereas those in the control group showed minimal change. The number of traffic violation tickets was reduced in the intervention group while the number remained unchanged in the control group. Improvements in road safety also carried over into home life.

Taken together, these results suggest that primary interventions designed to enhance workers' physical health and safety can be beneficial. Their efficacy and effectiveness, however, may depend on the specific design of the intervention. More research with stronger designs is needed to better establish the link between specific interventions and improvement in workers' physical health and safety.

Secondary Interventions to Improve Physical Health and Safety

Secondary interventions that are designed to promote workers' physical health and safety target specific at-risk populations (Tetrick & Quick, 2011). In this case, rather than trying to reach the entire population, these interventions are designed to reach workers in specific occupations or industries who are exposed to physical, chemical, and biological occupational hazards, or workers who engage in behaviors that may be damaging to their health (e.g., smoking). As mentioned earlier, it is common for organizations to conduct safety training to ensure that employees know the safety policies and regulations and how to use protective equipment. Training and education programs are also often used to promote healthy behaviors. Goal-setting for various safety and health target (e.g., being accident free) and distribution of rewards to individual employees when a goal is reached are also common. Finally, insurance companies could provide additional incentives to companies to enhance safety by adopting the experience-rating procedure. Such a procedure increases premiums for organizations that have a poor safety record and offers discounts for those that do not have accidents.

In terms of the efficacy of safety training, Rautiainen et al. (2008), in reviewing studies having randomized controlled designs, found that safety training had no effects on agricultural workers' risk of occupational injury. Bena, Berchialla, Coffano, Debernardi, and Icardi (2009) used an interrupted time series design to evaluate the effectiveness of training on injury prevention among construction workers. Although the training enhanced workers' safety knowledge, the intervention, unfortunately, did not result in changes in workers' actual injury rate. Research has also looked at efforts to promote the use of personal protective equipment. In a meta-analytic review, Verbeek, Kateman, Morata, Dreschler, and Mischke (2012) observed that "very low quality evidence of long-term evaluation studies... showed that the use of hearing protection devices in well-implemented [hearing loss prevention programs] was associated with less hearing loss" (p. S93). A meta-analysis of quasi-experimental studies reported that when training methods were more engaging and participative, safety and health training was linked to workers' knowledge acquisition and a reduction in accidents and injuries (Burke et al., 2006). These results suggest that the training design and delivery, in combination with content, are factors to consider when training is used as a secondary intervention to promote worker health and safety.

Regarding the effectiveness of providing incentives for safety and health, Rautiainen et al. (2008), in reviewing studies that employed interrupted time series designs, found that providing financial incentives decreased the injury frequency among agricultural workers immediately after the introduction of the intervention.

The effect, however, dissipated over time, a trend that suggests (a) a role for regular follow-ups after intervention delivery and (b) a need to allocate sufficient financial resources to support injury prevention efforts once the initial intervention has ended. Tompa, Trevithick, and McLeod's (2007) qualitative review indicates that across studies that used pre- and posttest designs, the introduction of experience ratings in insurance practice was associated with reduction in the frequency of injuries. Overall, providing financial incentives for reaching health and safety goals appears to be a viable way to promote workers' physical health and reduce injuries.

Tertiary Interventions to Improve Physical Health and Safety

Among tertiary interventions to support workers who have impaired health due to injuries or illnesses are found practices that either slow the development of impairment (e.g., smoking cessation or weight management programs) or promote a return to work among impaired workers (Tetrick & Quick, 2011). In their review of randomized controlled trials, Cahill, Hartmann-Boyce, and Perera (2015) found that worksite smoking cessation programs that use financial incentives help reduce smoking. In particular, individuals who received financial rewards or had their deposit returned to them for their abstinence were more likely to stop smoking. Cahill et al., however, cautioned that the long-term success of workplace smoking cessation programs would largely depend on sufficient funding for the incentives. As such, these programs may not be feasible if organizations lack resources to support the use of incentives.

In terms of promoting workers' return to work after a disability-related absence, de Boer et al. (2015), in their review of randomized controlled studies, found that a multidisciplinary approach appeared to yield the best results. In particular, interventions that involved vocational counseling, patient education and counseling, and biofeedback-assisted training increased cancer patients' return-to-work rates compared with care-as-usual control groups. In another review of workplace interventions to promote an earlier return to work, Franche et al. (2005) identified a number of intervention and organizational characteristics that appeared to support impaired workers. Intervention characteristics such as early contact with the impaired workers, a work accommodation offer, and involvement of the worker in return-to-work coordination efforts were related to shorter disability durations. Organizational characteristics such as supportive management and safety training were also positively associated with a faster return to work. Interestingly, Franche et al. (2005) noted that although the quality of workers' lives after they return to work is crucial to understanding the effectiveness of the intervention, research evidence concerning returning to work has been varied and difficult to integrate. Taken together, these results suggest that more research employing stronger designs is needed to evaluate the efficacy of return-to-work interventions.

Primary Interventions to Improve Psychological Health and Well-Being

Primary interventions to improve workers' psychological health and well-being may involve changes in organizational practices to reduce psychosocial stressors, as well as training for individual employees to improve their general capabilities to respond to different stressors. In the case of interventions for reducing psychosocial stressors, research has been inconsistent. Using a pre- and posttest quasi-experimental design,

Cydulka, Emerman, Shade, and Kubincane (1994) found that emergency medical personnel who volunteered to work a newly devised schedule (12-hour shifts on fewer days) did not experience less stress than did coworkers in the control group who worked the customary schedule (8-hour shifts on more days). Romig, Latif, Gill, Pronovost, and Sapirstein (2012) found that an intervention designed to reduce workload for health care workers had little effect on workers' burnout symptoms. Richardson and Rothstein's (2008) meta-analysis of experimental studies showed that primary interventions to encourage employee participation or improve coworker support had a nonsignificant effect on workers' psychological stress symptoms.

On the other hand, Ruotsalainen, Verbeek, Mariné, and Serra (2015) in their review identified two randomized controlled trials that showed that shorter work schedules reduced burnout symptoms in health care workers. A multiwave longitudinal study (De Raeve, Vasse, Jansen, ven den Brandt, & Kant, 2007) showed that, controlling for baseline decision latitude, increases in workers' latitude over 12 months predicted lower levels of after-work fatigue at 16 months. In a meta-analysis of randomized controlled studies that examined the efficacy of primary interventions, Montano, Hoven, and Siegrist (2014) showed that primary interventions reduced participants' perceived stress, and this effect was consistent across socioeconomic statuses although the research efforts could benefit from having more intervention studies involving workers employed in lower-status jobs.

Hasson et al. (2014) suggested that employees' perceptions regarding their having been exposed to an intervention may be as important as the nature of the intervention itself in promoting beneficial change. Specifically, although all employees in the study were exposed to an intervention designed to reduce psychosocial stressors, only when employees perceived that they have been exposed to a workplace intervention were they more likely to report lower workload and improved decision latitude and perceived support. These findings suggest that the use of employee perceptions of psychosocial stressors to evaluate the impact of an intervention may have a distorting effect.

Although our primary concern is improving working conditions, research has also emphasized developing worker resilience in relation to challenging conditions at work. Resilience is the ability to resist or recover from the impact of difficult conditions. Researchers have developed interventions (e.g., group programs on self-regulation, problem solving; one-on-one coaching) to enhance the resilience of workers. A qualitative review of resilience training found an overall positive effect on individual workers' general capability to respond to stress (Robertson, Cooper, Sarkar, & Curran, 2015). A meta-analysis also evaluated the effects of resilience training on workers' well-being (Vanhove, Herian, Perez, Harms, & Lester, 2016). As in the qualitative review by Robertson et al. (2015), most of the research included in Vanhove et al.'s (2016) meta-analysis were studies having experimental, quasi-experimental, and uncontrolled, pre- and postdesigns. The meta-analytic results showed that resilience training had a modest general positive effect on participants' well-being. Vanhove et al. (2016) further showed that although the positive effects weakened over time, the training appeared to still have a small but positive effect on well-being at 1-month follow-up or beyond. Echoing a finding by Robertson et al. (2015), Vanhove et al. (2016) found that one-on-one delivery of resilience training, usually in the format of coaching, resulted in significantly greater benefit compared with other types of delivery format (e.g., group based). Thus, much like the training programs to improve physical safety, effects of training as a primary intervention to improve psychological well-being may also depend on the design and delivery of the training.

Secondary and Tertiary Interventions to Improve Psychological Health and Well-Being

Secondary interventions aimed at improving psychological health and well-being target workers in specific occupations who are at risk for experiencing high levels of stress (Tetrick & Quick, 2011). Tertiary interventions, on the other hand, are designed to assist individuals who suffer severe stress symptoms and reduce these detrimental psychological effects of occupational exposures (Tetrick & Quick, 2011). Both types of interventions tend to be delivered to workers who are likely to experience burnout or other stress symptoms due to adverse psychosocial working conditions. It is not always possible to differentiate between the two types of interventions because the severity of existing symptoms determines whether the *same* intervention is solely preventative (secondary[1]) or treatment oriented (tertiary[2]). The two intervention categories will thus be discussed together. Unlike primary interventions that aim to lessen exposures to general stressors (e.g., reducing workload or increasing decision latitude) or enhance individuals' general resilience, secondary and tertiary interventions often involve more focused strategies to remove unique occupational stressors or to train workers to use coping strategies thought to alleviate the existing symptoms and reduce the likelihood of further aggravating an existing problem.

In terms of removing specific occupational stressors, Rydstedt, Johannsson, and Evans (1998) evaluated the effects of an intervention designed to remove stressors affecting bus drivers. By redesigning roads, bus routes, and traffic light programming, the intervention rerouted buses to reduce drivers' exposure to traffic congestion and reprogramed traffic lights such that buses were given priority at intersections. Using a pre–post quasi-experimental design, Rydstedt et al. (1998) found that, compared with the control drivers, drivers in the experimental group reported lower workload, higher perceived control, and lower average heart rate after the implementation of the intervention.

Other research focused on training workers to have better coping skills in order to enable them to better respond to stressors or stress symptoms. In a randomized controlled study, Bond and Bunce (2000) evaluated two interventions at a media organization. One was designed to improve emotion-focused coping skills by training workers to accept undesirable thoughts. The other was designed to improve problem-focused coping skills by training workers to come up with innovative ways to address stressors. Compared with control participants, who received no training, workers in both intervention groups reported lower postintervention levels of psychosomatic and depressive symptoms vis-à-vis baseline levels. Van Dierendonck, Schaufeli, and Buunk (1998), in a quasi-experiment, assessed the efficacy of a training intervention for staff providing direct care for the mentally disabled. The intervention was designed to increase their emotion-focused coping skills. The research team found that compared with the control group, staff who received training reported lower levels of burnout symptoms at a 6-month follow-up. In an earlier study using random assignment to experimental and no-treatment control conditions, Ganster, Mayes, Sime, and Tharp (1982) found that an intervention that included training for emotion-focused coping skills and relaxation techniques reduced depressive symptoms and epinephrine levels in social service employees. Ganster et al., however, were unable to later

---

[1] Symptoms exist but they are not severe.
[2] Symptoms are severe.

replicate the effects in the control participants. In their meta-analysis of experimental studies, Richardson and Rothstein (2008) found that cognitive-behavioral skills training interventions that resulted in the largest effect size in reducing participants' psychological stress symptoms.

Research on interventions designed to address the stress symptoms have demonstrated immediate benefits. For example, Wolever et al. (2012), in randomized controlled trial, found that insurance workers assigned to yoga or mindfulness meditation conditions showed improvement in perceived stress and reduced sleep difficulties at the end of the 12-week intervention period. In a randomized controlled trial involving university employees, Hartfiel, Havenhand, Khalsa, Clarke, and Krayer (2011) also found support for the benefits of yoga practices. Compared with a waitlist control group, participants who received the yoga intervention reported higher positive mood. In a meta-analysis of experimental studies, relaxation interventions were found to be beneficial in reducing participants' psychological stress symptoms (Richardson & Rothstein, 2008).

While the aforementioned studies focused on interventions to help workers respond to chronic stressors, it is helpful to examine research designed to evaluate the impact of interventions to help individuals exposed to acute stressors, such as a traumatic event. In particular, during psychological debriefing, individuals exposed to trauma are guided through a discussion of their experiences. The discussion is designed to promote emotional processing of the event in order to mitigate acute stress symptoms and to provide a sense of closure posttrauma (Rose, Brewin, Andrews, & Kirk, 1999). A review of randomized controlled studies, however, revealed that a single debriefing session after exposure to trauma did not reduce the likelihood of posttraumatic stress disorder (PTSD) onset, nor did it reduce PTSD symptom severity (Rose, Bisson, Churchill, & Wessely, 2002). Debriefing also did not significantly reduce psychological distress, anxiety, or depression after exposure. Taken together, Rose et al. cautioned against a single-session debriefing after exposure and recommended a "screen and treat" model. In other words, screen trauma-exposed individuals for early signs of a developing disorder (e.g., PTSD, depression) and provide individuals who screen positive a more extensive evidence-based treatment.

Overall, research shows that secondary and tertiary interventions benefit workers immediately after the interventions. However, longer-term follow-up is not always available to determine whether the intervention effects endure. More research with longer follow-up periods will provide evidence on the duration of effects.

SUMMARY

This chapter summarized interventions designed to support work–family balance, enhance workers' physical safety and health, and promote workers' psychological health and well-being. In terms of work–family balance, high-quality research evidence bearing on the efficacy of primary (e.g., flextime) and tertiary (e.g., EAPs) interventions is needed. There was, however, evidence suggesting that flexible work arrangements contribute to work–life balance. There is also evidence that some secondary interventions (e.g., training supervisors to be more family supportive) can be helpful in terms of work–life balance. For promoting physical safety and health, research suggests that primary (e.g., using feedback to train supervisors to communicate to subordinates in a way that integrates safety- and productivity-related concerns) and secondary interventions (e.g., insurance companies adopting the experience rating procedures) can benefit workers. More research, however, is needed to evaluate the tertiary interventions designed to promote a worker's return to work after injury or illness. Finally, mixed evidence was available for primary interventions (e.g., resilience training) to promote psychological health and well-being. Secondary and tertiary interventions (e.g., cognitive-behavioral interventions) appeared to alleviate the stress symptoms with short-term follow-up. Future research on interventions should focus on improving methodological rigor and consider the potential for the differential impact of interventions on workers, depending on job type.

REFERENCES

Addati, L., Cassirer, N., & Gilchrist, K. (2014). *Maternity and paternity at work: Law and practice across the world.* Geneva, Switzerland: International Labour Organization.

Allen, T. D., Johnson, R. C., Kiburz, K. M., & Shockley, K. M. (2013). Work-family conflict and flexible work arrangements: Deconstructing flexibility. *Personnel Psychology, 66,* 345–376. doi:10.1111/peps.12012

Arthur, A. R. (2000). Employee assistance programmes: The emperor's new clothes of stress management? *British Journal of Guidance & Counselling, 28,* 549–559. doi:10.1080/03069880020004749

Attridge, M. (2003). *EAP impact on work, stress and health: National data 1999–2002.* Presented at the biannual conference of the Work, Stress and Health Conference—APA/NIOSH, Toronto, Ontario, Canada.

Baltes, B. B., Briggs, T. E., Huff, J. W., Wright, J. A., & Neuman, G. A. (1999). Flexible and compressed workweek schedules: A meta-analysis of their effects on work-related criteria. *Journal of Applied Psychology, 84,* 496–513. doi:10.1037/0021-9010.84.4.496

Bena, A., Berchialla, P., Coffano, M. E., Debernardi, M. L. & Icardi, L. G. (2009). Effectiveness of the training program for workers at construction sites of the high-speed railway line between Torino and Novara: Impact on injury rates. *American Journal of Industrial Medicine, 52,* 965–972. doi:10.1002/ajim.20770

Berridge, J., & Cooper, C. (1994). The employee assistance programme: Its role in organizational coping and excellence. *Personnel Review, 23,* 4–20. doi:10.1108/00483489410072190

Berridge, J., Cooper, C., & Highley, C. (1997). *Employee assistance programmes and workplace counselling.* Chichester, UK: Wiley.

Beus, J. M., Payne, S. C., Bergman, M. E., & Arthur, W., Jr. (2010). Safety climate and injuries: An examination of theoretical and empirical relationships. *Journal of Applied Psychology, 95,* 713–727. doi:10.1037/a0019164

Bond, F. W., & Bunce, D. (2000). Mediators of change in emotion-focused and problem-focused worksite stress management interventions. *Journal of Occupational Health Psychology, 5,* 151–163. doi:10.1037/1076-8998.5.1.156

Bond, J. T., Galinsky, E., Kim, S. S., & Brownfield, E. (2005). *National study of employers.* New York, NY: Families and Work Institute.

Burke, M. J., Sarpy, S. A., Smith-Crowe, K., Chan-Serafin, S., Salvador, R. O., & Islam, G. (2006). Relative effectiveness of worker safety and health training methods. *American Journal of Public Health, 96,* 315–324. doi:10.2105/AJPH.2004.059840

Cahill, K., Hartmann-Boyce, J., & Perera, R. (2015). Incentives for smoking cessation. *Cochrane Database of Systematic Reviews, 2015*(5), 1–114. doi:10.1002/14651858.CD004307.pub5

Christian, M. S., Bradley, J. C., Wallace, J. C., & Burke, M. J. (2009). Workplace safety: A meta-analysis of the roles of person and situation factors. *Journal of Applied Psychology, 94,* 1103–1127. doi:10.1037/a0016172

Cydulka, R. K., Emerman, C. L., Shade, B., & Kubincane, J. (1994). Stress levels in EMS personnel: A longitudinal study with work-schedule modification. *Academic Emergency Medicine, 1,* 240–246. doi:10.1111/j.1553-2712.1994.tb02439.x

Davis, K. D., Lawson, K. M., Almeida, D. M., Kelly, E. L., King, R. B., Hammer, L., . . . McHale, S. M. (2015). Parents' daily time with their children: A workplace intervention. *Pediatrics, 135,* 875–882. doi:10.1542/peds.2014-2057 de Boer, A. G. E. M., Taskila, T. K., Tamminga, S. J., Feuerstein, M., Frings-Dresen, M. H. W., & Verbeek, J. H. (2015). Interventions to enhance return-to-work for cancer patients. *Cochrane Database of Systematic Reviews, 2013*(9), 1–79. doi:10.1002/14651858.CD007569.pub3

De Raeve, L., Vasse, W. M., Jansen, N. W. H., ven den Brandt, P. A., & Kant, I. (2007). Mental health effects of changes in psychosocial work characteristics: A prospective cohort study. *Journal of Occupational and Environmental Medicine, 49,* 890–899. doi:10.1097/JOM.0b013e31811eadd3

European Union. (2016, August). *European platform for investing in children.* Retrieved from http://europa.eu/epic/index_en.htm

Franche, R., Cullen, K., Clarke, J., Irvin, E., Sinclair, S., & Frank, J. (2005). Workplace-based return-to-work interventions: A systematic review of the quantitative literature. *Journal of Occupational Rehabilitation, 15,* 607–631. doi:10.1007/s10926-005-8038-8

Freak-Poli, R. L., Cumpston, M., Peeters, A., & Clemes, S. A. (2013). Workplace pedometer interventions for increasing physical activity. *Cochrane Database of Systematic Reviews, 2013*(4), 1–80. doi:10.1002/14651858.CD009209.pub2

Gajendran, R. S., & Harrison, D. A. (2007). The good, the bad, and the unknown about telecommuting: Meta-analysis of psychological mediators and individual consequences. *Journal of Applied Psychology, 92,* 1524–1541. doi:10.1037/0021-9010.92.6.1524

Ganster, D. C., Mayes, B. T., Sime, W. E., & Tharp, G. D. (1982). Managing organizational stress: A field experiment. *Journal of Applied Psychology, 67,* 533–542.

Garrett, R. K., & Danziger, J. N. (2007). Which telework? Defining and testing a taxonomy of technology-mediated work at a distance. *Social Science Computer Review, 25,* 27–47. doi:10.1177/0894439306293819

Grawitch, M. J., Gottschalk, M., & Munz, D. C. (2006). The path to a healthy workplace: A critical review linking healthy workplace practices, employee well-being, and organizational improvements. *Consulting Psychology Journal: Practice and Research, 58,* 129–147. doi:10.1037/1065-9293.58.3.129

Hammer, L. B., Johnson, R. C., Crain, T. L., Bodner, T., Kossek, E. E., Davis, K. D., . . . Berkman, L. (2016). Intervention effects on safety compliance and citizenship behaviors: Evidence from work, family, and health study. *Journal of Applied Psychology, 101,* 190–208. doi:10.1037/apl0000047

Hammer, L. B., Kossek, E. E., Anger, W. K., Bodner, T., & Zimmerman, K. L. (2011). Clarifying work-family intervention processes: The roles of work-family conflict and family supportive supervisor behaviors. *Journal of Applied Psychology, 96,* 134–153. doi:10.1037/a0020927

Hammer, L. B., Kossek, E. E., Yragui, N. L., Bodner, T. E., & Hanson, G. C. (2009). Development and validation of a multidimensional measure of family supportive supervisor behaviors (FSSB). *Journal of Management, 35,* 837–856.

Harlow, K. C. (2006). The effectiveness of a problem resolution and brief counseling EAP intervention. *Journal of Workplace Behavioral Health, 22,* 1–12. doi:10.1300/J490v22n01_01

Hartfiel, N., Havenhand, J., Khalsa, S. B., Clarke, G., & Krayer, A. (2011). The effectivenss of yoga for the improvement of well-being and resilience of stress in the workplace. *Scandinavian Journal of Work, Environment, & Health, 37,* 70–76. doi:10.5271/sjweh.2916

Hasson, H., Brisson, C., Guérin, S., Gilbert-Ouimet, M., Baril-Gingras, G., Vézina, M., & Bourbonnais, R. (2014). An organizational-level occupational health intervention: Employee perception of exposure to changes, and psychosocial outcomes. *Work & Stress, 28,* 179–197. doi:10.1080/20678373.2014.907370

Kelly, E. L., Kossek, E. E., Hammer, L. B., Durham, M., Bray, J., Chermack, K., . . . Kaskubar, D. (2008). Getting there from here: Research on the effects of work-family initiatives on work-family conflict and business outcomes. *The Academy of Management Annals, 2,* 305–349. doi:10.1080/19416520802211610

Kelly, E. L., Moen, P., Oakes, J. M., Fan, W., Okechukwu, C., Davis, K. D., . . . Casper, L. (2014). Changing work and work–family conflict: Evidence from the Work, Family, and Health Network. *American Sociological Review, 79,* 485–516. doi:10.1177/0003122414531435

Latack, J. C., & Foster, L. W. (1985). Implementation of compressed work schedules: Participation and job redesign as critical factors for employee acceptance. *Personnel Psychology, 38,* 75–92. doi:10.1111/j.1744-6570.1985.tb00542.x

Levy, P. E. (2013). *Industrial/organizational psychology: Understanding the workplace* (4th ed.). New York, NY: Palgrave Macmillan.

Macdonald, S., Lothian, S., & Wells, S. (1997). Evaluation of an employee assistance program at a transportation company. *Evaluation and Program Planning, 20,* 495–505. doi:10.1016/S0149-7189(97)00028-1

Macdonald, S., Wells, S., Lothian, S., & Shain, M. (2000). Absenteeism and other workplace indicators of employee assistance program clients and matched controls. *Employee Assistance Quarterly, 15,* 41–57. doi:10.1300/J022v15n03_04

McHale, S. M., Lawson, K. M., Davis, K. D., Casper, L., Kelly, E. L., & Buxton, O. (2015). Effects of a workplace intervention on sleep in employees' children. *Journal of Adolescent Health, 56*, 672–677. doi:10.1016/j.jadohealth.2015.02.014

Montano, D. Hoven, H., & Siegrist, J. (2014). A meta-analysis of health effects of randomized controlled worksite interventions: Does social stratification matter? *Scandinavian Journal of Work, Environment, & Health, 40*, 230–234. doi:10.5271/sjweh.3412

Naveh, E., & Katz-Navon, T. (2015). A longitudinal study of an intervention to improve road safety climate: Climate as an organizational boundary spanner. *Journal of Applied Psychology, 100*, 216–226. doi:10.1037/a0037613

Olson, R., Crain, T. L., Bodner, T., King, R. B., Hammer, L. B., Klein, L. C., . . . Buxton, O. M. (2015). A workplace intervention improves sleep: Results from the randomized controlled Work, Family & Health Study. *Sleep Health, 1*, 55–65. doi:10.1016/j.sleh.2014.11.003

Rautiainen, R., Lehtola, M. M., Day, L. M., Schonstein, E., Suutarinen, J., Salminen, S., & Verbeek, J. H. (2008). Interventions for preventing injuries in the agricultural industry. *Cochrane Database of Systematic Reviews, 2008*(1), 1–38. doi:10.1002/14651858.CD006398.pub2

Richardson, K. M., & Rothstein, H. R. (2008). Effects of occupational stress management intervention programs: A meta-analysis. *Journal of Occupational Health Psychology, 13*, 69–93. doi:10.1037/1076-8998.13.1.69

Robertson, I. T., Cooper, C. L., Sarkar, M., & Curran, T. (2015). Resilience training in the workplace from 2003 to 2014: A systematic review. *Journal of Occupational and Organizational Psychology, 88*, 533–562. doi:10.1111/joop.12120

Romig, M. C., Latif, A., Gill, R. S., Pronovost, P. J., & Sapirstein, A. (2012). Perceived benefit of a telemedicine consultative service in a highly staffed intensive care unit. *Journal of Critical Care, 27*(4), 426.e9–e16. doi:10.1016/j.jcrc.2011.12.007

Rose, S., Bisson, J., Churchill, R., & Wessely, S. (2002). Psychological debriefing for preventing posttraumatic stress disorder (PTSD). *Cochrane Database of Systematic Reviews, 2002*(2), 1–51. doi:10.1002/14651858.CD000560

Rose, S., Brewin, C., Andrews, A., & Kirk, M. (1999). A randomized controlled trial of psychological debriefing in victims of violent crime. *Psychological Medicine, 29*, 793–799.

Ruotsalainen, J. H., Verbeek, J. H., Mariné, A., & Serra, C. (2015). Preventing occupational stress in healthcare workers. *Cochrane Database of Systematic Reviews, 2015*(4), 1–155. doi:10.1002/14651858.CD002892.pub5

Rydstedt, L. W., Johannsson, G., & Evans, G. W. (1998). The human side of the road: Improving the working conditions of urban bus drivers. *Journal of Occupational Health Psychology, 3*, 161–171. doi:10.1037/1076-8998.3.2.161

Sauter, S. L., Hurrell, J. J., Fox, H. R., Tetrick, L. E., & Barling, J. (1999). Occupational health psychology: An emerging discipline. *Industrial Health, 37*, 199–211. doi:10.2486/indhealth.37.199

Schmidt, L. R. (1994). A psychological look at public health: Contents and methodology. In S. Maes, H. Leventhal, & M. Johnston (Eds.), *International review of health psychology* (Vol. 3, pp. 3–36). Chichester, UK: Wiley.

Shrestha, N., Kukkonen-Harjula, K. T., Verbeek, J. H., Ijaz, S., Hermans, V., & Bhaumik, S. (2016). Workplace interventions for reducing sitting at work. *Cochrane Database of Systematic Reviews, 2016*(3), 1–135. doi:10.1002/14651858.CD010912.pub3

Tetrick, L. E., & Quick, J. C. (2003). Prevention at work: Public health in occupational settings. In J. C. Quick & L. E. Tetrick (Eds.), *Handbook of occupational health psychology* (pp. 3–17). Washington, DC: American Psychological Association.

Tetrick, L. E., & Quick, J. C. (2011). Overview of occupational health psychology: Public health in occupational settings. In J. C. Quick & L. E. Tetrick (Eds.), *Handbook of occupational health psychology* (2nd ed., pp. 3–20). Washington, DC: American Psychological Association.

Tompa, E., Trevithick, S., & McLeod, C. (2007). Systematic review of the prevention incentives of insurance and regulatory mechanisms for occupational health and safety. *Scandinavian Journal of Work, Environment, & Health, 33*, 85–95. doi:10.5271/sjweh.1111

Van Dierendonck, D., Schaufeli, W., & Buunk, B. (1998). The evaluation of an individual burnout intervention program: The role of inequity and social support. *Journal of Applied Psychology, 83*, 392–407. doi:10.1037/0021-9010.83.3.392

Vanhove, A. J., Herian, M. N., Perez, A. L. U., Harms, P. D., & Lester, P. B. (2016). Can resilience be developed at work? *Journal of Occupational and Organizational Psychology, 89*, 278–307. doi:10.1111/joop.12123

Verbeek, J. H., Kateman, E., Morata, T. C., Dreschler, W., & Mischke, C. (2012). Interventions to prevent occupational noise-induced hearing loss. *Cochrane Database of Systematic Reviews, 2012*(10), 1–112. doi:10.1002/14651858.CD006396.pub3

Wolever, R., Bobinet, K., McCabe, K., MacKenzie, E., Fekete, E., Kusnick, C., & Baime, M. (2012). Effective and viable mind-body stress reduction in the workplace: A randomized controlled trial. *Journal of Occupational Health Psychology, 17,* 246–258. doi:0.1037/a0027278

Zohar, D., & Polachek, T. (2014). Discourse-based intervention for modifying supervisory communication as leverage for safety climate and performance improvement: A randomized field study. *Journal of Applied Psychology, 99,* 113–124. doi:10.1037/a0034096

ELEVEN

The Future of Occupational Health Psychology

I (I.S.S.) was the founding editor of the *Newsletter for the Society for Occupational Health Psychology (SOHP)*. In 2007, I solicited contributions for the newsletter's inaugural issue. I made sure to ask the then SOHP president, Peter Chen, to write an article that would go right on the first page of that first issue. I wanted him to underline for the newsletter's readers the importance of occupational health psychology (OHP), but in a personal way. Personal was what I got. Peter wrote a brief but moving memoir. He wrote what has been my favorite of all the articles I published over my term as editor. To me, Peter's article was a home run with the bases loaded.

He wrote about a job he once held at a company that was about to merge with another firm. One autumn afternoon, as Peter and a colleague walked over fallen leaves in the company parking lot, the colleague became distraught. The colleague recounted that he had just lost his job in a round of layoffs the merger precipitated. Peter stayed in the parking lot and talked with his colleague. After 30 minutes, the colleague experienced a stomachache.

Peter wrote that this incident was his "very first encounter with the reality of job stress" despite having "been working on job stress research for quite some time." He confessed that he felt ashamed and guilty because, although he enjoyed the research he had been conducting and experienced satisfaction publishing the fruits of that research, he missed, until that episode in the parking lot, the true meaning of what his research entailed. His confession set the stage for his resolution to do a better job applying knowledge OHP research produced to make the lives of working people better.

The future of OHP is closely tied to what Peter wrote. My colleagues in OHP and I do not ever want to lose the satisfaction we feel when we work hard conducting research on work, stress, and health. I think many readers of this book who are academics experience the satisfaction of conducting research and receiving an acceptance e-mail from a journal editor. Readers pursuing graduate degrees will soon experience this kind of satisfaction. But like Peter, we have to remember that ultimately, we want to make better—that is to say, healthier—the lives of people who work. A life without stress is impossible. We, however, want people to have jobs that are not excessively stressful, and that are not conducive to health problems such as depression or cardiovascular disease.

OHP is an exciting field with a bright future. One part of that bright future is in the excitement of conducting research that aims to uncover knowledge on the interplay of work and health. The other part of that bright future is in the application of that knowledge to making the lives of working people healthier.

THE FUTURE OF OHP, CHAPTER BY CHAPTER

This chapter is loosely organized, with broad exceptions, along the lines of the chapters in this book. Discussion of the future of research methodology (Chapter 2) will be threaded throughout the chapter. The first theme concerning OHP's future comes from Chapter 1, the chapter devoted to the history of OHP. I take up that theme right here in this section. In some of the remaining sections, I cover one main theme that is ripe for future research and one or more supplementary themes. For example, in the section on physical health, the main theme is research on recovery from the workday. Supplementary themes include research on the development of cerebrovascular disease and the targeting of specific samples that merit intensive study. Other sections (e.g., on specific occupations—Chapter 7) are organized a little differently, but important themes for future research are still underlined.

Chapter 1 underlined a certain trajectory to the history of OHP. What is it about the history of OHP that can help us make progress in the future? One answer is in the OHP-related organizations that emerged in the course of the discipline's history, the European Academy of Occupational Health Psychology (EA-OHP), the Society for Occupational Health Psychology (SOHP), and the International Commission on

Occupational Health's Scientific Committee on Work Organisation and Psychosocial Factors (ICOH-WOPS). Many of the individuals engaged in OHP research and practice are members of these organizations. The organizations, with their meetings, listservs, newsletters, and journals, promote communication among their members.

Readers of this book can register and attend the major conferences conducted by these organizations. Contributors to the conferences present on the latest developments in OHP research and practice. One series of conferences is conducted biennially by EA-OHP. Another series of biennial conferences is jointly conducted by the American Psychological Association (APA), the National Institute for Occupational Safety and Health (NIOSH), and SOHP. The EA-OHP and the APA/NIOSH/SOHP meetings are held in alternate years, making it possible to attend both in any 2-year span. The ICOH-WOPS conferences are on a different, and longer, cycle; those conferences are also well worth attending. The conferences will not only acquaint readers of this book with the latest developments in research and practice, but can also provide readers with an opportunity to meet and interact with OHP researchers and practitioners (this idea is reprised later in the chapter). Perhaps some readers will become researchers and practitioners themselves, and contribute to those very conferences. Readers interested in OHP should consider joining one of the three OHP-related organizations. By joining one of these organizations, readers will help support an institution that is important to sustaining OHP.

EA-OHP and SOHP are associated with important OHP-related journals. EA-OHP publishes *Work & Stress*. Although APA is the publisher of the *Journal of Occupational Health Psychology* (*JOHP*), SOHP plays an important editorial role in *JOHP*. SOHP will have launched a new journal, *Occupational Health Science*, in 2017. To stay abreast of the field, readers should consider subscribing to one or more journals, or at least monitoring the journals through databases such as PsycINFO and PubMed.

Mental Health

We know that workplace stressors in the form of excessive psychological demands, effort–reward imbalance, lack of autonomy, organizational injustice, and so forth contribute to depression, psychological distress, burnout, and more (see Chapter 3). It is worth noting that the Job Demands–Resources model (JD–R; Bakker & Demerouti, 2014; Demerouti, Bakker, Nachreiner, & Schaufeli, 2001) will play a role in future OHP research on the impact of psychosocial working conditions on mental health. The importance of the model's role is in its potential to integrate an array of factors such as psychological, physical, and organizational demands; job control; informational, emotional, and tangible support; effort–reward imbalance; organizational injustice; job insecurity, and so on. Conceptual difficulties that have to be resolved include the question of whether a factor such as lack of autonomy represents too little of a resource, the presence of a chronic stressor, or, perhaps, both. It can be anticipated that conceptual difficulties will be resolved, and that the future for the JD–R model will be bright.

Regardless of whether the research concerns the JD–R or the demand–control–support (DCS) model, most job stress research relies on generic measures of working conditions. There are, however, reasons to assess job- or situation-specific conditions. Beehr (1995) underscored the importance of developing job-specific measures, and suggested two reasons for taking a job-specific approach. First, heretofore overlooked stressors may be discovered. Second, generic stressors may take very specific forms in different organizations. Beehr noted that although research efforts employing stressor measures that are tailored to each specific job may become cumbersome, findings from such research are likely to more accurately reflect what is occurring in those jobs. Future research efforts, particularly efforts that employ computer-driven questioning, may be able to integrate generic and job-specific questions in such a way as to not impose too much of an extra burden on workers participating in research.

Money

Fred Ebb, the lyricist for the musical *Cabaret*, wrote "money makes the world go 'round." That is not the case if you don't have much. Financial stress is a topic that has been understudied in OHP (Sinclair & Cheung, 2016). It is well known that socioeconomic status (SES) is inversely related to health. Chapters 3 and 4 examined research on the adverse effects of unemployment and job insecurity. Financial or economic stress, however, can affect individuals who are employed, and even employed in stable jobs. Economic well-being buys resources (e.g., a home in a good neighborhood) that benefit health. Chapter 3 indicated that working conditions are associated with SES. For example, jobs that afford workers greater autonomy, on average, pay more. Sinclair and Cheung (2016) noted that clarifying (unconfounding) the relationship between working conditions and income (and the resource package income buys) as well as those factors' links to health outcomes will help to better specify the extent to which differences in working conditions and differences in income affect health.

Personality and Social Factors

In the future, OHP is likely to see advances in research that better integrate mental health outcomes and working conditions with assessments of individual differences. Research underlines this need. For example, it is a widely held view that very difficult working conditions (e.g., a teacher who has been confronted daily by disrespectful and defiant students) give rise to burnout. Burnout, however, is not purely a function of working conditions. Factors such as the personality dimension neuroticism, the symptoms of atypical depression[1] (e.g., hypersensitivity to social rejection), and a history of mood and anxiety disorders are associated with burnout (Bianchi, Schonfeld, & Laurent, 2015; Ronen & Baldwin, 2010; Rössler, Hengartner, Ajdacic-Gross, & Angst, 2015). Thus, a condition like burnout may be better thought to be a function of both external conditions and the individual's personal make-up and history. This kind of thinking carries over to research on other mental health outcomes (e.g., depression, anxiety, alcohol problems).

Social resources outside of work, such as social support from friends and relatives (Schonfeld, 2001), as well as individual differences in personality traits, such as conscientiousness and neuroticism (Lee, Sudom, & Zamorski, 2013), are likely to contribute to resilience or vulnerability that, along with job stressors, potentially affect mental health outcomes. For example, there is cross-sectional evidence that

---

[1] Despite its name, depression with atypical features is not rare. The features that distinguish it from, say, depression with melancholic features include the aforementioned hypersensitivity, mood reactivity (a depressed mood can brighten in response to a pleasant life event), and leaden paralysis.

the extent to which an individual has a proactive personality, that is, a tendency to feel empowered to act unhindered by situational constraints, tends to reduce the impact of family-to-work (but not work-to-family) stressors (Cunningham & De La Rosa, 2008).[2]

Job Crafting

Chapter 3 examined the impact of occupational coping on mental health. Research findings were described, at best, as equivocal. "Job crafting" is a related but broader concept than coping, and has roots in Schein's (1971) concept of role innovation.[3] Job crafting may offer more promise than coping. Job crafting refers to "the physical and cognitive changes individuals make in the task or relational boundaries of their work" (Wrzesniewski & Dutton, 2001, p. 179).

What is attractive about the idea of job crafting is that it connects with a fundamental idea in psychology. Jean Piaget (1947/1976), the biologist and father of developmental psychology, regarded adaptation as the foundation of intelligence. He posited that adaptation embraces the twin features of accommodation and assimilation. Accommodation refers to how an organism, a human being in this instance, has to change in order to adjust to the environment. A person in the workplace must follow rules and procedures, report on time, follow the supervisor's instructions, and so on. Assimilation, on the other hand, concerns how the person imposes changes on the environment and on how he or she cognizes the environment. Much of what happens at work reflects accommodation; job crafting, however, reflects the assimilation aspect of adaptation.

Much research on job crafting pertains to its relationship with task performance and work engagement, important topics in their own right, but largely not the subject matter of this book. There has been, however, research on job crafting and burnout. In a diary study involving Dutch workers in a variety of occupations, Demerouti, Bakker, and Halbesleben (2015) found that job crafting in the form of seeking challenges was related to reduced burnout, at least cross-sectionally (lagged effects were nonsignificant). Petrou, Demerouti, and Schaufeli (2015), in a longitudinal study of Dutch police officers experiencing organizational changes, found that the job crafting behavior of reducing demands, paradoxically, predicted greater burnout 1 year later. In addition, burnout at baseline predicted later demand reduction. By contrast, the job crafting behavior of seeking challenges predicted reduced burnout. A finding like the latter result shows promise. Job crafting, however, may at least be partly a function of how much decision latitude an organization affords a worker as well as preexisting mental health and personality factors. More research needs to be done with regard to the impact of job crafting on the well-being of workers, while integrating the role of decision latitude and preexisting psychological variables.

---

[2] Cunningham and De La Rosa's finding is consistent with Pearlin and Schooler's (1978) idea that the work role, in comparison with the role of spouse, is less amenable to successful coping (presuming proactive individuals are more likely to engage in active coping) because the work role is more impersonally organized (see Chapter 3).

[3] Role innovation involves the role occupant rejecting role norms and changing role practices. Schein suggested that role innovation is relatively rare, and largely limited to the liberal professions (e.g., medicine, law). By contrast, job crafting potentially applies to a broad cross section of occupations.

Physical Health

Interest in research on recovery from the stresses of the workday has grown in recent years, and is likely to continue to grow. Kompier, Taris, and van Veldhoven (2012) observed that there has been relatively little research on "the effects of everyday work stress on sleep quality and fatigue" (p. 239). Research in this area is important because sleep problems are related to lower performance at work; fatal, myocardial infarction; sickness absence; depression; and burnout (Åkerstedt, Nilsson, & Kecklund, 2009). Insomnia and sleepiness are also related to unsafe behaviors and nonfatal workplace accidents (DeArmond & Chen, 2009; Kao, Spitzmueller, Cigularov, & Wu, 2016).

There is evidence that job-related stressors, such as high workloads and job strain, spill over into home life. The continuing impact of the stressors impedes psychological detachment from work during after-work hours, disrupting recovery from the workday and contributing to difficulties at work the next day (Sonnentag & Fritz, 2015). For example, compared with teachers exposed to lower levels of job strain, teachers exposed to high levels of job strain are more likely to ruminate about work, particularly close to bedtime, and experience poorer sleep quality (Cropley, Dijk, & Stanley, 2006). Similar findings were obtained in research on workers in a wide variety of jobs (Kompier et al., 2012). Research on the benefits of vacations suggests that their capacity to reduce symptoms of burnout fades soon after the individual returns to a stressful job (Westman & Eden, 1997).

Exposure to stressors during the workday increases the risk of arousal after work (Sonnentag & Fritz, 2015). Although Chapter 4 looked at activity in the sympathetic nervous system in connection to arousal, there is evidence that exposure to job stressors is related to reduced activity in another component of the autonomic nervous system, the parasympathetic nervous system[4] (Clays et al., 2011). *Reduced* parasympathetic activation contributes to difficulties resting and recovering after a stressful day at work. After-work recovery and recovery via respite are fertile areas for future research.

Intermediate Pathways to CVD

Chapter 4 underlined the relationship of adverse psychosocial working conditions to cardiovascular disease (CVD), although these working conditions are not the sole cause of CVD. CVD can take years to develop. Researchers, however, can examine outcomes that are intermediate in the pathway from working conditions to CVD, for example, small elevations in blood pressure or cholesterol. Interventions that are aimed at benefiting worker mental health can have piggybacked on them assessments of the aforementioned biological markers. It is not far-fetched to think that an intervention that is designed to benefit mental health by providing workers with greater decision latitude may also lower blood pressure by a couple of milliliters of mercury.

OHP research on the relation of psychosocial working conditions to intermediate outcomes such as relatively small elevations in blood pressure does not negate the need for research on biological endpoints such as heart attack and stroke. Large-sample, longer-term, multiwave longitudinal research can more fully help investigators study intermediate *and* longer-term outcomes.

However, with regard to research methodology (Chapter 2), cross-sectional research remains a popular means for linking workplace stressors and outcomes. But

---

[4] The activation of the parasympathetic nervous system is important when the individual is at rest.

such research will not help add to our understanding of how psychosocial working conditions contribute causally to the aforementioned intermediate conditions, conditions that are links in a chain that lead to outcomes such as heart attack. Enthusiasm for longitudinal research, however, has grown. There have been many longitudinal studies that comprise two waves of data collection. Further growth in longitudinal research will be in the direction of launching studies that comprise three or more waves of data collection (Kelloway & Francis, 2013; Ployhart & Vandenberg, 2010). There are at least three reasons why the future OHP research should involve multiwave studies. First, a two-wave study is limited to showing linear change. By contrast, a multiwave study can ascertain whether change is linear or nonlinear. Second, the reliability of estimates of the rate of growth or change in a health-related dependent variable is greater in a multiwave than in a two-wave study (Willett, 1989). Third, when multiwave research is combined with hierarchical linear modeling (HLM; aka multilevel modeling), investigators have an opportunity to explore change in individual workers (Raudenbush & Bryk, 2002). Investigators can study in detail how the trajectory of change in blood pressure, depressive symptoms, or another health-related dependent variable varies among workers confronting particular job stressors, and apply HLM to evaluate factors that influence a particular trajectory of change. Thus, multiwave longitudinal studies hold a great deal of promise for future OHP research.

A knotty problem for multiwave as well as two-wave studies is that of ascertaining the "true" length of a causal time lag for stressors to work their effects on outcomes (Taris & Kompier, 2014) in a group of workers facing an identifiable set of job conditions. Progress, however, is being made with regard to the development of methods for ascertaining the length of between-wave time lags that is optimal for assessing the "maximum impact" of a particular stressor upon a health outcome (Dormann & Griffin, 2015), further strengthening longitudinal OHP research designs. Guthier (2016) applied Dormann and Griffin's (2015) method to a meta-analysis of the impact of job demands on burnout. Such research could be equally extended to biological outcomes such as blood pressure.

Stroke

A stroke, which is also called a "cerebrovascular accident," refers to cell death in a brain region. The cell death results from a lack of oxygen, a consequence of poor blood flow. The reduction in blood flow could result from conditions such as a hemorrhage (bleeding) or ischemia (a consequence of atherosclerosis or a clot blocking a vessel supplying a brain region with blood). It is a leading cause of death. It would have been natural for Chapter 4 to examine research on stroke given that the chapter's predominant theme is CVD, a disorder that is often mentioned with stroke. Research on the relationship of workplace psychosocial stressors to stroke, however, has been scarce. A meta-analysis (Huang et al., 2015) encompassing six prospective studies ($n > 130,000$) that met quality criteria (e.g., five of the six studies excluded individuals with baseline CVD) indicated that individuals with high-strain jobs were at a 22% higher adjusted risk for stroke over the follow-up period (unweighted median 10.5 years) compared with individuals with active jobs (high workload, high control), the reference category. Two large longitudinal studies (Toivanen, 2008; Virtanen & Notkola, 2002) found that low levels of job control predicted stroke. Gallo et al. (2006) found that involuntary job loss occurring in late career increased the risk of later stroke. It is anticipated that in the future, we will see more research on the relationship of psychosocial workplace factors to stroke.

Underrepresented Groups

Another kind of methodological gap needs to be closed. That gap concerns sampling. Most of the longitudinal research on the impact of psychosocial working conditions comes from Europe and North America. Longitudinal research from other parts of the world is needed. Moreover, within samples from Europe and North America, we need to ensure that groups that are often underrepresented (e.g., in the United States, African Americans and Hispanics) are included. In addition, research with cross-national samples would be helpful in understanding how stressors can have more or less of an impact in one cultural or national context than another (Liu, Nauta, Li, & Fan, 2010). There are, however, many trip wires that jeopardize the validity of such research, but tools exist to help ensure the equivalence of research procedures across cultural and national groups (see Spector, Liu, & Sanchez, 2015).

Workers Transitioning Into Retirement

There has been interest in samples comprising older workers, particularly older workers transitioning into retirement (Barnes-Farrell, 2003; Beehr, 1986; Beehr & Bennett, 2015; McGonagle, Fisher, Barnes-Farrell, & Grosch, 2015; Wang & Shultz, 2010). The aforementioned research makes clear that health plays a role in the decision to retire or assume a bridge job[5] after retiring from one's principal employment.

Higher SES is related to longevity (Brønnum-Hansen, & Baadsgaard, 2008; Chetty et al., 2016; Perenboom, van Herten, Boshuizen, & van den Bos, 2005; Tarkiainen, Martikainen, & Laaksonen, 2013) and, hence, the opportunity to enjoy a reasonably healthy retirement. The extent to which jobs are physically demanding is related to worse health in retirement (Wang & Shi, 2014). Some jobs are markedly associated with a shortened life span (Parker, 2011).[6] Psychological well-being in retirement is adversely affected by the experience of unemployment just before retirement as well as the stressfulness of the job from which an individual retired (Wang & Shi, 2014).

Work can affect functioning in retirement in other ways as well. Jobs having more intense mental demands are related to higher levels of cognitive functioning before retirement and greater resistance to cognitive decline after (Fisher et al., 2014). A line of future longitudinal and experimental research that identifies preretirement working conditions—particularly conditions affecting blue collar and service workers—that contribute to a transition to a physically and cognitively healthy retirement would be invaluable.

Aggression in the Workplace

Another area of research OHP can address is that of the origins of workplace aggression. Chapter 5 described risk factors for workplace aggression. Evidence is beginning to accumulate regarding factors that influence individuals to act in a rude and uncivil manner. Factors associated with engaging in rude/uncivil behaviors include having been a target of such behavior and organizational policies that are tolerant of incivility (Gallus, Bunk, Matthews, Barnes-Farrell, & Magley, 2014). There is also evidence that some individuals engage in rude/hostile workplace behavior for reasons

---

[5] A bridge job is a paying job some individuals take after retiring from their principal job but before they fully withdraw from the labor force.
[6] See the later discussion of correctional officers.

of retaliation and power assertion, although some individuals indicate no reason at all (Bunk, Karabin, & Lear, 2011).

We, however, need more knowledge about the transactions that take place that culminate in episodes of incivility and more outright aggression, including behaviors a worker directs against a coworker and against clients, patients, students, and customers. To get a footing in this tricky terrain, future qualitative research (see Chapter 2) would be helpful, particularly research that examines aggression from the point of view of perpetrators, an understudied group. In attempting to understand the social reality of bullies, Bloch (2012) conducted a qualitative study in which she interviewed individuals who bullied coworkers. The research does not justify bullying. Rather, it gives us clues to its sources. She examined what led perpetrators to think ill of their targets, how perpetrators classify their targets morally, actions the bullies took, emotions they experienced, and so on. Qualitative research—I include interview studies and close observational research—may be helpful in obtaining a preliminary map of the transactions and contextual factors that culminate in workplace aggression. That preliminary map could help guide later quantitatively organized longitudinal studies and prevention-oriented interventions.

Work-Related Mistreatment via the Internet

A relatively new avenue of work-related aggression needs to be explored. Although the mistreatment of others via the Internet has, for many years, been associated with middle- and high school students, online mistreatment has also begun to emerge as a work-related condition. A phenomenon that has come to be known as "cyber incivility" in which supervisors and coworkers, intentionally or not, communicate rude messages to other workers has become a concern (Giumetti, McKibben, Hatfield, Schroeder, & Kowalski, 2012). Giumetti et al. found that the intensity of cyber incivility initiated by supervisors is concurrently related to elevated levels of burnout in employees, including employees who were low in neuroticism.[7]

Organizational Climate and Leadership

Safety climate (Chapter 6) refers to the extent to which employees perceive that safety is a priority relative to other organizational goals. Leitão and Greiner's (2016) epidemiology-based review of 17 studies involving industrial organizations indicates that safety climate, particularly safety climate as measured at the group level, is associated with reduced numbers of injuries and accidents. Because the preponderance of the research was cross-sectional, and only a few studies had sufficient controls on confounding factors, the results do not provide clear evidence of a causal link between safety climate and accident risk. Although the results were largely supportive of the idea that safety climate affects injury risk, Leitão and Greiner recommended for the future (a) observational longitudinal research with "rigorous control for confounding factors" and (b) intervention research aimed at reducing injury risk by way of strengthening safety climate.

Another concern regarding the impact of safety climate is that the principles and vision that upper management espouses with regard to safety may or may not align with the procedures line managers require of their workers when confronted

---

[7] Giumetti et al. also found that compared to employees with low levels of neuroticism, coworkers with high and intermediate levels of neuroticism were more vulnerable to cyber incivility.

with heavy demands. What line managers require, more than upper management's principles, influences how workers make sense of their workplace situation. Zohar (2010) suggested that research on shared worker sense-making in arriving at commonly held perceptions of safety climate is a fertile area for research.

Industry-Specific Research

Zohar (2010) also advanced the view that we would benefit from more industry-specific safety climate measures. Industry-specific measures could supplement the more commonly used generic measures—akin to this notion is the idea raised earlier in the chapter regarding the use of measures of workplace-specific stressors (Beehr, 1995). An example of an industry-specific safety scale would be a measure of safety climate in the trucking industry. A scale administered to a trucker could include highly concrete items such as "My dispatcher insists that I do not use in-vehicle communication devices while driving." The use of such measures would "offer opportunities for eliciting and testing hypotheses regarding processes underlying climate emergence" (p. 1521).

Safety climate is not the only set of shared workplace perceptions. There is innovation climate, service climate, and so forth. Zohar suggested that it would be helpful from the standpoint of theory development if more research effort were applied to understanding the interconnections of safety climate with other climate dimensions.

Leadership

The relationship of organizational leadership to safety outcomes (Chapter 6) is a promising avenue of research. One OHP research path could begin with Barling, Loughlin, and Kelloway's (2002) idea of safety-specific transformational leadership. Another promising avenue of research could begin with Dollard and Bakker's (2010) idea of psychological safety climate, which links leadership and climate. That linkage originates with an organization's top leadership setting priorities that bear on protecting the *psychological* well-being of the individuals who work for the organization. The concern is how the leadership's priorities flow through an organization. In addition, leadership that affords workers freedom to discuss safety concerns directly with managers, a research area that has not received enough attention, is related to lower accident risk (Kath, Marks, & Ranney, 2010). Research in these leadership areas is likely to secure more attention in the near future.

Research on Specific Occupations

This section renews the examination of some occupations noted in Chapter 7, namely, that of combat soldiers, police officers, and firefighters. The section looks at other occupational categories as well. These include correctional officers and the self-employed.

Combat Soldiers

Chapter 7 examined a number of occupational groups, one of which was the military. The chapter noted that an unfortunate trend in the U.S. military has been the increasing rate of suicide, through the period during which the wars in Iraq and Afghanistan were waged. In contrast to the U.S. findings, rates of suicide in the U.K. military between 1984 and 2007 were significantly lower (with one exception) than contemporaneous rates in the general U.K. population, controlling for gender and age

(Fear et al., 2009). In contrast to the trend in the U.S. military, in the U.K. military there was no evidence of a similar trend of an increasing rate of suicide during the period in which British troops served in Iraq and Afghanistan. In addition, the rate of probable posttraumatic stress disorder (PTSD; 4%) was lower in returning British troops, including combat troops, serving in the Iraq and Afghanistan theaters (Fear et al., 2010[8]), compared with the rate in U.S. troops (e.g., 14% from the report by Tanielian & Jaycox, 2008). Moreover, in the British study, the rates of PTSD in deployed and nondeployed soldiers did not differ. This is not to say that British troops were without elevated risk for problems. Rates of alcohol misuse were higher in deployed (16%) than in nondeployed British troops (11%; Fear et al., 2010) and rates of elevated General Health Questionnaire (GHQ) scores[9] were higher in deployed U.K. military than in U.K. civilians (Goodwin et al., 2015). Future OHP research that capitalizes on cross-national comparisons may be able to identify specific differences (e.g., organizational differences, differences in the nature of leadership) that provide clues that will help us to better identify protective factors that could prevent psychiatric casualties in the U.S. military. Some potential protective factors that characterize the U.K. forces are shorter deployments, lower troop-to-leader ratios, and lower casualty and fatality rates.

Ursano et al. (2015) identified a number of risk factors for attempted suicide in U.S. enlisted soldiers, an event that is predictive of future completed suicide. Among the risk factors identified were a first deployment (especially the first months) and pre-enlistment mental disorder. Ursano et al. (2015) suggested that this knowledge could aid in the surveillance of soldiers who are at risk. Such surveillance is especially important because firearms are a part of military life. There is a good deal of evidence indicating that the availability of firearms is related to increased suicide risk in civilian life (e.g., Anestis & Anestis, 2015). In addition, after a soldier is released from psychiatric hospitalization, there is an elevated risk of completed suicide as well as other adverse outcomes, including accidental death, a suicide attempt, and rehospitalization (Kessler et al., 2015). Future research on mental health in the military could help in implementing early warning systems to identify soldiers in need of help before a suicidal gesture is made. Kessler et al. recommended posthospitalization interventions for soldiers with the highest prehospitalization suicide risk.

Imaging studies of cases of mild traumatic brain injury (TBI) often fail to show brain abnormalities, although military personnel so diagnosed experience problems such as sleep disturbance, difficulty concentrating, memory difficulties, and depression. The way has been opened, however, to better understand the impact of combat exposure on TBI and PTSD. A recent postmortem study (Shively et al., 2016) that builds on the World War I research by Mott (described in Chapter 1) examined the brains of male members of the U.S. military who had been exposed to blasts of explosives; some died a short time after a blast (4 days to 2 months) and others, later (7 months to 9 years). The latter group also showed evidence of PTSD. The research team found scarring in astroglial cells of the brains of the men who were exposed to blasts. Among other functions, astroglial cells provide nutrients to neurons and help maintain the ion balance between neurons and the extraneuronal environment. The

---

[8] Figure 5 in the paper by Fear et al. (2010) provides a comparison of rates of probable PTSD obtained from a variety of returning U.K. and U.S. military study samples.
[9] See Chapter 3 for a description of the GHQ.

research team found evidence of the beginning of scarring in men who died soon after blast exposure, and more scarring in the brains of men who were blast exposed but lived more than 6 months postblast.

The scarring was found in a number of sites, including the boundaries between gray matter and white matter, the hippocampus (associated with memory and learning), the hypothalamus (as mentioned in Chapter 4, related to regulation of the fight–flight response), the temporal cortex (a recognition center), amygdala (decision-making, emotion regulation, memory), and more. Control cases, which included civilians who had experienced blunt trauma, had been opioid abusers, or had died from other causes (e.g., CVD), did not show the scarring evident in the blast-exposed cases.

It is important to realize that although the military provides soldiers with protective equipment, the blast wave still constitutes a great danger. The wave can affect unprotected parts of the torso, and then propagate its force to the brain. The blast can also cause debris to fly at great penetrating velocities. The research thus more specifically linked blast-related trauma to changes in the brain and implicitly to PTSD. Shively et al.'s (2016) study will likely accelerate brain research on TBI and PTSD. With new medical insights into the neurological substrate of TBI and PTSD, treatments for the sufferers can be developed.

Police Officers and Firefighters

In the section on combat soldiers, I underlined international comparisons of the U.S. and the U.K. militaries. Although international comparisons have methodological challenges (e.g., national differences in the rates at which screening for a disorder takes place), comparative data can help efforts in identifying health disparities and their sources (Banks, Marmot, Oldfield, & Smith, 2006). Chapter 7 contrasted the mortality rates for U.S. and U.K. police officers. One clear difference between the two nations is that firearms are more widely available in the United States. That difference is reflected in the vastly higher rates at which U.S. police officers are killed in the line of duty. One partial solution in which OHP researchers could play a role would be to testify before legislatures in order to motivate U.S. lawmakers to arrive at ways to make firearms less freely available (e.g., barring felons and individuals with serious mental disorders from obtaining a firearm). Chapter 7 also indicated that the fatality rates for firefighters in the United States have been higher than the rates in the United Kingdom. Unlike the case of police officers, the reasons for cross-national differences in firefighter fatality rates do not immediately emerge from the data. Future OHP research involving international comparisons may provide clues that can be used to identify ways to make firefighting safer.

Correctional Officers

Although Chapter 7 contained a section devoted to police officers, an occupational group allied to police officers, namely, correctional officers (COs), was not covered in that chapter. In the future, it would be helpful if as much effort were applied to research on COs as the effort devoted to research on police officers. COs are men and women who work under very stressful conditions. A French study (Neveu, 2007) found that COs' mean score on the CES-D[10] was almost 18; a score of 16 is considered a marker of elevated risk for clinical depression (Schonfeld, 1990).

---

[10] See Chapter 3 for a description of this measure of depressive symptoms.

The health of COs is at risk. Because many deal with inmates who have committed heinous crimes, the safety of COs is in jeopardy. Between 1999 and 2008, there were 113 fatalities (homicides, suicides, accidents, etc.) among COs in the United States, a rate of about 11 per year (Konda, Tiesman, Reichard, & Hartley, 2013). The injury rate, including injuries resulting from nonfatal assaults, is also high compared to other occupational groups (Konda et al., 2013). A study conducted in Florida found that the average age at death among COs was 62.4 years, about 12 years less than the average for Florida residents in general (Parker, 2011).

Recently emerging OHP-related research (Cherniack, Dussetschleger, Henning, El Ghaziri, & Warren, 2015; El Ghaziri, 2015; Fritz, Guros, Hammer, Shepherd, & Meier, 2015; Violanti, 2015) helps us better understand the stress process as it unfolds in COs' work lives, and what they bring home from work. Understanding the stress process can contribute to efforts to make the lives of COs healthier and better. More of this kind of research is expected in the future.

I add a thought connected to the aforementioned research on COs, a thought that underlines an idea I mentioned early in this chapter. I learned about the research on COs at a recent APA/NIOSH/SOHP conference that I attended. Although research on COs is not the area in which I conduct research, I was pleased that I had an opportunity to learn about the research and talk to John Violanti, an investigator who has been engaged in that research. I think that if the readers of this book were to attend an EA-OHP, APA/NIOSH/SOHP, or ICOH-WOPS conference, they would have similar opportunities to learn about advances in OHP research, and interact with investigators who are conducting that research.

The Self-Employed

I turn to a highly diverse but understudied group of workers not covered in Chapter 7, but whom OHP research may be able to benefit, namely, individuals who are self-employed. They constitute more than 10% of the workforce in Canada (Statistics Canada, 2014), the European Union (Teichgraber, 2013), and the United States (Hipple, 2010). A large fraction of workers in the developing world, particularly women, is self-employed (Gindling & Newhouse, 2014). The diversity of jobs among the self-employed is vast, and includes software and hardware specialists, many different types of artists and designers, painters (artists *and* house painters), consultants of a rainbow of stripes, hair stylists, writers, musicians, plumbers, electricians, vending machine operators, private tutors, *bricoleurs*, and much more. Although the self-employed have been studied by economists, they have largely not been the subject of OHP research (Schonfeld & Mazzola, 2015). The self-employed, particularly individuals who are self-employed in solo businesses, are subject to considerable economic insecurity and are exposed to unfair reputational threat and customer and contractor betrayal (Schonfeld & Mazzola). In the developing world, self-employment is often characterized by its precariousness (Mandelman, & Montes Rojas, 2007).

The self-employed, moreover, are disadvantaged in other ways as well. When an economy enters a recession, the self-employed are doubly affected. First, they lose business like almost everyone else. Second, organizationally employed individuals who lose their jobs or are moved to part-time positions often join the ranks of the self-employed, further tightening the competition for whatever business remains (Cichocki, 2012; Hipple, 2010).

Unlike the organizationally employed, who often have a certain amount of support from coworkers and supervisors as well as human resource departments, individuals who are self-employed in solo businesses often lack such support (Schonfeld & Mazzola, 2015). The self-employed pose a challenge for OHP. OHP researchers and practitioners may be able to help develop ways to make the lives of the self-employed less stressful, particularly given that economies around the world increasingly rely on freelancers and contract workers.

Teaming With Workers to Develop Research Ideas

Chapter 7 covered occupations such as teaching, nursing, and agricultural work. With regard to the serious stressors affecting incumbents in specific kinds of work, OHP researchers may not by themselves be able to arrive at workable solutions to the problems facing those job incumbents. A preferred method would be for researchers to team up with the workers in a combined effort to identify solutions. Chapter 2 described a quasi-experiment conducted by Bond and Bunce (2001) in which the investigators evaluated the impact of job reorganization on a work unit comprising British government administrative employees. The intervention itself was shaped by the employees, who collaboratively investigated work-related problems, and then arrived at and implemented a consensus intervention plan. The plan involved increasing employees' control over their work. The investigators found that the workers in the planning-and-implementation group showed better mental health and lower absence rates than workers in the comparison group. Thus, there is promise for research in which investigators team up with members of an occupational group in developing interventions aimed at improving worker health by changing psychosocial working conditions.

Safety

Chapter 8 examined research on safety. One particular concern covered in the chapter is the relationship of shift work and long hours to accident risk. Night shift work and more hours on the job are related to accident risk (Baker, Olson, & Morisseau, 1994; Folkard & Tucker, 2003). These findings are relevant to many jobs, but none more so than medicine. Many physicians, particularly young doctors and medical students (who also have clinical duties), work 80 or more hours a week (Lamberg, 2002). Rodriguez-Jareño et al.'s (2014) literature review indicated that long working hours for doctors, residents, and medical students are related to risk of needle-stick injuries (also see Ayas et al., 2006) and road accidents. More research is needed to investigate mortality risk and other kinds of accidents including those that compromise patient health. However, there is enough evidence to suggest that shorter work days are in order; future OHP research can help in this area.

Worker Empowerment and Safety

Dictatorships are the worst form of government. Some workplaces are run like dictatorships. Workers have little in the way of power or freedom to express their views. Workplace safety, however, can be enhanced when workers feel empowered to discuss safety concerns with supervisors and managers. Kath et al. (2010), in a study involving nonmanagerial employees who worked in railroad repair shops, found that the perceived seriousness with which management concerns itself with safety was the factor most closely related to a worker's confidence that he or she can raise safety concerns with supervisors. The next most important factor was the quality of supervisor–employee relationships. Connected to a worker's feeling the freedom to raise safety concerns with supervisors is the idea of psychological empowerment at the workplace, a concept that refers to the worker's sense of competence and self-determination at the job. Ford and Tetrick (2011) found that psychological empowerment is associated with the use of safety equipment among hospital workers. The investigators also found that the extensiveness of hazards at work were inversely related to psychological empowerment. Future longitudinal and experimental research should look closely at factors that increase worker empowerment in the area of safety.

Work–Family Balance

Chapter 9 underlined research on work–family conflict (WFC), and its opposite of work–family enhancement (WFE). WFC and WFE contribute to work–family balance (Greenhaus & Allen, 2011). Greenhaus and Allen provided a useful model (described in Chapter 9) that can help guide future research on work–family balance. Research on WFC, however, is considerably more abundant than research on WFE. With increasing interest in what has been termed "positive psychology," more research interest in WFE is anticipated in the future. The impact of stressors occurring at work is not limited to the employee, but has the potential to carry over to a spouse or child (e.g., Stellman et al., 2008). Although there has been some research on the impact of WFC and WFE on spouses and children (e.g., Ferguson, 2012; Ilies et al., 2007), more research is warranted.

Families Responsible for Other Kinds of Care

WF research has examined families in which demands for dependent care involve children under age 18 and spouses who are ill. Work-related conflicts for single parents are also deserving of study. Given increases in longevity, it would be helpful to have more research on working families that have responsibilities for caring for aging parents (Matthews, Mills, Trout, & English, 2014). Moreover, given changes in how we view families, the research could be further extended to include cohabiting heterosexual couples (Matthews, Del Priore, Acitelli, & Barnes-Farrell, 2006) and married and cohabiting gay couples.

The Self-Employed

A little earlier in this concluding chapter, an occupational category relevant to work–family balance was mentioned. The category of self-employment, as noted earlier, is not a specific occupation; it embraces a great many different jobs. With the growing number of individuals who are self-employed, the question of work–family balance is an important topic for research. For many of the self-employed in solo businesses, it is sometimes not clear where work ends and family life begins (Schonfeld & Mazzola, 2015). Research on the boundary conditions between work and personal life (Bulger, Matthews, & Hoffman, 2007) in different types of self-employment is important. How does WFC play out in the self-employed? What are its antecedents and consequences? What about WFE? How does it play out? What are its antecedents and consequences? Because of the great diversity of jobs among the self-employed, does work–family balance differ by job type? These are questions future OHP research can answer.

Physicians

There are some occupations that require individuals to work extremely long hours. As mentioned earlier, in the context of a brief discussion of research on reducing accidents, physicians work extremely long hours. It is important to understand how the long hours that some jobs demand affect work–family balance. One accepts that such jobs shrink the amount of time available for family life. OHP research can tell us about the extent to which the effect is deleterious, and what hospitals, clinics, and state regulators can do to make work–family balance better for those who regularly work long hours. Preliminary evidence indicates that physicians, especially surgeons and obstetricians, are dissatisfied with the balance between work and the rest of life (Shanafelt et al., 2012).

Interventions in the Workplace

Research on health-related interventions in the workplace (Chapter 10) is challenging. Even at the level of national and transnational policies designed to improve psychosocial risk management, there are obstacles to both implementation and evaluation (Leka, Jain, Zwetsloot, & Cox, 2010). With regard to researcher attempts to initiate interventions, Kompier et al. (1998) observed that upper-level management is not likely to deem "sound scientific research" to be a goal of their company, and may even view research as a nuisance. Researchers will also have to think about the cost of the most humane, well-intentioned interventions, and consider working with economists to demonstrate to managers that a planned health-related intervention will profit the company (Kompier et al., 1998).

In biomedical research, the ideal—"the gold standard"— approach to assessing the efficacy of a health-related intervention is the randomized controlled trial (RCT), that is, the true experiment. Cox, Karanika, Griffiths, and Houdmont (2007) advanced the idea that it is misplaced to judge the quality of research on workplace interventions against the RCT, with its random allocation of participants to experimental and control groups. Cox et al. and Grant and Wall (2009) showed that quasi-experimental designs are more amenable to the reality of intervention research in modern organizations. In modern organizations, investigators' command over the research endeavor is limited by factors such as the diverse goals and motivations of employees and managers. Moreover, obstacles in the structure of many workplaces prevent the random allocation of workers to experimental and control groups, underlining the importance of quasi-experimental designs. Cox et al. suggested that "if a large number of studies, none of them ideal but differing in their inadequacies, present the same results then there might be an argument that those results might be accepted if they are theoretically and practically credible" (p. 356).

It should also be underlined that RCTs are not without weaknesses. Many RCTs that have been aimed at reducing workplace stress have been limited to assessing outcomes almost immediately after the intervention or within a few weeks of the intervention's conclusion (Richardson & Rothstein, 2008). Clearly, longer-term follow-up assessments are needed to assess the durability of the effects of interventions.

Within the context of intervention research within a complex, always-evolving work organization, Griffiths (1999) stressed the importance of investigators including qualitative methods among their research tools. She advanced the idea that it is unlikely that standard natural-science (i.e., experimental) methods, without the help of qualitative methods, can explain ongoing processes that mediate the relationship between an intervention and the hypothesized outcomes. Future investigators should build into intervention research a qualitative component that looks deeply into the processes that the intervention sets in motion. Qualitative methods can also be helpful in understanding local conditions such as the sympathies and antipathies of managers regarding the intervention.

Learning From Failure

A health-related intervention in the workplace is subject to the risk of failure, a risk that is inherent in the undertaking, even if the intervention is well executed (Semmer, 2006). Semmer's warning is important because it underlines an idea that we acquired early in life, namely, that we should learn from our failures and our mistakes. Learning from the failures of interventions, however, is often difficult because research reports on failed interventions rarely get published. Either investigators are embarrassed by such failures or, more likely, there is a bias against publishing unhappy results.

A recent volume by Karanika-Murray and Biron (2015) shows that we can profit from learning about derailments of past interventions. Efforts to examine why interventions fail are important for the purpose of developing successful future interventions. Karanika-Murray and Biron underscored a number of ways in which health-related interventions in the workplace can derail. First, there are a multitude of workplace factors over which investigators have no control. For example, the commitment of the leadership of an organization to the intervention can dim over time because of changing economic conditions. Second, research in fields that bear on workplace interventions develop "in silo"; in other words, there is a certain amount of separation among the fields with which researchers are affiliated, leading to a degree of conflict regarding what constitutes the proper research design and evidence of success. Because of the prestige of the biomedical sciences, research methods that took hold in those sciences (e.g., the RCT) may make the quasi-experimental methods often used in OHP intervention research look weak (although such criticism is overblown [Grant & Wall, 2009]). Even if the OH psychologist conducts a true experiment, he or she may mistakenly assume that the work environment, the context for the intervention and control conditions, is more stable than it actually is. A stable environment is an important assumption of RCTs. Work environments are rarely stable.

Karanika-Murray and Biron (2015) suggested that interventions can fail for many other reasons. First, the theory underlying the intervention is flawed in such a way that creating an intervention that is faithful to the theory fails to have an effect on worker health. Second, the content of the intervention may not have been implemented the way it should be. Third, the workplace context could modify or undermine the intervention (e.g., critical stakeholders are unenthusiastic about the intervention). Fourth, something goes wrong in the process of the delivery of the intervention. And so on. Karanika-Murray and Biron's book is punctuated with examples of failed interventions. Although one of many, Sørensen (2015) provided a key example of an intervention aimed at improving the well-being of knowledge workers (e.g., consultant engineers) that failed because events (e.g., changes in ownership, management changes) unrelated to the intervention torpedoed it.

Nielsen and Abildgaard (2013) underscored the importance of middle managers (line managers) as "drivers of change." Researchers planning interventions must enlist middle managers' cooperation. Their passive (or active) resistance can undermine an intervention. Nielsen (2013) also emphasized the importance of viewing the employees who are targets of an intervention as more than passive recipients. Researchers should capitalize on employees' local knowledge when developing an intervention. Greater employee participation in the process of fashioning and implementing an intervention could help in increasing the chances of success (Kompier et al., 1998).

Total Worker Health™

In many companies, employee safety and health are managed in a fragmented way, with one department providing an employee assistance program and another concerning itself with exposure to toxic conditions (Schill & Chosewood, 2013). The work environment has largely served as a setting in which health-oriented researchers and practitioners can easily reach workers for the purpose of implementing individually oriented interventions; the work environment itself has largely not been a target to be changed (Semmer, 2006). In addition, when workers are reached through intervention efforts, those efforts are likely to represent secondary and tertiary prevention activities such as health promotion and screening programs (Cooper & Cartwright, 1994). The implementation of secondary and tertiary prevention efforts is more common than the implementation of primary prevention activities, which require change at the level of the organization or work environment, a more difficult goal for interventionists.

An effort has begun to develop better ways to integrate workplace health and safety measures. In 2004, NIOSH and its partners began to explore approaches to improving worker health that potentially could be more beneficial than past approaches (NIOSH, 2012). A number of ideas emerged in 2004 in a NIOSH-sponsored conference. These ideas included improving communication between researchers and practitioners who share the goal of improving worker health. The conference referenced both occupational safety and health (OSH) and worksite health promotion (HP). OSH refers to efforts at the level of the organization or the work environment that are aimed at reducing exposures to hazards "that can lead to work-related injury, illness, and disability." These efforts include reducing exposures to toxic chemicals, minimizing ergonomic hazards, and getting workers to wear safety-related equipment. Interventions include substituting safer chemicals for more toxic ones and job redesign. HP refers to interventions that attempt to reduce health-compromising behaviors (e.g., getting workers to quit smoking or control their weight) and to promote healthful behaviors (e.g., adopting a healthful diet or engaging in physical activity). In other words, primary prevention is integrated into secondary and tertiary prevention campaigns.

Because both OSH and HP interventions are aimed at worker health, the idea emerged that a multifaceted approach could provide a synergy with effects that are greater than the sum of its component parts (Hammer & Sauter, 2013). More concretely, worker health can be aided by integrating organizational- and workplace-level approaches with worker-level approaches (Semmer, 2006). Organizational-level approaches derive from OSH interventions. HP avenues are embodied in approaches such as employee assistance programs.

A programmatic strategy advanced by NIOSH that combines OSH and HP ideas became known as Total Worker Health™ (TWH), a name that emerged in 2011. The idea behind the program is that evidence-based practices bearing on the physical and organizational facets of the workplace as well as the health behaviors of workers can be integrated and harnessed to advance workers' physical and mental health. There are several reasons to expect that integration of OSH and HP approaches is particularly effective. First, causes of disorders are ordinarily multifactorial, with organizational *and* personal risk factors contributing additively or interactively (Schulte, Pandalai, Wulsin, & Chun, 2012) as in the combination of workplace exposures to toxic aerosols and cigarette consumption. Second, blue collar workers may mistakenly believe that involuntary worksite exposures are more dangerous than health behaviors such as smoking and excessive alcohol consumption, and thus may concern themselves more with worksite exposures than with altering health behaviors (Schulte et al., 2012; Sorensen et al., 2002). Linking OSH-related reductions in workplace exposures and HP-related efforts to change harmful health behaviors is thought to increase the credibility of efforts to reduce harmful health behaviors and increase worker motivation to change (Sorensen et al., 2002). In 2013, the biennial Work, Stress, and Health conference that is sponsored by APA, NIOSH, and SOHP was devoted to TWH.

Sorensen et al. (2002), in a rare, early example of a TWH-type approach, combined an HP condition (e.g., worksite tobacco control messaging, self-help activities to manage cigarette consumption) and an OSH condition (e.g., reduction of exposure to hazardous substances at the worksite). In their study, which involved 15 industrial sites, workers in the combined OSH/HP condition were more likely to quit smoking than workers in the HP condition. A review (Anger et al., 2015) of 17 extant studies (nine were randomized trials) that evaluated the impact of TWH-type interventions that integrate OSH and HP approaches indicates that such interventions can improve worker health and safety.

The ultimate goal of OHP is to protect and improve the health of people who work. The apotheosis of that goal is the intervention. The future promises more efforts to advance TWH interventions.

FINAL THOUGHTS

> *Now, in Russia, they got it mapped out so that everyone pulls for everyone else . . . that's the theory, anyway. But what I know about is Texas, and down here . . . you're on your own.*
>
> —The Coen brothers, *Blood Simple* (1984)

I begin this final section of this last chapter by describing the experience of an individual.[11] His experience underlines a growing problem, namely, that of job insecurity and the general precariousness of work. He lives in Brooklyn, not Texas, although the story would resonate there too. He holds a bachelor's degree in chemistry. He worked for many years at an industrial paint factory, directing the entire manufacturing process. One of the factory's biggest customers was also a manufacturer, but a manufacturer of all varieties of steel cabinets (e.g., steel shelving to hold equipment, cabinets to cover fuses and circuit breakers). The cabinet manufacturer eventually stopped doing business with the paint manufacturer. Given the growth of international trade, the cabinet manufacturer began to obtain steel, manufactured *and* prepainted, from a factory in a developing country at a cost that was less than what the manufacturer paid for the steel previously purchased from U.S. firms. Of course, the U.S. steel needed to

---

[11] The individual involved gave me permission to describe his story.

be painted. The cabinet manufacturer laid off several blue collar employees who had previously been engaged in painting the steel purchased from U.S. companies. The paint manufacturer continued to lose business, and laid off employees as the business shrank. Eventually the director found himself working for free. After a few months, the paint company dissolved, and whatever was left of the director's job also dissolved.

I deliberately chose to describe what happened to a well-educated individual. He is what economists would call a "member of the primary labor market," the labor market comprising more highly trained individuals. Economic conditions are even more difficult for workers in the secondary labor market (Kalleberg, 2009), the labor market for workers who can be found in the service sector, lower skilled manufacturing (e.g., the men who painted the steel shelving), and retail.

Karl Polanyi (2001/1944) wrote of a "double movement" in economic history. One movement involves a drive to extend the market economy into every corner of the earth, with a minimum of regulation (classical economic liberalism). The other is the movement toward "social protection," the purpose of which has been to safeguard individuals and societies from the "pernicious effects" of market excesses. For a period of time, especially with the advent of the New Deal in the United States and the development, after the Second World War, of the welfare state in European nations, the second movement has been ascendant. In parts of Europe, North America, and elsewhere, the first movement has in the last few decades reasserted itself. Markets have expanded and regulation diminished. Many people in today's workforce "are on their own." Powerful forces have acted to make work more precarious. Bourdieu (1998) described the growth of temporary and interim positions. He wrote of an intense competition for work that mirrors the competition between firms, a competition that echoes Hobbes's state of nature ("d'une véritable lutte de tous contre tous"). Kalleberg (2009) described the transformation of employment relationships such that workers can be easily added to, and just as easily dropped from, a company's workforce in the name of economic flexibility.

A great deal of the OHP-related research described in Chapters 3 and 4 underscores the adverse effects unemployment and job insecurity have on mental and physical health. To slightly reinterpret Polanyi (2001/1944), these kinds of job conditions "could not exist for any length of time without annihilating the human and natural substance of society" (p. 3). OHP-related research has done much to document the baleful effects of unemployment and job insecurity, which include psychological distress, depression, suicide, and heart disease.

Although OHP has been accumulating experience intervening in workplaces to make them more healthful, that experience does not directly bear on reducing unemployment and job insecurity. Nevertheless, OHP has an important role to play in terms of bearing witness to the adverse health effects of unemployment and job insecurity, including testifying before national and local legislatures and regulatory bodies regarding these health effects.

More than bearing witness, occupational health psychologists can collaborate with economists, sociologists, and business, labor, and political leaders in developing plans to mitigate, and prevent, the adverse health effects precarious economic conditions bring about. With knowledge of these adverse health effects, researchers and business, labor, and political leaders should collaborate to develop ways to reduce the general amount of insecurity to which working people are exposed. What that collaboration would eventually look like (e.g., an FDR-like "brain trust"?) is not clear. Whatever shape the leadership of that effort takes, occupational health psychologists should be partners in that effort.

REFERENCES

Åkerstedt, T., Nilsson, P. M., & Kecklund, G. (2009). Sleep and recovery. In S. Sonnentag, P. L. Perrewé, D. C. Ganster, S. Sonnentag, P. L. Perrewé, & D. C. Ganster (Eds.), *Current perspectives on job-stress recovery* (pp. 205–247). Bingley, UK: JAI Press/Emerald.

Anestis, M. D., & Anestis, J. C. (2015). Suicide rates and state laws regulating access and exposure to handguns. *American Journal of Public Health, 105,* 2049–2058. doi:10.2105/AJPH.2015.302753

Anger, W. K., Elliot, D. L., Bodner, T., Olson, R., Rohlman, D. S., Truxillo, D. M., . . . Montgomery, D. (2015). Effectiveness of Total Worker Health interventions. *Journal of Occupational Health Psychology, 20,* 226–247. doi:10.1037/a0038340

Ayas, N. T., Barger, L. K., Cade, B. E., Hashimoto, D. M., Rosner, B., Cronin, J. W., . . . Czeisler, C. A. (2006). Extended work duration and the risk of self-reported percutaneous injuries in interns. *Journal of the American Medical Association, 296,* 1055–1062. doi:10.1001/jama.296.9.1055

Baker, K., Olson, J., & Morisseau, D. (1994). Work practices, fatigue, and nuclear power plant safety performance. *Human Factors, 36,* 244–257. doi:10.1177/001872089403600206

Bakker, A. B., & Demerouti, E. (2014). Job demands-resources theory. In P. Y. Chen & C. L. Cooper (Eds.), *Work and wellbeing: A complete reference guide* (Vol. 3, pp. 37–64). Chichester, UK: Wiley.

Banks, J., Marmot, M., Oldfield, Z., & Smith, J. P. (2006). Disease and disadvantage in the United States and in England. *Journal of the American Medical Association, 295*(17), 2037–2045. doi:10.1001/jama.295.17.2037

Barling, J., Loughlin, C., & Kelloway, E. K. (2002). Development and test of a model linking safety-specific transformational leadership and occupational safety. *Journal of Applied Psychology, 87,* 488–496. doi:10.1037/0021-9010.87.3.488

Barnes-Farrell, J. L. (2003). Beyond health and wealth: Attitudinal and other influences on retirement decision-making. In G. A. Adams & T. A. Beehr (Eds.), *Retirement: Reasons, processes, and results* (pp. 159–187). New York, NY: Springer Publishing Company.

Beehr, T. A. (1986). The process of retirement: A review and recommendations for future investigation. *Personnel Psychology, 39,* 31–55. doi:10.1111/j.1744-6570.1986.tb00573.x

Beehr, T. A. (1995). *Psychological stress in the workplace.* London, UK: Routledge.

Beehr, T. A., & Bennett, M. M. (2015). Working after retirement: Features of bridge employment and research directions. *Work, Aging and Retirement, 1,* 112–128. doi:10.1093/workar/wau007

Bianchi, R., Schonfeld, I. S., & Laurent, E. (2015). Interpersonal rejection sensitivity predicts burnout: A prospective study. *Personality and Individual Differences, 75,* 216–219. doi:10.1016/j.paid.2014.11.043

Bloch, C. (2012). How do perpetrators experience bullying at the workplace? *International Journal of Work Organisation and Emotion, 5*(2), 159–177.

Bond, F. W., & Bunce, D. (2001). Job control mediates change in a work reorganization intervention for stress reduction. *Journal of Occupational Health Psychology, 6,* 290–302. doi:10.1037/1076-8998.6.4.290

Bourdieu, P. (1998). *Contre-feux.* Paris, France: Liber-Raison d'agir.

Brønnum-Hansen, H., & Baadsgaard, M. (2008). Increase in social inequality in health expectancy in Denmark. *Scandinavian Journal of Public Health, 36,* 44–51. doi:10.1177/1403494807085193

Bulger, C. A., Matthews, R. A., & Hoffman, M. E. (2007). Work and personal life boundary management: Boundary strength, work/personal life balance, and the segmentation-integration continuum. *Journal of Occupational Health Psychology, 12,* 365–375. doi:10.1037/1076-8998.12.4.365

Bunk, J. A., Karabin, J., & Lear, T. (2011). Understanding why workers engage in rude behaviors: A social interactionist perspective. *Current Psychology, 30,* 74–80. doi:10.1007/s12144-011-9102-5

Chen, P. (2007). Personal reflection: The meaning of occupational health psychology. *Newsletter of the Society of Occupational Health Psychology, 1,* 1.

Cherniack, M., Dussetschleger, J., Henning, R., El Ghaziri, M., & Warren, N. (2015, May). *Health Improvement through Employee Control (HITEC2): Adapting the participatory action research to Corrections.* APA/NIOSH/SOHP Work, Stress, and Health Conference, Atlanta, GA.

Chetty, R., Stepner, M., Abraham, S., Lin, S., Scuderi, B., Turner, N., . . . Cutler, D. (2016). The association between income and life expectancy in the United States, 2001–2014. *Journal of the American Medical Association, 315*(16), 1750–1766. doi:10.1001/jama.2016.4226

Cichocki, S. (2012). Self-employment and the business cycle: Evidence from Poland. *Post-Communist Economies, 24,* 219–239. doi:10.1080/14631377.2012.675157

Clays, E., De Bacquer, D., Crasset, V., Kittel, F., de Smet, P., Kornitzer, M., . . . De Backer, G. (2011). The perception of work stressors is related to reduced parasympathetic activity. *International Archives of Occupational and Environmental Health, 84,* 185–191. doi:10.1007/s00420-010-0537-z

Coen, J., & Coen, E. (1984). *Blood simple* [Motion picture]. U.S.: River Road Productions Foxton Entertainment.

Cooper, C. L., & Cartwright, S. (1994). Healthy mind; healthy organization: A proactive approach to occupational stress. *Human Relations, 47*, 455–471. doi:10.1177/001872679404700405

Cox, T., Karanika, M., Griffiths, A., & Houdmont, J. (2007). Evaluating organizational-level work stress interventions: Beyond traditional methods. *Work & Stress, 21*, 348–362. doi:10.1080/02678370701760757

Cropley, M., Dijk, D., & Stanley, N. (2006). Job strain, work rumination, and sleep in school teachers. *European Journal of Work and Organizational Psychology, 15*, 181–196. doi:10.1080/13594320500513913

Cunningham, C. L., & De La Rosa, G. M. (2008). The interactive effects of proactive personality and work-family interference on well-being. *Journal of Occupational Health Psychology, 13*, 271–282. doi:10.1037/1076-8998.13.3.271

DeArmond, S., & Chen, P. Y. (2009). Occupational safety: The role of workplace sleepiness. *Accident Analysis and Prevention, 41*, 976–984. doi:10.1016/j.aap.2009.06.018

Demerouti, E., Bakker, A. B., & Halbesleben, J. B. (2015). Productive and counterproductive job crafting: A daily diary study. *Journal of Occupational Health Psychology, 20*, 457–469. doi:10.1037/a0039002

Demerouti, E., Bakker, A. B., Nachreiner, F., & Schaufeli, W. B. (2001). The job demands-resources model of burnout. *Journal of Applied Psychology, 86*, 499–512. doi:10.1037/0021-9010.86.3.499

Dollard, M. F., & Bakker, A. B. (2010). Psychosocial safety climate as a precursor to conducive work environments, psychological health problems, and employee engagement. *Journal of Occupational and Organizational Psychology, 83*, 579–599. doi:10.1348/096317909X470690

Dormann, C., & Griffin, M. A. (2015). Optimal time lags in panel studies. *Psychological Methods, 21*. doi:10.1037/met0000041

El Ghaziri, M. (2015, May). *The organized workforce in corrections: An invisible key to officer health and well-being.* Paper presented at APA/NIOSH/SOHP Work, Stress, and Health Conference, Atlanta, GA.

Fear, N. T., Jones, M., Murphy, D., Hull, L., Iversen, A. C., Coker, B., . . . Wessely, S. (2010). What are the consequences of deployment to Iraq and Afghanistan on the mental health of the UK armed forces? A cohort study. *The Lancet, 375*(9728), 1783–1797. doi:10.1016/S0140-6736(10)60672-1

Fear, N. T., Ward, V. R., Harrison, K., Davison, L., Williamson, S., & Blatchley, N. F. (2009). Suicide among male regular UK Armed Forces personnel, 1984–2007. *Occupational and Environmental Medicine, 66*, 438–441. doi:10.1136/oem.2008.040816

Ferguson, M. (2012). You cannot leave it at the office: Spillover and crossover of coworker incivility. *Journal of Organizational Behavior, 33*, 571–588. doi:10.1002/job.774

Fisher, G. G., Stachowski, A., Infurna, F. J., Faul, J. D., Grosch, J., & Tetrick, L. E. (2014). Mental work demands, retirement, and longitudinal trajectories of cognitive functioning. *Journal of Occupational Health Psychology, 19*, 231–242. doi:10.1037/a0035724

Folkard, S., & Tucker, P. (2003). Shift work, safety and productivity. *Occupational Medicine, 53*, 95–101. doi:10.1093/occmed/kqg047

Ford, M. T., & Tetrick, L. E. (2011). Relations among occupational hazards, attitudes, and safety performance. *Journal of Occupational Health Psychology, 16*, 48-66. doi:10.1037/a0021296

Fritz, C., Guros, F., Hammer, L. B., Shepherd, B., & Meier, D. (2015, May). *Always on alert: Work-related hypervigilance and employee outcomes in corrections.* Paper presented at APA/NIOSH/SOHP Work, Stress, and Health Conference, Atlanta, GA.

Gallo, W. T., Teng, H. M., Falba, T. A., Kasl, S. V., Krumholz, H. M., & Bradley, E. H. (2006). The impact of late career job loss on myocardial infarction and stroke: A 10 year follow up using the Health and Retirement Survey. *Occupational and Environmental Medicine, 63*, 683–687. doi:10.1136/oem.2006.026823

Gallus, J. A., Bunk, J. A., Matthews, R. A., Barnes-Farrell, J. L., & Magley, V. J. (2014). An eye for an eye? Exploring the relationship between workplace incivility experiences and perpetration. *Journal of Occupational Health Psychology, 19*, 143–154. doi:10.1037/a0035931

Gindling, T., & Newhouse, D. (2014). Self-employment in the developing world. *World Development, 56*, 313–331. doi:10.1016/j.worlddev.2013.03.003

Giumetti, G. W., McKibben, E. S., Hatfield, A. L., Schroeder, A. N., & Kowalski, R. M. (2012). Cyber incivility @ work: The new age of interpersonal deviance. *Cyberpsychology, Behavior, and Social Networking, 15*, 148–154. doi:10.1089/cyber.2011.0336

Goodwin, L., Wessely, S., Hotopf, M., Jones, M., Greenberg, N., Rona, R. J., . . . Fear, N. T. (2015). Are common mental disorders more prevalent in the UK serving military compared to the general working population? *Psychological Medicine, 45*, 1881–1891. doi:10.1017/S0033291714002980

Grant, A. M., & Wall, T. D. (2009). The neglected science and art of quasi-experimentation: Why-to, when-to, and how-to advice for organizational researchers. *Organizational Research Methods, 12*, 653–686. doi:10.1177/1094428108320737

Greenhaus, J. H., & Allen, T. D. (2011). Work–family balance: A review and extension of the literature. In J. C. Quick & L. E. Tetrick (Eds.), *Handbook of occupational health psychology* (2nd ed., pp. 165–183). Washington, DC: American Psychological Association.

Griffiths, A. (1999). Organizational interventions: Facing the limits of the natural science paradigm. *Scandinavian Journal of Work, Environment & Health, 25*, 589–596. doi:org/10.1037/a0034508

Guthier, G. (2016). *Things we can learn from longitudinal studies about the relationship between job demands and burnout.* Paper presented at the Psychology Department colloquium, The City College of the City University of New York, New York, NY.

Hammer, L. B., & Sauter, S. (2013). Total Worker Health and work-life stress. *Journal of Occupational and Environmental Medicine, 55*(12, Suppl.), S25–S29. doi:10.1097/JOM.0000000000000043

Hipple, S. (2010). Self-employment in the United States. *Monthly Labor Review, 133*, 17–32.

Huang, Y., Xu, S., Hua, J., Zhu, D., Liu, C., Hu, Y., . . . Xu, D. (2015). Association between job strain and risk of incident stroke: A meta-analysis. *Neurology, 85*, 1648–1654. doi:10.1212/WNL.0000000000002098

Ilies, R., Schwind, K. M., Wagner, D. T., Johnson, M. D., DeRue, D. S., & Ilgen, D. R. (2007). When can employees have a family life? The effects of daily workload and affect on work-family conflict and social behaviors at home. *Journal of Applied Psychology, 92*, 1368–1379. doi:10.1037/0021-9010.92.5.1368

Kalleberg, A. L. (2009). Precarious work, insecure workers: Employment relations in transition. *American Sociological Review, 74*, 1–22. doi:10.1177/000312240907400101

Kao, K., Spitzmueller, C., Cigularov, K., & Wu, H. (2016). Linking insomnia to workplace injuries: A moderated mediation model of supervisor safety priority and safety behavior. *Journal of Occupational Health Psychology, 21*, 91–104. doi:10.1037/a0039144

Karanika-Murray, M., & Biron, C. (2015). *Derailed organizational interventions for stress and well-being: Confessions of failure and solutions for success.* Dordrecht, The Netherlands: Springer.

Kath, L. M., Marks, K. M., & Ranney, J. (2010). Safety climate dimensions, leader–member exchange, and organizational support as predictors of upward safety communication in a sample of rail industry workers. *Safety Science, 48*, 643–650. doi:10.1016/j.ssci.2010.01.016

Kelloway, E. K., & Francis, L. (2013). Longitudinal research and data analysis. In R. R. Sinclair, M. Wang, & L. E. Tetrick (Eds.), *Research methods in occupational health psychology: Measurement, design, and data analysis* (pp. 374–394). New York, NY: Routledge/Taylor & Francis Group.

Kessler, R. C., Warner, C. H., Ivany, C., Petukhova, M. V., Rose, S., Bromet, E. J., . . . Ursano, R. J. (2015). Predicting suicides after psychiatric hospitalization in US Army soldiers: The Army Study to Assess Risk and Resilience in Service Members (Army STARRS). *JAMA Psychiatry, 72*, 49–57. doi:10.1001/jamapsychiatry.2014.1754

Kompier, M. J., Geurts, S. E., Gründemann, R. M., Vink, P., & Smulders, P. W. (1998). Cases in stress prevention: The success of a participative and stepwise approach. *Stress Medicine, 14*, 155–168. doi:10.1002/(SICI)1099-1700(199807)14:33.0.CO;2-C

Kompier, M. J., Taris, T. W., & van Veldhoven, M. (2012). Tossing and turning: Insomnia in relation to occupational stress, rumination, fatigue, and well-being. *Scandinavian Journal of Work, Environment & Health, 38*, 238–246. doi:10.5271/sjweh.3263

Konda, S., Tiesman, H., Reichard, A., & Hartley, D. (2013). U.S. correctional officers killed or injured on the job. *Corrections Today, 75*(5), 122–125.

Lamberg, L. (2002). Long hours, little sleep: Bad medicine for physicians-in-training? *Journal of the American Medical Association, 287*(3), 303–306.

Lee, J. C., Sudom, K. A., & Zamorski, M. A. (2013). Longitudinal analysis of psychological resilience and mental health in Canadian military personnel returning from overseas deployment. *Journal of Occupational Health Psychology, 18*, 327–337. doi:10.1037/a0033059

Leitão, S., & Greiner, B. A. (2016). Organisational safety climate and occupational accidents and injuries: An epidemiology-based systematic review. *Work & Stress, 30*, 71–90. doi:10.1080/02678373.2015.1102176

Leka, S., Jain, A., Zwetsloot, G., & Cox, T. (2010). Policy-level interventions and work-related psychosocial risk management in the European Union. *Work & Stress, 24*, 298–307. doi:10.1080/02678373.2010.519918

Liu, C., Nauta, M. M., Li, C., & Fan, J. (2010). Comparisons of organizational constraints and their relations to strains in China and the United States. *Journal of Occupational Health Psychology, 15*, 452–467. doi:10.1037/a0020721

Mandelman, F. S., & Montes Rojas, G. V. (2007). Microentrepreneurship and the business cycle: Is self-employment a desired outcome? *Working Paper Series (Federal Reserve Bank of Atlanta), 15*, 1–39.

Matthews, R. A., Del Priore, R. E., Acitelli, L. K., & Barnes-Farrell, J. L. (2006). Work-to-relationship conflict: Crossover effects in dual-earner couples. *Journal of Occupational Health Psychology, 11*, 228–240. doi:10.1037/1076-8998.11.3.228

Matthews, R. A., Mills, M. J., Trout, R. C., & English, L. (2014). Family-supportive supervisor behaviors, work engagement, and subjective well-being: A contextually dependent mediated process. *Journal of Occupational Health Psychology, 19*, 168–181. doi:10.1037/a0036012

McGonagle, A. K., Fisher, G. G., Barnes-Farrell, J. L., & Grosch, J. W. (2015). Individual and work factors related to perceived work ability and labor force outcomes. *Journal of Applied Psychology, 100*, 376–398. doi:10.1037/a0037974

Nielsen, K. (2013). Review article: How can we make organizational interventions work? Employees and line managers as actively crafting interventions. *Human Relations, 66*, 1029–1050. doi:10.1177/0018726713477164

Nielsen, K., & Abildgaard, J. S. (2013). Organizational interventions: A research-based framework for the evaluation of both process and effects. *Work & Stress, 27*, 278–297. doi:10.1080/02678373.2013.812358

Neveu, J. (2007). Jailed resources: Conservation of resources theory as applied to burnout among prison guards. *Journal of Organizational Behavior, 28*, 21–42. doi:10.1002/job.393

NIOSH. (2012). *Research Compendium: The NIOSH Total Worker Health™ Program: Seminal Research Papers 2012.* (DHHS [NIOSH] Publication No. 2012–146). Washington, DC: U.S. Department of Health and Human Services, Public Health Service, Centers for Disease Control and Prevention. Retrieved from www.cdc.gov/niosh/docs/2012-146

Parker, J. R. (2011). *Florida mortality study: Florida law enforcement and correctional officers compared to Florida general population.* Retrieved from www.floridastatefop.org/pdf_files/floridamortalitystudy.pdf

Pearlin, L. I., & Schooler, C. (1978). The structure of coping. *Journal of Health and Social Behavior, 19*, 2–21. doi:10.2307/2136319

Perenboom, R. M., van Herten, L. M., Boshuizen, H. C., & van den Bos, G. M. (2005). Life expectancy without chronic morbidity: Trends in gender and socioeconomic disparities. *Public Health Reports, 120*(1), 46–54.

Petrou, P., Demerouti, E., & Schaufeli, W. B. (2015). Job crafting in changing organizations: Antecedents and implications for exhaustion and performance. *Journal of Occupational Health Psychology, 20*, 470–480. doi:10.1037/a0039003

Piaget, J. (1976). *The psychology of intelligence* (M. Piercy & D. E. Berlyne, Trans.). Totowa, NJ: Littlefield, Adams. (Original work published 1947)

Ployhart, R. E., & Vandenberg, R. J. (2010). Longitudinal research: The theory, design, and analysis of change. *Journal of Management, 36*, 94–120. doi:10.1177/0149206309352110

Polanyi, K. (2001). *The great transformation: The political and economic origins of our time.* Boston, MA: Beacon. (Original work published 1944)

Raudenbush, S. W., & Bryk, A. S. (2002). *Hierarchical linear models: Applications and data analysis methods* (2nd ed.). Thousand Oaks, CA: Sage.

Richardson, K. M., & Rothstein, H. R. (2008). Effects of occupational stress management intervention programs: A meta-analysis. *Journal of Occupational Health Psychology, 13*, 69–93. doi:10.1037/1076-8998.13.1.69

Rodriguez-Jareño, M. C., Demou, E., Vargas-Prada, S., Sanati, K. A., Skerjanc, A., Reis, P. G., . . . Serra, C. (2014). European Working Time Directive and doctors' health: A systematic review of the available epidemiological evidence. *BMJ Open, 4*(7), e004916. doi:10.1136/bmjopen-2014-004916

Ronen, S., & Baldwin, M. W. (2010). Hypersensitivity to social rejection and perceived stress as mediators between attachment anxiety and future burnout: A prospective analysis. *Applied Psychology, 59*, 380–403. doi:10.1111/j.1464-0597.2009.00404.x

Rössler, W., Hengartner, M., Ajdacic-Gross, V., & Angst, J. (2015). Predictors of burnout: Results from a prospective community study. *European Archives of Psychiatry and Clinical Neuroscience, 265*, 19–25. doi:10.1007/s00406-014-0512-x

Schein, E. H. (1971). Occupational socialization in the professions: The case of role innovation. *Journal of Psychiatric Research, 8*, 521–530. doi:10.1016/0022-3956(71)90041-0

Schill, A. L., & Chosewood, L. C. (2013). The NIOSH Total Worker Health™ program: An overview. *Journal of Occupational and Environmental Medicine, 55*(12, Suppl.), S8–S11. doi:10.1097/JOM.0000000000000037

Schonfeld, I. S. (1990). Psychological distress in a sample of teachers. *Journal of Psychology, 124*, 321–338. doi:10.1080/00223980.1990.10543227

Schonfeld, I. S. (2001). Stress in 1st-year women teachers: The context of social support and coping. *Genetic, Social, and General Psychology Monographs, 127*(2), 133–168.

Schonfeld, I. S., & Mazzola, J. J. (2015). A qualitative study of stress in individuals self-employed in solo businesses. *Journal of Occupational Health Psychology, 20*, 501–513. doi:org/10.1037/a0038804

Schulte, P. A., Pandalai, S., Wulsin, V., & Chun, H. (2012). Interaction of occupational and personal risk factors in workforce health and safety. *American Journal of Public Health, 102*, 434–448. doi:10.2105/AJPH.2011.300249

Semmer, N. (2006). Job stress interventions and the organization of work. *Scandinavian Journal of Work, Environment & Health, 32*, 515–527. doi:10.5271/sjweh.1056

Shanafelt, T. D., Boone, S., Tan, L., Dyrbye, L. N., Sotile, W., Satele, D., . . . Oreskovich, M. R. (2012). Burnout and satisfaction with work-life balance among US physicians relative to the general US population. *Archives of Internal Medicine, 172*, 1377–1385. doi:10.1001/archinternmed.2012.3199

Shively, S. B., Horkayne-Szakaly, I., Jones, R. V., Kelly, J. P., Armstrong, R. C., & Perl, D. P. (2016). Characterisation of interface astroglial scarring in the human brain after blast exposure: A post-mortem case series. *The Lancet Neurology, 5*, 944–953. doi:10.1016/S1474-4422(16)30057-6

Sinclair, R. R., & Cheung, J. H. (2016). Money matters: Recommendations for financial stress research in occupational health psychology. *Stress and Health, 32*, 181–193. doi:10.1002/smi.2688

Sonnentag, S., & Fritz, C. (2015). Recovery from job stress: The stressor-detachment model as an integrative framework. *Journal of Organizational Behavior, 36*(Suppl. 1), S72–S103. doi:10.1002/job.1924

Sorensen, G., Stoddard, A. M., LaMontagne, A. D., Emmons, K., Hunt, M. K., Youngstrom, R., . . . Christiani, D. C. (2002). A comprehensive worksite cancer prevention intervention: Behavior change results from a randomized controlled trial (United States). *Cancer Causes & Control, 13*(6), 493–502.

Sørensen, O. H. (2015). Organizational changes torpedoing the intervention. In M. Karanika-Murray & C. Biron (Eds.), *Derailed organizational interventions for stress and well-being: Confessions of failure and solutions for success* (pp. 79–86). Dordrecht, The Netherlands: Springer.

Spector, P. E., Liu, C., & Sanchez, J. I. (2015). Methodological and substantive issues in conducting multinational and cross-cultural research. *Annual Review of Organizational Psychology and Organizational Behavior, 2*, 101–131. doi:10.1146/annurev-orgpsych-032414-111310

Statistics Canada. (2014). *Table 2: Employment by class of worker and industry, Canada, seasonally adjusted.* Retrieved from www.statcan.gc.ca/pub/71-001-x/2013012/t002-eng.htm

Stellman, J. M., Smith, R. P., Katz, C. L., Sharma, V., Charney, D. S., Herbert, R., . . . Southwick, S. (2008). Enduring mental health morbidity and social function impairment in World Trade Center rescue, recovery, and cleanup workers: The psychological dimension of an environmental health disaster. *Environmental Health Perspectives, 116*, 1248–1253. doi:10.1289/ehp.11164

Tanielian, T., & Jaycox, L. H. (2008). *A comprehensive study of the post-deployment health-related needs associated with post-traumatic stress disorder, major depression, and traumatic brain injury among service members returning from Operations Enduring Freedom and Iraqi Freedom.* Santa Monica, CA: Rand.

Taris, T. W., & Kompier, M. J. (2014). Cause and effect: Optimizing the designs of longitudinal studies in occupational health psychology. *Work & Stress, 28*, 1–8. doi:10.1080/02678373.2014.878494

Tarkiainen, L., Martikainen, P., & Laaksonen, M. (2013). The changing relationship between income and mortality in Finland, 1988–2007. *Journal of Epidemiology and Community Health, 67*, 21–27. doi:10.1136/jech-2012-201097

Teichgraber, M. (2013). Statistics in focus: Labour market and labour force statistics. *European Union Labour Force Survey—Annual results 2012.* Retrieved from http://epp.eurostat.ec.europa.eu/statistics_explained/index.php/Labour_market_and_labour_force_statistics

Toivanen, S. (2008). Job control and the risk of incident stroke in the working population in Sweden. *Scandinavian Journal of Work, Environment & Health, 34*(1), 40–47.

Ursano, R. J., Kessler, R. C., Stein, M. B., Naifeh, J. A., Aliaga, P. A., Fullerton, C. S., . . . Heeringa, S. G. (2015). Suicide attempts in the US Army during the wars in Afghanistan and Iraq, 2004 to 2009. *Journal of the American Medical Association: Psychiatry, 72*, 917–926. doi:10.1001/jamapsychiatry.2015.0987

Violanti, J. M. (2015, May). Correctional officer suicide: Recent national data. APA/NIOSH/SOHP Work, Stress, and Health Conference, Atlanta, GA.

Virtanen, S. V., & Notkola, V. (2002). Socioeconomic inequalities in cardiovascular mortality and the role of work: A register study of Finnish men. *International Journal of Epidemiology, 31*(3), 614–621.

Wang, M., & Shi, J. (2014). Psychological research on retirement. *Annual Review of Psychology, 65*, 209–233. doi:10.1146/annurev-psych-010213-115131

Wang, M., & Shultz, K. S. (2010). Employee retirement: A review and recommendations for future investigation. *Journal of Management, 36*, 172–206. doi:10.1177/0149206309347957

Westman, M., & Eden, D. (1997). Effects of a respite from work on burnout: Vacation relief and fade-out. *Journal of Applied Psychology, 82,* 516–527. doi:10.1037/0021-9010.82.4.516

Willett, J. B. (1989). Some results on reliability for the longitudinal measurement of change: Implications for the design of studies of individual growth. *Educational and Psychological Measurement, 49,* 587–602. doi:10.1177/001316448904900309

Wrzesniewski, A., & Dutton, J. E. (2001). Crafting a job: Revisioning employees as active crafters of their work. *Academy of Management Review, 26,* 179–201. doi:10.5465/AMR.2001.4378011

Zohar, D. (2010). Thirty years of safety climate research: Reflections and future directions. *Accident Analysis and Prevention, 42,* 1517–1522. doi:10.1016/j.aap.2009.12.019

Index